DOWN SYNDROME

Edited by **Subrata Kumar Dey**

Down Syndrome
http://dx.doi.org/10.5772/46009
Edited by Subrata Kumar Dey

Contributors

Kazuko Kudo, Melanie Pritchard, Érika Cristina Pavarino, Joice Matos Biselli, Eny Maria Goloni Bertollo, Walter Pinto Júnior, Francisco Javier Ordonez, Volney Sheen, Jie Lu, A K M Mamunur Rashid, George Grouios, Antonia Ypsilanti, Irene Koidou, Darija Mateja Strah, Maja Pohar-Perme, Ksenija Gersak, Ferdinando Di Cunto, Gaia Berto, Gislaine Czlusniak, Ana Paula Teitelbaum, Sujoy Ghosh, Subrata Kumar Dey, Jaana Marttala

Published by InTech
Janeza Trdine 9, 51000 Rijeka, Croatia

Publishing Process Manager Dejan Grgur
Technical Editor InTech DTP team
Cover InTech Design team

Additional hard copies can be obtained from orders@intechopen.com

Down Syndrome, Edited by Subrata Kumar Dey
p. cm.
ISBN 978-953-51-1036-1

For EU product safety concerns:
IN TECH d.o.o., Prolaz Marije Krucifikse Kozulić 3, 51000 Rijeka, Croatia,
info@intechopen.com or visit our website at intechopen.com.

Meet the editor

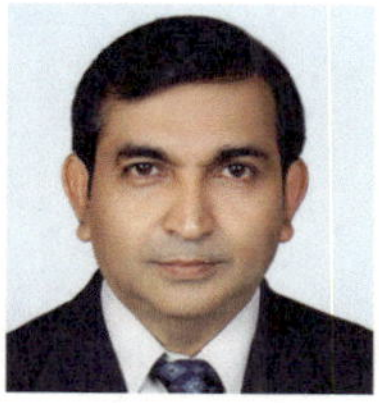

Dr. Subrata Dey is the Director of School of Biotechnology and Biological Sciences and Professor of Biotechnology and Human Molecular Genetics at the West Bengal University of Technology. His laboratory has long been involved in research on Molecular Genetics of Down syndrome. His current research interests include the identification of genes involved in the development of Congenital heart disease and Alzheimer's disease in both Down syndrome and healthy individuals. His group also studies the mechanism of radiation induced genomic instability and radioprotection. Dr. Dey has been teaching courses in Genetics, Molecular Biology, Evolution and Developmental Biology for more than thirty years. He is also the founding Director of Centre for Genetic Studies. Dr. Dey is the author of many scientific papers and has edited two books on Down syndrome.

Contents

Preface IX

Section 1 Prenatal Diagnosis and Genetic Counseling 1

Chapter 1 **Down Syndrome: Clinical and Genetic Aspects, Genetic Counseling and Prenatal Screening and Diagnosis 3**
Érika Cristina Pavarino, Joice Matos Biselli, Walter Pinto Junior and Eny Maria Goloni Bertollo

Chapter 2 **Increased Fetal Nuchal Translucency Thickness and Normal Karyotype: Prenatal and Postnatal Outcome 21**
Ksenija Gersak, Darija M. Strah and Maja Pohar-Perme

Chapter 3 **Prenatal Screening and Diagnosis 35**
Jaana Marttala

Section 2 Diseases in Children with Down Syndrome 63

Chapter 4 **Control of Dental Biofilm and Oral Health Maintenance in Patients with Down Syndrome 65**
Ana Paula Teitelbaum and Gislaine Denise Czlusniak

Chapter 5 **How to Design an Exercise Program TO Reduce Inflammation in Obese People With Down Syndrome 83**
Francisco J. Ordonez, Gabriel Fornieles, Alejandra Camacho, Miguel A. Rosety, Antonio J Diaz, Ignacio Rosety, Natalia Garcia and Manuel Rosety-Rodriguez

Chapter 6 **Heart Diseases in Down Syndrome 95**
A. K. M. Mamunur Rashid

Chapter 7 **Myeloid Leukemia Associated with Down Syndrome 107**
Kazuko Kudo

Section 3 Genetics of Down Syndrome 115

Chapter 8 **Molecular Pathways of Down Syndrome Critical Region Genes 117**
Ferdinando Di Cunto and Gaia Berto

Chapter 9 **Risk Factors for Down Syndrome Birth: Understanding the Causes from Genetics and Epidemiology 149**
Sujay Ghosh and Subrata Kumar Dey

Chapter 10 **RCAN1 and Its Potential Contribution to the Down Syndrome Phenotype 173**
Melanie A. Pritchard and Katherine R. Martin

Section 4 Neural Development in Down Syndrome 207

Chapter 11 **Laterality Explored: Atypical Hemispheric Dominance in Down Syndrome 209**
George Grouios, Antonia Ypsilanti and Irene Koidou

Chapter 12 **Genetic and Epigenetic Mechanisms in Down Syndrome Brain 237**
Jie Lu and Volney Sheen

Preface

This book provides recent developments and advances in research on Down syndrome. It covers a wide range of topics, including investigations on prenatal diagnosis and screening, genetic counseling, neoplastic disease, congenital heart disease, dentistry and oral health, obesity, molecular genetics and neurological disorders in Down syndrome. It is also a resource for scientists and research workers who wish to learn more about Down syndrome. To date, well over one hundred chromosome syndromes have been reported. Whilst on an individual basis many of these are rare, together they make a major contribution to human morbidity and mortality. Chromosome aneuploidies are now known to account for a large proportion of spontaneous pregnancy loss and childhood disability, and can also contribute to the genesis of a significant proportion of malignancy. Trisomy 21 in humans, commonly referred as Down syndrome, is the most common genetic cause of mental retardation and most frequent autosomal trisomies in liveborns. In approximately ninety five percent of cases , the extra chromosome occurs as a result of meiotic nondisjunction or abnormal segregation of chromosome. The cause of nondisjunction of chromosome 21 is largely unknown. Although several hypotheses have been suggested, it is still unclear as to whether particular gene loci on chromosome 21 are sufficient to cause Down syndrome and its associated features. The risk factors associated with the birth of Down syndrome are enigmatic. The overall maternal risk factors for Down syndrome birth are multifactorial and include both genetic and environmental factors.

This book is organized into four sections. All sections include chapters on recent advances in research on Down syndrome. The editor endeavored to keep the big picture and overarching philosophy of the review articles in focus while editing the text and illustrations for consistent use of scientific terminology and level of exposition.

The first section deals with our present knowledge on common diseases in Down syndrome. The second one discusses the present status of investigations on molecular genetics of Down syndrome. The third section covers the recent investigations on neurological disorders in Down syndrome, and the concluding section focuses on prenatal diagnosis, screening and genetic counseling in Down syndrome.

This book provides a concise yet comprehensive source of current information on Down syndrome. Research workers, scientists, medical graduates and pediatricians will find the book Down syndrome an excellent source for reference and review.

The editor wants to acknowledge the superb assistance of staff members and management of InTech Publisher. In particular, Mr. Dejan Grgur for co-ordination and editorial assistance. We are grateful to all contributing authors and scientists who made this book possible by providing valuable research and review articles. Finally, I would like to dedicate this book to children with Down syndrome who need our love and care to lead a healthy life.

Dr. Subrata Dey
Director,
School of Biotechnology & Biological Sciences,
West Bengal University of Technology,
India

Section 1

Prenatal Diagnosis and Genetic Counseling

Chapter 1

Down Syndrome: Clinical and Genetic Aspects, Genetic Counseling and Prenatal Screening and Diagnosis

Érika Cristina Pavarino, Joice Matos Biselli,
Walter Pinto Junior and Eny Maria Goloni Bertollo

Additional information is available at the end of the chapter

http://dx.doi.org/10.5772/52950

1. Introduction

1.1. Clinical and genetic aspects

Down syndrome (DS) or trisomy 21 is the most common genetic disorder with a prevalence of 1 in 660 live births [1]. In 1959, Lejeune and colleagues discovered the genetic basis of DS and named as trisomy of chromosome 21, which is the smallest human autosomal chromosome [2]. Trisomy 21 can occur as three types of chromosomal abnormalities: free trisomy 21, translocation or mosaicism. Free trisomy 21 is characterized by the presence of three complete copies of chromosome 21, occurring in about 90-95% of DS cases [3-5]. More than 90% of the cases of chromosomal nondisjunction are of maternal origin, mainly during meiosis I, about 5% involve an additional paternal extra chromosome and a small proportion (2%) is consequence of post-zygotic mitotic non-disjunction [6]. Translocations are attributed to 1-7% of the cases, with Robertsonian translocation involving chromosomes 14 and 21 being the most common type. Mosaicism, characterized by some cells containing 46 chromosomes and others with 47 chromosomes (with an extra chromosome 1), is reported in 1-7% of DS cases [3-5].

DS phenotype is complex and varies among individuals, who may present a combination of dysmorphic features and developmental delay [7]. The intellectual disability is a characteristic observed in all cases and the most frequent clinical features include muscular hypotonia (99%), diastasis of the muscle rectus of abdomen (90%), upslanted palpebral fissures (90%), microcephaly (85%), flat occipital (80%), joint hyperextension (80%), broad hands with short fingers (70%), short stature (60%), clinodactyly of fifth finger (50%), epicanthal fold (40%), low-set ears (50%), single palmar crease (40%), atlantoaxial instability (15%) and label-femoral instability (10%) [8]. On average, 50-70% of children with DS have congenital heart defects, such as ventricular septal defect, atrial septal defect, tetralogy of Fallot, patent ductus arteriosus and atrioventricular septal defect [3,4,9]. There are also ocular problems, such as refractive errors, nystagmus, abnormalities of the retina, among others [10]. About 80% of cases present hearing loss, which can be conductive, sensorineural, or mixed [11]. Thyroid dysfunction, particularly hypothyroidism [9], periodontal diseases [10], upper airway obstruction [12] and hypogonadism [14] are more frequent in individuals with DS than in the general population. Other important clinical aspects of DS include immunodeficiency [15], increased risk for hematological disorders and leukemia [16] and early onset of Alzheimer's disease [17].

The development of secondary sexual characteristics in DS is similar to other adolescents. The fetal oogenesis of women with the syndrome appears to be normal and, therefore, they are capable of reproduction [18]. On the other hand, men have diminished reproductive capacity, showing testicular histology compatible with oligospermia and, frequently, hypogonadism [19]. However, there have been reports of men with Down syndrome who have fathered pregnancies [20].

2. Genetic counseling

Genetic counseling can be defined as a communication process that takes care of the human problems associated with the occurrence or recurrence of a genetic disease in a family with the purpose of providing individuals and families comprehensive understanding of all the implications related to genetic disease under discussion, the options that the current medicine offers for therapy or for reducing the risk of occurrence or recurrence of the disease and psychotherapeutic support [21,22].

For DS, a well-established risk factor is advanced maternal age at conception [23,24]. The estimated risk for fetal trisomy 21 for a woman aged 20 years at 12 weeks of gestation is about 1 in 1000, and the risk of such woman delivering an affected baby at term is 1 in 1500. The risk for this aneuploidy for a woman aged 35 years at 12 weeks of gestation is about 1 in 250 and the risk of delivering an affected baby at term is 1 in 350 [25].

Although there is considerable variation in the physical features of individuals with DS, most individuals present with a range of characteristics that enable clinical diagnosis of the syndrome [3,4,7]. However, cytogenetic investigation of individuals who present with clinical characteristics of DS is fundamental to establish a precise diagnosis, which may have implications in the genetic counseling process, once it is very important in determining the recurrence risk of the syndrome. In addition, the karyotype analysis of affected individuals identifies cases that may have been inherited making necessary the investigation of the parents' karyotypes. In this case, the cytogenetic investigation of the genitors is essential to establish the risk of recurrence of the syndrome in future generations. Thus, all individuals with a diagnosis suggestive of DS should be referred to a genetic counseling service.

Accurate estimation of recurrence risks depends upon the verification of the individual's karyotype. Cases of free trisomy 21 and mosaicism generally do not recur in siblings of individuals with DS. For women with maternal age <35 at previous trisomy 21, the revised risk is the age-related risk times 3.5. For those with maternal age ≥35 at previous trisomy 21, the revised risk is the age-related risk times 1.7 [26]. So, these risk times implies that other factors might influence the risk for DS in young mothers [27]. On the other hand, translocation may be recurrent. If neither parent carries a balanced translocation, the DS recurrence risk is low, probably similar to that of free trisomy 21. However, if one of the parents is the carrier of a balanced translocation, the risk of recurrence is dependent on the type of translocation and the sex of the carrier parent. In the case of Robertsonian translocations involving chromosome 13, 14, 15 or 22 and the chromosome 21, the recurrence risk at time of amniocentesis is of up to 17% when the mother is the carrier and of up to 1.4% when the carrier of this balanced translocation is the father. On the other hand, if one of the parents is the carrier of a balanced translocation involving two chromosomes 21, the recurrence risk of DS is 100% [26]. Thus, once diagnosed as a case of DS due to a translocation, a karyotype analysis of both parents is recommended.

For an individual with DS, the theoretical chance to have a child with DS is 50%, and 66% when both partners have DS. However, empiric risks are difficult to estimate, once the reproduction rates are low. Empiric data indicate a 30–50% chance of a woman with DS have a child with DS [26]. However, considering that the rate of fetal death between 11 weeks and term is about 43% for trisomy 21 [28], the chance of birth of a child with DS decreases. For individuals with mosaicism, the maximum theoretical recurrence risk is as high as 50%, but is dependent upon the proportion of trisomic gonadal cells and whether the other partner has DS as well [26].

Genetic counseling is also important to guide the parents about caring for the child with DS. Because individuals with DS often experience delays in reaching various developmental milestones, early intervention with speech therapy, occupational therapy, and physical therapy is recommended as it maximizes long-term outcomes [29]. As healthcare has improved for individuals with DS, the average life expectancy has increased by more than 30 years, from an average of 25 years of age in 1983 to almost 60 years of age in 2000 [30]. A study performed between 1985–2004 in England showed that the one-year survival of live births with DS increased, especially in babies with cardiovascular malformations, reaching almost 100% [31], and a more recent study showed that the 25-year survival of DS individuals is about 87.5% [32].

Genetic counselors should balance the negative aspects of DS, such as birth defects, medical complications, and developmental delay, with positive aspects like available treatments, therapies, and the ability for people with DS and their families to enjoy a high quality of life [33].

3. Prenatal screening and diagnosis

There are several methods that allow the early detection of DS in prenatal phase. At this point, it is not possible avoid congenital malformations or genetic diseases, but the objective is its early detection, looking for emotional and psychological preparation for parents and family and adequate medical support and monitoring for the child's birth. Furthermore, early detection allows treatment of malformations of the complications that may occur, preventing or attenuating their evolution through surgical correction in utero.

There are some methods used to screen fetus with DS that allow the prenatal diagnosis of the syndrome. Among the screening methods are the nuchal translucency test, the measurement of maternal serum concentrations of various fetoplacental products and fetal ultrasound. The nuchal translucency (NT) test is the measurement of the fluid filled fold at the back of the fetal neck in the first trimester of pregnancy, performed through transabdominal or transvaginal sonography. The test is performed between the 11th and 13th weeks of gestation and the minimum fetal crown–rump length (CRL) should be 45 mm and the maximum 84 mm. Fetal NT increases with CRL and therefore it is essential to take gestation into account when determining whether a given NT thickness is increased [25]. The excess skin in the fetus may be the consequence of excessive accumulation of subcutaneous fluid behind the fetal neck which could be visualized by ultrasonography as increased NT in the third month of intrauterine life [34]. Nowadays, it is well established that the measurement of fetal NT thickness provides effective and early screening for trisomy 21 and other major aneuploidies, such as Edwards syndrome (trisomy 18) and Patau syndrome (trisomy 13) [34-36] besides for screening of congenital heart disease [37]. In case of abnormality in NT measurement, additional tests are needed to elucidate the cause of increased nuchal fold.

Pregnancies with fetal aneuploidies are associated with altered maternal serum concentrations of various fetoplacental products, including alpha-fetoprotein (AFP), free chorionic gonadotropin (β-hCG), unconjugated estriol (uE3), inhibin A (INH-A) and pregnancy associated plasma protein-A (PAPP-A) [38-42]. The measurement of concentrations of maternal serum AFP, β-hCG and uE3, the triple test, is one of a range of screening tests that are used to identify pregnant women whose fetus is likely to be affected by trisomy 21 and who should then be offered a diagnostic test. AFP is produced in the yolk sac and fetal liver, while uE3 and hCG are produced by the placenta. Elevated β-hCG concentration and low levels of AFP and uE3 suggests the presence of a fetus with DS [38-40]. The test is performed in second trimester of pregnancy and the values should be adjusted to gestational age. The expected detection rate and false-positive rate are about 73 - 78% and 7.5 - 9%, respectively [43].

The incorporation of INH-A into maternal serum DS screening in the second trimester, along with AFP, hCG and uE3, is named quadruple test. INH-A is a glycoprotein mainly secreted from the corpus luteum and the placenta [44] and its concentration is raised in the serum of pregnant women carrying a fetus with DS [42]. The quadruple test presents expected detection rate and false-positive rate about 79 - 82% and 6.5 - 7.8%, respectively [43]. The measurement of PAPP-A is also used as a screening gestations of fetus with DS in the first trimester, once the maternal serum concentration of this protein are reduced in these women [41]. The measurement of PAPP-A at 10–14 weeks of pregnancy is used to screen for fetal DS during the first trimester of pregnancy [45,47].

The fetal ultrasound is also considered a method of screening for DS, once any change in the development of organs or structures is easily visualized. The objective is the detection of major and soft markers of aneuploidy, including alterations in central nervous system, face, neck, heart, gastrointestinal tract, genitourinary tract among others [47]. Besides increased nuchal translucency in the first trimester, alterations commonly detected in DS in the second trimester of gestation include lack of visualization of the nasal bone [48], reduced femur and humerus, mild pyelectasis, hyperechoic bowel and echogenic intracardiac focus [47,49].

Importantly, any suspect result of the markers mentioned implies the genetic analysis of the fetus, the only way to accurate diagnosis. The methods for obtaining fetal cells for analysis vary with gestational age. Among the invasive methods for obtaining fetal cells, chorionic villus sampling (CVS) allows diagnosis in the first trimester of pregnancy (between the 10th and 13th weeks of gestation) [50]. The procedure involves aspiration of trophoblastic tissue under continuous ultrasound monitoring, performed via trans-cervical or trans-abdominal. Studies have showed that the risk miscarriage associated to this procedure is about 0.6-1.1% [51,52] and the procedure is not recommended for pregnant women that present bleeding due to an increase in the procedure-related fetal loss rate [51].

The amniocentesis is the method indicated for obtaining fetal cells after 15 weeks of gestation [53]. This requires taking a small sample of amniotic fluid transabdominally under ultrasound guidance. The procedure-related fetal loss rate is about 0.4-0.8 % [51,52]. After 20th week of gestation, the option is percutaneous umbilical blood sampling or cordocentesis, which involves direct sampling of fetal blood from the umbilical cord. The procedure-related loss rate is about 1.0-1.5% and cordocentesis with placenta penetration had a significantly higher rate of fetal loss [54-56].

Considering the risks which accompany invasive methods for obtaining fetal cells [51,52,56], the use of noninvasive methods could be a good option. Several methods to develop a noninvasive prenatal test for trisomy 21 and other aneuploidies have been investigated, including the use of cell-free fetal nucleic acids [57-60] and nucleated red blood fetal cells present in maternal peripheral blood [61,62]. Although studies have showed that noninvasive methods for obtaining fetal cells allow noninvasive prenatal diagnosis for a variety of genetic conditions and may in future form part of national antenatal screening programs for DS and other common genetic disorders, a major obstacle in the widespread application of noninvasive methods for obtaining fetal cells in clinical diagnostics is still that fetal cells / DNA constitutes a small percentage of total cell / DNA in maternal blood and the inconsistencies in enrichment strategies of these fetal samples [62,63].

After obtaining fetal cells, conventional karyotype analysis has been used for the past few decades as the gold standard for the prenatal diagnosis of numerical and major structural chromosomal abnormalities. Nevertheless, it is labor intensive and requires skilled chromosomal analysis with an average reporting time of 14 days. However, the availability of molecular techniques such as fluorescence in situ hybridization (FISH) has allowed the prenatal diagnosis of most frequent trisomies (21, 13, 18) and aneuploidy of sex chromosomes quickly and accurately, obtaining result from one to two days [64,65]. In addition, the technique of polymerase chain reaction quantitative fluorescent (QF-PCR), besides other molecular techniques such as the multiplex ligation-dependent probe amplification (MLPA) test and DNA sequencing, can also be used for a rapid diagnosis of aneuploidies [66-68]. It has been showed that QF-PCR technique presents 95.4% sensitivity, 100% specificity, 99.5% efficiency and is less laborious than the FISH technique, less time consuming, and some results were obtained in eight hours. The sensitivity, specificity, and efficiency of the assay for detecting DS using this technique are about 95.4%, 100%, and 99.5%, respectively [69]. Molecular techniques also enable the diagnosis of pre-implantation embryos in assisted reproduction [70].

It is important to note that the examinations of prenatal diagnosis should not be offered without the guidance of a geneticist to explain the risks to the parents and especially the implications of possible results. Early diagnosis helps couples to program for the treatment of the consequences of the syndrome diagnosed, preventing further damage and making possible the early stimulation of the patients, aiming their better integration into society.

4. Gene expression and DS phenotype

In a recent review of chromosome 21 content, 552 genes were identified in the long arm of the chromosome (21q) [71], including 161 protein-coding genes cataloged in the Reference Sequence database of the National Center for Biotechnology Information (NCBI). The remaining 391 gene models are referred to as novel genes or non-cataloged genes, which could be protein-coding genes or functional RNA genes. Considering that the genetic basis of DS is the presence of three copies of chromosome 21, the first and most commonly accepted hypothesis for DS phenotype is that the genes in triplicate are overexpressed and, thus, the dosage imbalance of genes on chromosome 21 is responsible for the molecular dysfunctions in DS [72]. Among the genes present in chromosome 21, may be highlighted some described in the literature with overexpression associated with phenotypes of DS, most influencing the structure or function of the central nervous system (Table 1). Location of these genes on chromosome 21 is presented in Figure 1.

Gene symbol*	Gene location*	Candidate gene for	Reference
APP	21q21.3	Neurodegeneration	[73,74]
BACH1	21q22.11	Alzheimer's disease-like neuropathological changes	[75]
DOPEY2	21q22.2	Functional brain alterations and mental retardation	[76]
DSCAM	21q22.2	Mental retardation and the precocious dementia	[77]
DYRK1A	21q22.13	Leukemogenesis	[78]
		Impaired brain development	[79]
		Early onset of neurofibrillary degeneration	[80]
ERG	21q22.3	Alzheimer's disease-like neuropathological changes	[75]
OLIG2	21q22.11	Developmental brain defects	[81]
SIM2	21q22.13	Impairment of learning and memory	[82]
		Pathogenesis of mental retardation	[83]
SOD1	21q22.11	Neurodegeneration	[84]
PCP4	21q22.2	Abnormal neuronal development	[85]

* http://www.ncbi.nlm.nih.gov/gene

Table 1. Chromosome 21 gene-located with overexpression in DS influencing the structure or function of the central nervous system.

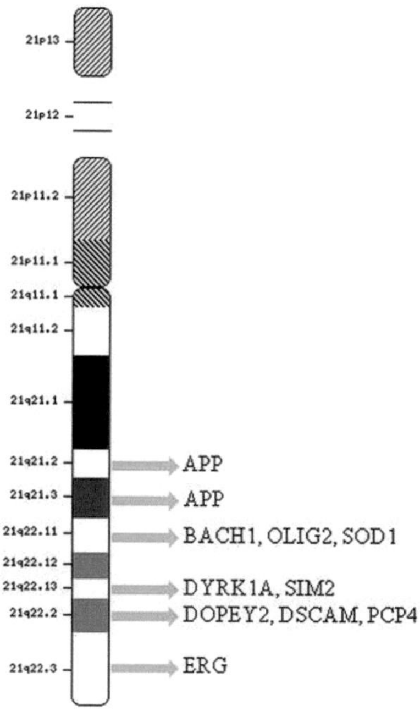

Figure 1. Location of genes overexpressed in DS influencing the structure or function of the central nervous system. Figure adapted from the NCBI Map Viewer database (http://www.ncbi.nlm.nih.gov/mapview/).

However, although elevated levels of gene expression on chromosome 21 in trisomy 21 tissues have been reported in several studies, there are evidences that increased copy number does not always correspond with increased gene expression level or even less with increased gene function [86,87]. In addition, studies have showed up- or downregulation of genes located on disomic chromosomes, indicating that the phenotype is due to an unstable environment resulting from the dosage imbalance of the hundreds of genes on chromosome 21 which determines a non-specific disturbance of genomic regulation and expression [88-90].

Besides altered pattern of gene expression, regulatory mechanisms are also altered in trisomy 21. Individuals with DS present altered pattern of DNA methylation in genes present in two or three copies with functional consequences in gene expression [91,92]. More recent studies have shown that trisomy 21 results in altered expression of microRNAs, small molecules of noncoding RNA involved in post-transcriptional gene regulation, which could result in abnormal expression of specific proteins and contribute to the DS phenotype [93-97]

The complete sequencing of chromosome 21 provided basis for the identification of candidate genes for DS phenotype manifestations. Currently, there are several genes located on chromosome 21 associated to DS phenotype and the involvement of other genes still will be elucidated with advances of genomics and proteomics. The knowing of these gene functions and their contribution for DS phenotype are fundamental for the understanding of the syndrome and for providing basis for the planning of therapeutic strategies that could contribute to improve the quality of life of DS individuals.

5. Conclusion

Although individuals with trisomy 21 present several characteristics that make possible the clinical diagnosis of DS, the confirmation of the diagnosis by cytogenetic analysis is essential to establish the recurrence risks of the syndrome. We highlight the importance of the prenatal diagnosis of DS to provide the needed healthcare for the child, to prepare the family emotional and psychologically and to plan early intervention therapies. The successful control of pharmacological and clinical problems of patients with DS is the biggest medical challenge and depends on the understanding of unbalanced metabolism induced by high expression of the genes located on chromosome 21.

Acknowledgments

The authors acknowledge support from FAPESP (São Paulo Research Foundation), CNPq (National Council for Scientific and Technological Development) and CAPES (Coordination for the Improvement of Higher Education Personnel).

Author details

Érika Cristina Pavarino[1,2*], Joice Matos Biselli[1], Walter Pinto Junior[3] and Eny Maria Goloni Bertollo[1,2]

*Address all correspondence to: erika@famerp.br

1 Department of Molecular Biology, Sao Jose do Rio Preto Medical School (FAMERP), Genetics and Molecular Biology Research Unit (UPGEM), Sao Jose do Rio Preto, Brazil

2 Ding-Down multidisciplinary group, Sao Jose do Rio Preto Medical School (FAMERP), Sao Jose do Rio Preto, Brazil

3 Medical and Forensic Genetics Ltd, Campinas, Brazil

References

[1] Jones, K.L. Smith's recognizable patterns of human malformation. 6th ed. Philadelphia: Elsevier Saunders, 2006.

[2] Neri G, Opitz JM. Down syndrome: comments and reflections on the 50th anniversary of Lejeune's discovery. Am J Med Genet A. 2009 Dec;149A(12):2647-54. http://onlinelibrary.wiley.com/doi/10.1002/ajmg.a.33138/abstract (accessed 20 July 2012).

[3] Ahmed I, Ghafoor T, Samore NA, Chattha MN. Down syndrome: clinical and cytogenetic analysis. J Coll Physicians Surg Pak. 2005 Jul;15(7):426-9.

[4] Azman BZ, Ankathil R, Siti Mariam I, Suhaida MA, Norhashimah M, Tarmizi AB, et al. Cytogenetic and clinical profile of Down syndrome in Northeast Malaysia. Singapore Med J. 2007 Jun;48(6):550-4. http://smj.sma.org.sg/4806/4806a10.pdf (accessed 7 June 2012).

[5] Biselli JM, Goloni-Bertollo EM, Ruiz MT, Pavarino-Bertelli EC. Cytogenetic profile of Down syndrome cases seen by a general genetics outpatient service in Brazil. Down's syndrome, research and practice, 2008 Feb; 12(3). http://www.down-syndrome.org/reports/2010/ (accessed 5 June 2012).

[6] Vraneković J, Božović IB, Grubić Z, Wagner J, Pavlinić D, Dahoun S, et al. Down syndrome: parental origin, recombination, and maternal age. Genet Test Mol Biomarkers. 2012 Jan;16(1):70-3.

[7] Pavarino Bertelli EC, Biselli JM, Bonfim D, Goloni-Bertollo EM. Clinical profile of children with Down syndrome treated in a genetics outpatient service in the southeast of Brazil. Rev Assoc Med Bras. 2009 Sep-Oct;55(5):547-52. http://www.scielo.br/scielo.php?script=sci_arttext&pid=S0104-42302009000500017&lng=en&nrm=iso&tlng=en (accessed 5 June 2012)

[8] Mustacchi Z. Síndrome de Down. In: Mustacchi Z, Peres S. Genética Baseada em Evidências Síndromes e Heranças. São Paulo: CID Editora, 2000. p817-894.

[9] Mıhçı E, Akçurin G, Eren E, Kardelen F, Akçurin S, Keser I, et al. Evaluation of congenital heart diseases and thyroid abnormalities in children with Down syndrome. Anadolu Kardiyol Derg. 2010 Oct;10(5):440-5. http://www.anakarder.com/yazilar.asp?yaziid=1739&sayiid= (accessed 20 June 2012).

[10] Morgan J. Why is periodontal disease more prevalent and more severe in people with Down syndrome? Spec Care Dentist. 2007 Sep-Oct;27(5):196-201.

[11] Stirn Kranjc B. Ocular abnormalities and systemic disease in down syndrome. Strabismus. 2012 Jun;20(2):74-7. http://informahealthcare.com/doi/abs/10.3109/09273972.2012.680234 (accessed 20 June 2012).

[12] Raut P, Sriram B, Yeoh A, Hee KY, Lim SB, Daniel ML. High prevalence of hearing loss in Down syndrome at first year of life. Ann Acad Med Singapore. 2011 Nov; 40(11):493-8. http://www.annals.edu.sg/pdf/40VolNo11Nov2011/V40N11p493.pdf (accessed 20 June 2012).

[13] Mitchell RB, Call E, Kelly J. Ear, nose and throat disorders in children with Down syndrome. Laryngoscope. 2003 Feb;113(2):259-63. http://onlinelibrary.wiley.com/doi/10.1097/00005537-200302000-00012/abstract (accessed 15 June 2012).

[14] Grinspon RP, Bedecarrás P, Ballerini MG, Iñiguez G, Rocha A, Mantovani Rodrigues Resende EA, et al. Early onset of primary hypogonadism revealed by serum anti-

Müllerian hormone determination during infancy and childhood in trisomy 21. Int J Androl. 2011 Oct;34(5 Pt 2):e487-98. http://onlinelibrary.wiley.com/doi/10.1111/j.1365-2605.2011.01210.x/abstract (accessed 5 July 2012).

[15] Ram G, Chinen J. Infections and immunodeficiency in Down syndrome. Clin Exp Immunol. 2011 Apr;164(1):9-16. http://www.ncbi.nlm.nih.gov/pmc/articles/PMC3074212/?tool=pubmed (accessed July 2012).

[16] Bruwier A, Chantrain CF. Hematological disorders and leukemia in children with Down syndrome. Eur J Pediatr. 2011 Nov 24. DOI: 10.1007/s00431-011-1624-1. http://www.springerlink.com/content/a8730m24l57uu14g/?MUD=MP (accessed 3 June 2012).

[17] Lockrow JP, Fortress AM, Granholm AC. Age-related neurodegeneration and memory loss in down syndrome. Curr Gerontol Geriatr Res. 2012;2012:463909. http://www.ncbi.nlm.nih.gov/pmc/articles/PMC3318235/?tool=pubmed (accessed 20 June 2012).

[18] Jagiello GM, Fang JS, Nogawa T, Sung WK, Ducayen MB, Bowne W. Chromosome 21 behavior during fetal oogenesis in Down's syndrome. Obstet Gynecol. 1987 Dec; 70(6):878-83.

[19] Mercer ES, Broecker B, Smith EA, Kirsch AJ, Scherz HC, Massad CA. Urological manifestations of Down syndrome. J Urol. 2004 Mar;171(3):1250-3.

[20] Pradhan, M., Dalal, A., Khan, F., & Agrawal, S. Fertility in men with Down syndrome: A case report. Fertil Steril. 2006 Dec;86(6):1765.e1-3. http://www.fertstert.org/article/S0015-0282(06)03067-6/abstract (accessed 20 June 2012).

[21] Epstein CJ. Genetic Counseling: Statement of the American Society of Human GeneticsAd Hoc Committee on Genetic Counseling. Am J Hum Genet. 1975; 27(2): 241-242.

[22] Pinto Junior, W. Diagnóstico pré-natal. Ciênc. saúde coletiva. 2002; 7(1):139-157. http://redalyc.uaemex.mx/pdf/630/63070113.pdf. (accessed 18 June 2012).

[23] Jyothy A, Kumar KS, Mallikarjuna GN, Babu Rao V, Uma Devi B, Sujatha M, et al. Parental age and the origin of extra chromosome 21 in Down syndrome. J Hum Genet. 2001;46(6):347-50. http://www.nature.com/jhg/journal/v46/n6/full/jhg200164a.html. (accessed 20 June 2012).

[24] Allen EG, Freeman SB, Druschel C, Hobbs CA, O'Leary LA, Romitti PA, et al. Maternal age and risk for trisomy 21 assessed by the origin of chromosome nondisjunction: a report from the Atlanta and National Down Syndrome Projects. Hum Genet. 2009 Feb;125(1):41-52. http://www.ncbi.nlm.nih.gov/pmc/articles/PMC2833410/?tool=pubmed (accessed 6 June 2012).

[25] Nicolaides KH. Screening for fetal aneuploidies at 11 to 13 weeks. Prenat Diagn. 2011 Jan;31(1):7-15. http://onlinelibrary.wiley.com/doi/10.1002/pd.2637/abstract (accessed 18 June 2012).

[26] Sheets KB, Crissman BG, Feist CD, Sell SL, Johnson LR, Donahue KC, et al. Practice guidelines for communicating a prenatal or postnatal diagnosis of Down syndrome: recommendations of the national society of genetic counselors. J Genet Couns. 2011 Oct;20(5):432-41. http://www.springerlink.com/content/a238112117611644/ (accessed 18 June 2012).

[27] Pavarino EC, Zampieri BL, Biselli JM, Goloni-Bertollo EM. Abnormal Folate Metabolism and Maternal Risk for Down Syndrome. In: Dey S., editor. Genetics and Etiology of Down Syndrome. Rijeka, Croácia: InTech; 2011. p. 97-120. Available from http://www.intechopen.com/books/genetics-and-etiology-of-down-syndrome/abnormal-folate-metabolism-and-maternal-risk-for-down-syndrome (accessed 15 June 2012).

[28] Morris JK, Wald NJ, Watt HC. Fetal loss in Down syndrome pregnancies. Prenat Diagn. 1999 Feb;19(2):142-5. http://onlinelibrary.wiley.com/doi/10.1002/(SICI)1097-0223(199902)19:2% 3C142::AID-PD486% 3E3.0.CO;2-7/abstract (accessed 30 July 2012).

[29] Rihtman T, Tekuzener E, Parush S, Tenenbaum A, Bachrach SJ, Ornoy A. Are the cognitive functions of children with Down syndrome related to their participation? Dev Med Child Neurol. 2010 Jan;52(1):72-8. http://onlinelibrary.wiley.com/doi/10.1111/j.1469-8749.2009.03356.x/abstract (accessed 20 June 2012).

[30] Glasson EJ, Sullivan SG, Hussain R, Petterson BA, Montgomery PD, Bittles AH. The changing survival profile of people with Down's syndrome: Implications for genetic counselling. Clin Genet. 2002 Nov;62(5):390-3. http://onlinelibrary.wiley.com/doi/10.1034/j.1399-0004.2002.620506.x/abstract (accessed 12 July 2012).

[31] Irving C, Basu A, Richmond S, Burn J, Wren C. Twenty-year trends in prevalence and survival of Down syndrome. Eur J Hum Genet. 2008 Nov;16(11):1336-40. http://www.nature.com/ejhg/journal/v16/n11/full/ejhg2008122a.html (accessed 15 July 2012).

[32] Wang Y, Hu J, Druschel CM, Kirby RS. Twenty-five-year survival of children with birth defects in New York State: a population-based study. Birth Defects Res A Clin Mol Teratol. 2011 Dec;91(12):995-1003. http://onlinelibrary.wiley.com/doi/10.1002/bdra.22858/abstract (accessed 18 June 2012).

[33] Bryant LD, Murray J, Green JM, Hewison J, Sehmi I, Ellis A. Descriptive information about Down syndrome: A content analysis of serum screening leaflets. Prenat Diagn. 2001 Dec;21(12):1057-63. http://onlinelibrary.wiley.com/doi/10.1002/pd.179/abstract (accessed 5 July 2012).

[34] Nicolaides KH, Azar G, Byrne D, Mansur C, Marks K. Fetal nuchal translucency: ultrasound screening for chromosomal defects in first trimester of pregnancy. BMJ. 1992 Apr 4;304(6831):867-9. http://www.ncbi.nlm.nih.gov/pmc/articles/PMC1882788/?tool=pubmed (accessed 18 June 2012).

[35] Pandya PP, Kondylios A, Hilbert L, Snijders RJ, Nicolaides KH. Chromosomal defects and outcome in 1015 fetuses with increased nuchal translucency. Ultrasound

Obstet Gynecol. 1995 Jan;5(1):15-9. http://onlinelibrary.wiley.com/doi/10.1046/j.1469-0705.1995.05010015.x/abstract (accessed 18 June 2012).

[36] Mendoza-Caamal EC, Grether-González P, Hernández-Gómez M, Guzmán-Huerta M, Aguinaga-Ríos M. Birth defects associated with increased nuchal translucency. Ginecol Obstet Mex. 2010 Oct;78(10):533-9.

[37] Mogra R, Alabbad N, Hyett J. Increased nuchal translucency and congenital heart disease. Early Hum Dev. 2012 May;88(5):261-7. http://www.earlyhumandevelopment.com/article/S0378-3782(12)00063-1/abstract (accessed 18 June 2012).

[38] Merkatz IR, Nitowsky HM, Macri JN, Johnson WE. An association between low m7ternal serum alpha-fetoprotein and fetal chromosomal abnormalities. Am J Obstet Gynecol. 1984 Apr 1;148(7):886-94.

[39] Bogart MH, Pandian MR, Jones OW. Abnormal maternal serum chorionic gonadotropin levels in pregnancies with fetal chromosome abnormalities. Prenat Diagn. 1987 Nov;7(9):623-30.

[40] Canick JA, Knight GJ, Palomaki GE, Haddow JE, Cuckle HS, Wald NJ. Low second trimester maternal serum unconjugated oestriol in pregnancies with Down's syndrome. Br J Obstet Gynaecol. 1988 Apr;95(4):330-3.

[41] Brambati B, Macintosh MC, Teisner B, Maguiness S, Shrimanker K, Lanzani A, et al. Low maternal serum levels of pregnancy associated plasma protein A (PAPP-A) in the first trimester in association with abnormal fetal karyotype. Br J Obstet Gynaecol. 1993 Apr;100(4):324-6.

[42] Aitken DA, Wallace EM, Crossley JA, Swanston IA, van Pareren Y, van Maarle M, et al. 1996. Dimeric inhibin A as a marker for Down's syndrome in early pregnancy. N Engl J Med. 1996 May 9;334(19):1231-6. http://www.nejm.org/doi/full/10.1056/NEJM199605093341904 (accessed 1 July 2012).

[43] Benn PA. Advances in prenatal screening for Down syndrome: I. General principles and second trimester testing. Clin Chim Acta. 2002 Sep;323(1-2):1-16. http://www.sciencedirect.com/science/article/pii/S0009898102001869 (accessed 26 July 2012).

[44] Minami S, Yamoto M, Nakano R. Sources of inhibin in early pregnancy. Early Pregnancy. 1995 Mar;1(1):62-6.

[45] Malone FD, Canick JA, Ball RH, Nyberg DA, Comstock CH, Bukowski R, et al. First-trimester or second-trimester screening, or both, for Down's syndrome. N Engl J Med. 2005 Nov 10;353(19):2001-11. http://www.nejm.org/doi/full/10.1056/NEJMoa043693 (accessed 18 June 2012).

[46] Kagan KO, Wright D, Baker A, Sahota D, Nicolaides KH. Screening for trisomy 21 by maternal age, fetal nuchal translucency thickness, free beta-human chorionic gonadotropin and pregnancy-associated plasma protein-A. Ultrasound Obstet Gynecol. 2008

Jun;31(6):618-24. http://onlinelibrary.wiley.com/doi/10.1002/uog.5331/abstract (accessed 16 July 2012).

[47] Raniga S, Desai PD, Parikh H. Ultrasonographic soft markers of aneuploidy in second trimester: are we lost? MedGenMed. 2006 Jan 11;8(1):9. http://www.ncbi.nlm.nih.gov/pmc/articles/PMC1681991/?tool=pubmed (accessed 18 June 2012).

[48] Mazzoni GT Jr, Cabral AC, de Lima Faria MM, Castro MJ, de Carvalho Pires M, Johnson DS, et al. Ultrasound evaluation of the fetal nasal bone: what is the most appropriate first-trimester cut-off point for aneuploidy screening? Arch Gynecol Obstet. 2012 May;285(5):1263-70. http://www.springerlink.com/content/w04724766836n9x2/ (accessed 18 June 2012).

[49] Bromley B, Lieberman E, Shipp TD, Benacerraf BR. The genetic sonogram: a method of risk assessment for Down syndrome in the second trimester. J Ultrasound Med. 2002 Oct;21(10):1087-96; quiz 1097-8. http://www.jultrasoundmed.org/content/21/10/1087.long (accessed 6 July 2012).

[50] Simpson JL. Invasive procedures for prenatal diagnosis: Any future left? Best Pract Res Clin Obstet Gynaecol. 2012 Jun 30. DOI: 10.1016/j.bpobgyn.2012.05.007. http://www.sciencedirect.com/science/article/pii/S1521693412000934 (accessed 18 June 2012).

[51] Enzensberger C, Pulvermacher C, Degenhardt J, Kawacki A, Germer U, Gembruch U, et al. Fetal Loss Rate and Associated Risk Factors After Amniocentesis, Chorionic Villus Sampling and Fetal Blood Sampling. Ultraschall Med. 2012 May 23. DOI: 10.1055/s-0031-1299388. https://www.thieme-connect.com/DOI/DOI?10.1055/s-0031-1299388 (accessed 15 July 2012).

[52] Dhaifalah I, Zapletalova J. Safety and risks associated with screening for chromosomal abnormalities during pregnancy Ceska Gynekol. 2012 Summer;77(3):236-241.

[53] Alfirevic Z, Sundberg K, Brigham S. Amniocentesis and chorionic villus sampling for prenatal diagnosis. Cochrane Database Syst Rev. 2003;(3):CD003252. http://onlinelibrary.wiley.com/doi/10.1002/14651858.CD003252/abstract;jsessionid=9599AB64C84E30EF63AFAB4D48359C0F.d03t02 (accessed 7 July 2012).

[54] Tongsong T, Wanapirak C, Kunavikatikul C, Sirirchotiyakul S, Piyamongkol W, Chanprapaph P. Fetal loss rate associated with cordocentesis at midgestation. Am J Obstet Gynecol. 2001 Mar;184(4):719-23. http://www.ajog.org/article/S0002-9378(01)74471-7/abstract (accessed 18 June 2012).

[55] Liao C, Wei J, Li Q, Li L, Li J, Li D. Efficacy and safety of cordocentesis for prenatal diagnosis. Int J Gynaecol Obstet. 2006 Apr;93(1):13-7. http://www.ijgo.org/article/S0020-7292(06)00013-0/abstract (accessed 18 June 2012).

[56] Boupaijit K, Wanapirak C, Piyamongkol W, Sirichotiyakul S, Tongsong T. Effect of placenta penetration during cordocentesis at mid-pregnancy on fetal outcomes. Pre-

nat Diagn. 2012 Jan;32(1):83-7. http://onlinelibrary.wiley.com/doi/10.1002/pd.2916/abstract (accessed 5 June 2012).

[57] Wright CF, Burton H. The use of cell-free fetal nucleic acids in maternal blood for non-invasive prenatal diagnosis. Hum Reprod Update. 2009 Jan-Feb;15(1):139-51. http://humupd.oxfordjournals.org/content/15/1/139.long (accessed 18 June 2012).

[58] Chiu RHK, Akolekar R, Zheng YWL, Leung TY, Sun H, Chan KCA, et al. Non-invasive prenatal assessment of trisomy 21 by multiplexed maternal plasma DNA sequencing: large scale validity study. BMJ. 2011 Jan 11;342:c7401. http://www.ncbi.nlm.nih.gov/pmc/articles/PMC3019239/?tool=pubmed (accessed 7 June 2012).

[59] Canick JA, Kloza EM, Lambert-Messerlian GM, Haddow JE, Ehrich M, van den Boom D, et al. DNA sequencing of maternal plasma to identify Down syndrome and other trisomies in multiple gestations. Prenat Diagn. 2012 Aug;32(8):730-4. http://onlinelibrary.wiley.com/doi/10.1002/pd.3892/abstract (accessed 7 June 2012).

[60] Ashoor G, Syngelaki A, Wagner M, Birdir C, Nicolaides KH. Chromosome-selective sequencing of maternal plasma cell-free DNA for first-trimester detection of trisomy 21 and trisomy 18. Am J Obstet Gynecol. 2012 Apr;206(4):322.e1-5. http://www.ajog.org/article/S0002-9378(12)00060-9/abstract (accessed 1 July 2012).

[61] Yang YH, Kim SH, Yang ES, Kim SK, Kim IK, Park YW, et al. Prenatal diagnosis of fetal trisomy 21 from maternal peripheral blood. Yonsei Med J. 2003 Apr 30;44(2):181-6. http://www.eymj.org/DOIx.php?id=10.3349/ymj.2003.44.2.181 (accessed 18 June 2012).

[62] Sifakis S, Papantoniou N, Kappou D, Antsaklis A. Noninvasive prenatal diagnosis of Down syndrome: current knowledge and novel insights. J Perinat Med. 2012 Feb 13;40(4):319-27. http://www.degruyter.com/view/j/jpme.2012.40.issue-4/jpm-2011-0282/jpm-2011-0282.xml;jsessionid=0E0E90A7F0EAF0618F024D6215251415 (accessed 18 June 2012).

[63] Choolani M, Mahyuddin AP, Hahn S. The promise of fetal cells in maternal blood. Best Pract Res Clin Obstet Gynaecol. 2012 Jul 12. DOI: 10.1016/j.bbr.2011.03.031. http://www.sciencedirect.com/science/article/pii/S152169341200106X (accessed 6 June 2012).

[64] Jia CW, Wang SY, Ma YM, Lan YL, Si YM, Yu L, et al. Fluorescence in situ hybridization in uncultured amniocytes for detection of aneuploidy in 4210 prenatal cases. Chin Med J (Engl). 2011 Apr;124(8):1164-8. http://www.cmj.org/Periodical/paperlist.asp?id=LW2011420367338008724&linkintype=pubmed (accessed 20 June 2012).

[65] Ho SS, Chua C, Gole L, Biswas A, Koay E, Choolani M. Same-day prenatal diagnosis of common chromosomal aneuploidies using microfluidics-fluorescence in situ hybridization. Prenat Diagn. 2012 Apr;32(4):321-8. http://onlinelibrary.wiley.com/doi/10.1002/pd.2946/abstract (accessed 5 July 2012).

[66] Hills A, Donaghue C, Waters J, Waters K, Sullivan C, Kulkarni A, et al. QF-PCR as a stand-alone test for prenatal samples: the first 2 years' experience in the London region. Prenat Diagn. 2010 Jun;30(6):509-17. http://onlinelibrary.wiley.com/doi/10.1002/pd.2503/abstract (accessed 29 July 2012).

[67] Faas BHW, Cirigliano V, Bui TH. Rapid methods for targeted prenatal diagnosis of common chromosome aneuploidies. Semin Fetal Neonatal Med. 2011 Apr;16(2):81-7. http://www.sfnmjournal.com/article/S1744-165X(11)00004-7/abstract (accessed 12 July 2012).

[68] Canick JA, Kloza EM, Lambert-Messerlian GM, Haddow JE, Ehrich M, van den Boom D, et al. DNA sequencing of maternal plasma to identify Down syndrome and other trisomies in multiple gestations. Prenat Diagn. 2012 Aug;32(8):730-4. http://onlinelibrary.wiley.com/doi/10.1002/pd.3892/abstract;jsessionid=8345A09565F7EB0EE80CE1EE242D45CA.d03t01 (accessed 18 June 2012).

[69] Lee MH, Ryu HM, Kim DJ, Lee BY, Cho EH, Yang JH, et al. Rapid prenatal diagnosis of Down syndrome using quantitative fluorescent PCR in uncultured amniocytes. J Korean Med Sci. 2004 Jun;19(3):341-4. http://www.ncbi.nlm.nih.gov/pmc/articles/PMC2816832/?tool=pubmed (accessed 18 June 2012).

[70] Zhang Y, Xu CM, Zhu YM, Dong MY, Qian YL, Jin F, et al. Preimplantation genetic diagnosis for Down syndrome pregnancy. J Zhejiang Univ Sci B. 2007 Jul;8(7):515-21. http://www.ncbi.nlm.nih.gov/pmc/articles/PMC1906599/?tool=pubmed (accessed 18 June 2012).

[71] Sturgeon X, Gardiner KJ. Transcript catalogs of human chromosome 21 and orthologous chimpanzee and mouse regions. Mamm Genome. 2011 Jun;22(5-6):261-71. http://www.springerlink.com/content/q35t330n314v6107/ (accessed 15 June 2012).

[72] Antonarakis SE, Lyle R, Chrast R, Scott HS. Differential gene expression studies to explore the molecular pathophysiology of Down syndrome. Brain Res Brain Res Rev. 2001 Oct;36(2-3):265-74. http://www.sciencedirect.com/science/article/pii/S0165017301001035 (accessed 15 July 2012).

[73] Millan Sanchez M, Heyn SN, Das D, Moghadam S, Martin KJ, Salehi A. Neurobiological elements of cognitive dysfunction in down syndrome: exploring the role of APP. Biol Psychiatry. 2012 Mar 1;71(5):403-9. http://www.biologicalpsychiatryjournal.com/article/S0006-3223(11)00822-5/abstract (accessed 18 June 2012).

[74] Moncaster JA, Pineda R, Moir RD, Lu S, Burton MA, Ghosh JG, et al. Alzheimer's disease amyloid-beta links lens and brain pathology in Down syndrome. PLoS One. 2010 May 20;5(5):e10659. http://www.ncbi.nlm.nih.gov/pmc/articles/PMC2873949/?tool=pubmed (accessed 20 June 2012).

[75] Shim KS, Ferrando-Miguel R, Lubec G. Aberrant protein expression of transcription factors BACH1 and ERG, both encoded on chromosome 21, in brains of patients with Down syndrome and Alzheimer's disease. J Neural Transm Suppl. 2003;(67):39-49.

[76] Rachidi M, Delezoide AL, Delabar JM, Lopes C. A quantitative assessment of gene expression (QAGE) reveals differential overexpression of DOPEY2, a candidate gene for mental retardation, in Down syndrome brain regions. Int J Dev Neurosci. 2009 Jun;27(4):393-8. http://www.sciencedirect.com/science/article/pii/S0736574809000197 (accessed 20 July 2012).

[77] Saito Y, Oka A, Mizuguchi M, Motonaga K, Mori Y, Becker LE, et al. The developmental and aging changes of Down's syndrome cell adhesion molecule expression in normal and Down's syndrome brains. Acta Neuropathol. 2000 Dec;100(6):654-64. http://www.springerlink.com/content/gbjxfuyf3d4lk98p/ (accessed 20 July 2012).

[78] Malinge S, Bliss-Moreau M, Kirsammer G, Diebold L, Chlon T, Gurbuxani S, et al. Increased dosage of the chromosome 21 ortholog Dyrk1a promotes megakaryoblastic leukemia in a murine model of Down syndrome. J Clin Invest. 2012 Mar 1;122(3): 948-62. http://www.ncbi.nlm.nih.gov/pmc/articles/PMC3287382/?tool=pubmed (accessed 15 June 2012).

[79] Mazur-Kolecka B, Golabek A, Kida E, Rabe A, Hwang YW, Adayev T, et al. Effect of DYRK1A activity inhibition on development of neuronal progenitors isolated from Ts65Dn mice. J Neurosci Res. 2012 May;90(5):999-1010. http://onlinelibrary.wiley.com/doi/10.1002/jnr.23007/abstract. (accessed 15 June 2012).

[80] Wegiel J, Kaczmarski W, Barua M, Kuchna I, Nowicki K, Wang KC, et al. Link between DYRK1A overexpression and several-fold enhancement of neurofibrillary degeneration with 3-repeat tau protein in Down syndrome. J Neuropathol Exp Neurol. 2011 Jan;70(1):36-50. http://www.ncbi.nlm.nih.gov/pmc/articles/PMC3083064/?tool=pubmed (accessed 20 June 2012).

[81] Chakrabarti L, Best TK, Cramer NP, Carney RS, Isaac JT, Galdzicki Z, et al. Olig1 and Olig2 triplication causes developmental brain defects in Down syndrome. Nat Neurosci. 2010 Aug;13(8):927-34. http://www.ncbi.nlm.nih.gov/pmc/articles/PMC3249618/?tool=pubmed (accessed 3 July 2012).

[82] Meng X, Peng B, Shi J, Zheng Y, Chen H, Zhang J, et al. Effects of overexpression of Sim2 on spatial memory and expression of synapsin I in rat hippocampus. Cell Biol Int. 2006 Oct;30(10):841-7. http://www.cellbiolint.org/cbi/030/0841/cbi0300841.htm (accessed 20 July 2012).

[83] Rachidi M, Lopes C, Charron G, Delezoide AL, Paly E, Bloch B, et al. Spatial and temporal localization during embryonic and fetal human development of the transcription factor SIM2 in brain regions altered in Down syndrome. Int J Dev Neurosci. 2005 Aug;23(5):475-84. http://www.sciencedirect.com/science/article/pii/S0736574805000638 (accessed 20 July 2012).

[84] Shin JH, London J, Le Pecheur M, Weitzdoerfer R, Hoeger H, Lubec G. Proteome analysis in hippocampus of mice overexpressing human Cu/Zn-superoxide dismutase 1. Neurochem Int. 2005 Jun;46(8):641-53. http://www.sciencedirect.com/science/article/pii/S0197018605000434 (accessed 20 July 2012).

[85] Mouton-Liger F, Thomas S, Rattenbach R, Magnol L, Larigaldie V, Ledru A, et al. PCP4 (PEP19) overexpression induces premature neuronal differentiation associated with Ca(2+) /calmodulin-dependent kinase II-δ activation in mouse models of Down syndrome. J Comp Neurol. 2011 Oct 1;519(14):2779-802. http://onlinelibrary.wiley.com/doi/10.1002/cne.22651/abstract (accessed 20 July 2012).

[86] Aït Yahya-Graison E, Aubert J, Dauphinot L, Rivals I, Prieur M, Golfier G, et al. Classification of human chromosome 21 gene-expression variations in Down syndrome: impact on disease phenotypes. Am J Hum Genet. 2007 Sep;81(3):475-91. http://www.ncbi.nlm.nih.gov/pmc/articles/PMC1950826/?tool=pubmed (accessed 9 July 2012).

[87] Kahlem P, Sultan M, Herwig R, Steinfath M, Balzereit D, Eppens B, et al. Transcript level alterations reflect gene dosage effects across multiple tissues in a mouse model of down syndrome. Genome Res. 2004 Jul;14(7):1258-67. http://www.ncbi.nlm.nih.gov/pmc/articles/PMC442140/?tool=pubmed (accessed 29 July 2012).

[88] Saran NG, Pletcher MT, Natale JE, Cheng Y, Reeves RH. Global disruption of the cerebellar transcriptome in a Down syndrome mouse model. Hum Mol Genet. 2003 Aug 15;12(16):2013-9. http://hmg.oxfordjournals.org/content/12/16/2013.long (accessed 20 July 2012).

[89] FitzPatrick DR. Transcriptional consequences of autosomal trisomy: primary gene dosage with complex downstream effects. Trends Genet. 2005 May;21(5):249-53. http://www.sciencedirect.com/science/article/pii/S0168952505000582 (accessed 29 June 2012).

[90] Dauphinot L, Lyle R, Rivals I, Dang MT, Moldrich RX, Golfier G, et al. The cerebellar transcriptome during postnatal development of the Ts1Cje mouse, a segmental trisomy model for Down syndrome. Hum Mol Genet. 2005 Feb 1;14(3):373-84. http://hmg.oxfordjournals.org/content/14/3/373.long (accessed 29 June 2012).

[91] Kuromitsu J, Yamashita H, Kataoka H, Takahara T, Muramatsu M, Sekine T, et al. A unique downregulation of h2-calponin gene expression in Down syndrome: a possible attenuation mechanism for fetal survival by methylation at the CpG island in the trisomic chromosome 21. Mol Cell Biol. 1997 Feb;17(2):707-12. http://www.ncbi.nlm.nih.gov/pmc/articles/PMC231796/?tool=pubmed (accessed 29 June 2012).

[92] Kerkel K, Schupf N, Hatta K, Pang D, Salas M, Kratz A, et al. Altered DNA methylation in leukocytes with trisomy 21. PLoS Genet. 2010 Nov 18;6(11):e1001212. http://www.ncbi.nlm.nih.gov/pmc/articles/PMC2987931/?tool=pubmed (accessed 29 June 2012).

[93] Sethupathy P, Borel C, Gagnebin M, Grant GR, Deutsch S, Elton TS, et al. Human microRNA-155 on chromosome 21 differentially interacts with its polymorphic target in the AGTR1 3' untranslated region: a mechanism for functional single-nucleotide

polymorphisms related to phenotypes. Am J Hum Genet. 2007 Aug;81(2):405-13. http://www.ncbi.nlm.nih.gov/pmc/articles/PMC1950808/?tool=pubmed (accessed 6 June 2012).

[94] Kuhn DE, Nuovo GJ, Martin MM, Malana GE, Pleister AP, Jiang J, et al. Human chromosome 21-derived miRNAs are overexpressed in down syndrome brains and hearts. Biochem Biophys Res Commun. 2008 Jun 6;370(3):473-7. http://www.ncbi.nlm.nih.gov/pmc/articles/PMC2585520/?tool=pubmed (accessed 15 June 2012).

[95] Elton TS, Sansom SE, Martin MM. Trisomy-21 gene dosage over-expression of miRNAs results in the haploinsufficiency of specific target proteins. RNA Biol. 2010 Sep-Oct;7(5):540-7. http://www.ncbi.nlm.nih.gov/pmc/articles/PMC3073250/?tool=pubmed (accessed 26 June 2012).

[96] Kuhn DE, Nuovo GJ, Terry AV Jr, Martin MM, Malana GE, Sansom SE, et al. Chromosome 21-derived microRNAs provide an etiological basis for aberrant protein expression in human Down syndrome brains. J Biol Chem. 2010 Jan 8;285(2):1529-43. http://www.ncbi.nlm.nih.gov/pmc/articles/PMC2801278/?tool=pubmed (accessed 15 June 2012).

[97] Keck-Wherley J, Grover D, Bhattacharyya S, Xu X, Holman D, Lombardini ED, et al. Abnormal microRNA expression in Ts65Dn hippocampus and whole blood: contributions to Down syndrome phenotypes. Dev Neurosci. 2011;33(5):451-67. http://content.karger.com/produktedb/produkte.asp?DOI=10.1159/000330884 (accessed 15 June 2012).

Chapter 2

Increased Fetal Nuchal Translucency Thickness and Normal Karyotype: Prenatal and Postnatal Outcome

Ksenija Gersak, Darija M. Strah and
Maja Pohar-Perme

Additional information is available at the end of the chapter

http://dx.doi.org/10.5772/53112

1. Introduction

Nuchal translucency (NT) is the assessment of the amount of fluid behind the neck of the fetus, also known as the nuchal fold. An anechoic space is visible and measurable sonographically in all fetuses between the 11th and the 14th week of the pregnancy (Figure 1). Underlying pathophysiological mechanisms for nuchal fluid collection under the skin include cardiac dysfunction, venous congestion in the head and neck, altered composition of the extracellular matrix, failure of lymphatic drainage, fetal anemia or hypoproteinemia and congenital infection [1]. The abnormal accumulation of nuchal fluid decreases after the 14th week.

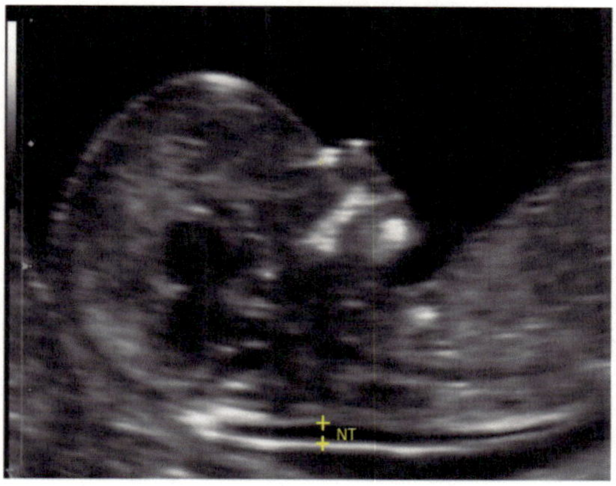

Figure 1. Normal nuchal translucency thickness (NT)

1.1. Increased NT in chromosomally abnormal fetuses

The association between the increased NT and the chromosomal abnormalities has been well documented (Figure 2). It helps us identify the high-risk fetuses for trisomy 21 and other chromosomal abnormalities [2,3].

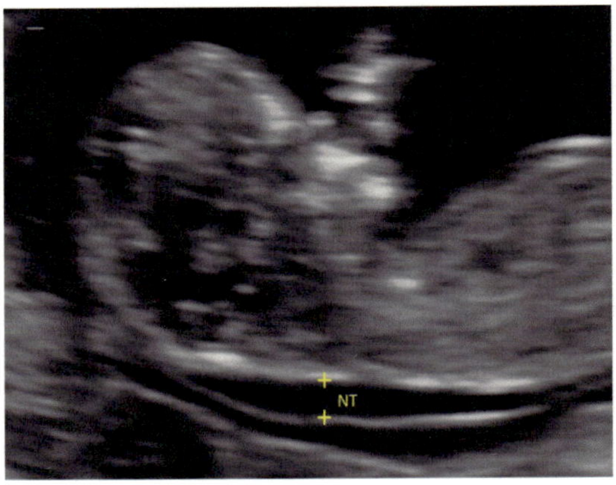

Figure 2. Increased nuchal translucency thickness (NT)

The findings of numerous studies suggest that an effective first trimester screening for trisomy 21 can be obtained by the combination of maternal age and measurement of fetal NT [4-11]. At a risk cut-off of 1 in100, the detection rate of trisomy 21 is about 75%, at a false positive rate of about 2%. The detection rate can be improved to 85% by the additional assessment of the fetal nasal bone and even more by the Doppler assessment of blood flow across the tricuspid valve or blood flow in the ductus venosus, which has increased the detection rate to about 95% at a false positive rate of 2.5% [11].

Our retrospective study of the first trimester screening for trisomy 21 in 5-year period from 2005 to 2010 by employing the combination of maternal age, sonographic measurement of the fetal NT thickness and assessment of the fetal nasal bone, included 13,049 pregnant women [12]. The sample represented an unselected population of women with singleton pregnancies. The cut-off risk for trisomy 21 was set at 1 in 300. The distribution of maternal age of the examined women was compared to the age distribution in the pregnant population in Slovenia for the same time interval (2005-2010). The balance between the false positive rate and the detection rate was studied and the trends were inspected graphically. The cut-off risk that would yield 5% false positives was calculated for trisomy 21. The average gestation was 12 4/7 weeks (range from 11 1/7 weeks to 14 0/7 weeks). The average fetal CRL was 63.2 mm (from 45 mm to 83 mm). The average NT thickness was 1.7 mm (range from 0.9 mm to 13.4 mm). The NT was above the 95th centile of the normal range for the CRL in 75% (15 out of 20) of trisomy 21 pregnancies and in 64% (16 out of 25) pregnancies with other chromosomal abnormalities. At the time of the testing the estimated risk for trisomy 21 was 1 in 300 or higher in 3% of all the pregnancies (394 out of 13,049), considering the calculation based on FMF program. Three hundred and sixty cases (2.8%) turned out to be false positive. At the invasive testing, chromosomal abnormalities were identified in 8.6% of high risk cases (34 out of 394), which represented one case of fetal chromosomal abnormality, detected per 12 invasive diagnostic procedures. Consequently we believe that the effective screening for trisomy 21 can be achieved in the first trimester of pregnancy by the combination of maternal age, sonographic measurement of the fetal NT thickness and assessment of the fetal nasal bone, with detection rate of 85% at a false positive rate of less than 3%.

Karyotype	n
Trisomy 21	20
Trisomy 18	10
Trisomy 13	2
45,X (Turner syndrom)	3
47,XXY	2
Mosaic structure	3
Unbalanced structural rearrangements	5
Total	45

Table 1. Chromosomal abnormalities in fetuses and newborns in our sample of 13,049 women with singleton pregnancies [12].

1.2. Increased NT in chromosomally normal fetuses

The NT can be increased also in chromosomally normal fetuses. When the karyotype is normal, the fetus is still at a significant risk of adverse pregnancy outcome e.g. fetal loss, structural abnormalities, particularly cardiac defects, various genetic syndromes and delayed neurodevelopment [9,13]. The prevalence of fetal abnormalities and adverse pregnancy outcomes increases with the thickness of NT.

The impact of the increased nuchal fluid collection, seen during the ultrasound examination, raises the parents' great anxiety about future fetal development [13]. The risks of adverse pregnancy outcomes have to be discussed with the parents and an objective counseling has to be offered to them together with detailed ultrasound examinations later in the pregnancy. But even in the absence of clear fetal abnormalities, some couples request pregnancy termination in such circumstances [14].

Therefore, the aim of this study was to evaluate the pregnancy outcomes of fetuses with increased NT thickness and normal karyotype in an unselected pregnant population.

2. Subjects and methods

2.1. Study design

The retrospective study included unselected population of pregnant women of Caucasian ethnic origin appointed for the first trimester ultrasound screening examination at a single outpatient clinic between January 4, 2005 and April 30, 2010. Included in the study population were only singleton pregnancies with live fetus from the 11th to the 14th week of gestation with the CRL of 45-83 mm.

Before the screening they had all received counseling by their level one gynecologists and an information leaflet about the ultrasound examination and the aim of the screening. In the majority of cases the examination of early fetal morphology and other measurements was performed transabdominally within 20 minutes. In less than 1% of the cases a transvaginal ultrasound examination had to be carried out.

For the examinations we used 2-5 MHz and 3.7-9.3 MHz transducers GE Healthcare Voluson 730 Pro, Milwaukee, USA, 4–6 MHz, 4–7 MHz, 5–9 MHz and 7–9 MHz transducers Acuson S2000, Siemens Medical Solution, Mountain View CA, USA.

The measurement of fetal NT followed the criteria recommended by the Fetal Medicine Foundation (FMF). The increased NT thickness was defined as a measurement above the 95th percentile for the normal range. Risks were calculated according to the FMF program, following its guidelines [15,16].

The women with an increased risk for chromosomal anomalies (≥ 1:300) calculated on the basis of maternal age, NT and fetal crown-rump length (CRL) were offered invasive testing for fetal karyotyping. The karyotyping was performed by using chorionic villus sampling or amniocentesis in three cytogenetic laboratories.

The fetuses with increased fetal NT and normal karyotype were followed by detailed structural ultrasound evaluation between the 20th and the 24th week of gestation. Fetal echocardiography was performed in cases in which NT exceeded 3.5 mm.

After an informed consent had been signed, pregnancy outcomes were obtained from the participating women by written questionnaires. In cases of non-responders or uncertainty, telephone contact with the parents was established. The length of follow-up ranged from 18 months to 5 years.

2.2. Exclusion criteria

The exclusion criteria were the loss to follow-up, the chromosomal abnormalities or no information on karyotype in a fetal loss.

2.3. Classification of adverse outcome

Adverse pregnancy outcome was defined as fetal loss (miscarriage, intrauterine death, termination of pregnancy), and as liveborn infant with structural abnormality, genetic disorders and/or neurodevelopmental delay diagnosed before or after delivery. Stillbirth <22 weeks of pregnancy was defined as miscarriage, and stillbirth ≥22 weeks of pregnancy or birth of a child of at least 500 g weight without vital signs as intrauterine fetal death.

2.4. Statistical analysis

Descriptive statistics were used to describe our sample. Means, standard deviations and ranges are reported for continuous variables, numbers and proportions are reported for categorical variables. Statistical analysis was performed using R statistical package, version 2.14.

3. Results

3.1. Study population

The sample represented 11,980 unselected pregnant women appointed for the first trimester ultrasound screening examination at a single outpatient clinic between January 4, 2005 and April 30, 2010.

Five hundred and fifty-eight fetuses had an increased fetal NT and normal karyotype (558/11,980; 4.7%). In 46 cases (46/558; 8.2%) the outcome of the pregnancy was unknown; therefore 512 singleton pregnancies were included in the further analysis.

The mean maternal age was 30.2 years (range from 17 to 46 years, SD=4.8). There were 421 out of 512 pregnancies (82.2%) conceived naturally and 91 (17.8%; 91/512) after in vitro fertilization. The mean NT ≥95th percentile was of 2.5 mm (range from 1.3 to 13.4 mm).

3.2. Fetal loss

The fetal loss was registered in 36 pregnancies (36/512; 7%). Twelve women (2.3%; 12/512) had miscarriage, 19 pregnancies (3.7%; 19/512) were terminated at parental request or due to the finding of structural abnormalities, and 1% of pregnancies (5/512) ended with intrauterine death. The outcomes with respect to the NT thickness are presented in Table 2. Table 3 provides details on all the types of fetal loss. The most common causes of termination were hydrops fetalis, increased NT or cystic hygroma (Figure 3).

NT (mm)	≤ 3.4	3.5-4.4	4.5-5.4	5.5-6.4	≥ 6.5	Total
Outcome						
Delivery	436	34	5	1	0	476 (93%)
Miscarriage	11	0	1	0	0	12 (2.3%)
Intrauterine death	1	3	0	0	1	5 (1%)
Termination	8	2	3	2	4	19 (3.7%)
Total	456	39	9	3	5	512

Table 2. Outcome of pregnancies with respect to the NT thickness.

Fetal loss	n	NT (mm)
Miscarriage (unspecified)	10	2.1/2.2/2.3/2.5/2.6/ 2.9/2.9/3.0/3.0/4.6
Spontaneous abortion after amniocentesis	2	2.5/3.0
Intrauterine death (unspecified)	4	3.0/3.5/3.7/4.2
Intrauterine death/tetralogy of Fallot	1	7.8
Termination:	19	
Hydrops fetalis	5	2.7/3.7/6.4/7.4/12.0
Increased NT	4	2.9/3.0/5.0/5.2
Cystic hygroma	3	12.2/13.4
Hydrocephalus	2	2.5/4.9
VSD/valve anomaly	1	3.7
Dandy-Walker malformation	1	5.6
Diaphragmatic hernia	1	3.2
Renal dysplasia	1	2.2
Neurofibromatosis type I (inherit)	1	2.1

Table 3. Fetal loss with respect to the NT thickness.

3.3. Liveborn infants with abnormalities

Four hundred and seventy-six pregnancies ended with delivery of a viable infant (93%). Among them we found 48 newborns (9.5%; 48/476) with either single or multiple abnormalities. The clinical findings in 476 liveborn infants with respect to the NT thickness are presented in Table 4. There were 8 cases (1.7%, 8/476) born with heart defects, other structural abnormalities were found in 30 newborns (6.3%; 30/476). During the first year of life some genetic syndromes or neurodevelopmental delay were recorded in 10 cases (2.1%; 10/476). All abnormalities were found in the group of newborns with mildly enlarged NT, between 95th percentiles to 4.4 mm. Among healthy babies, there was no NT thicker than 6.4 mm. Table 5 describes the disorders of 48 babies in more detail.

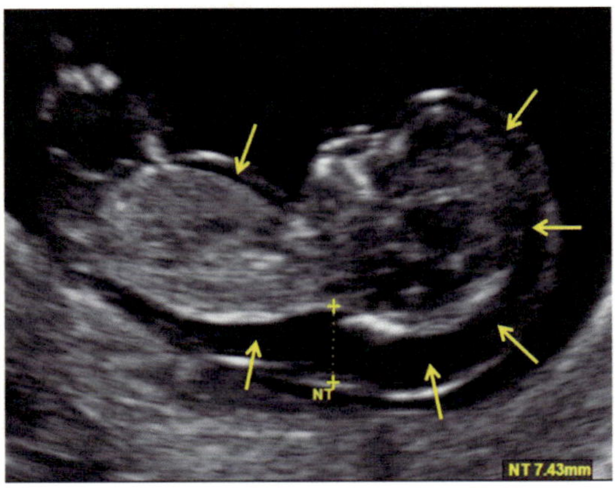

Figure 3. Hydrops fetalis

	NT (mm)≤ 3.4	3.5-4.4	4.5-5.4	5.5-6.4	≥ 6.5	Total
Clinical findings						
Healthy	393	29	5	1	0	431
Heart defect	6	2	0	0	0	8
Structural abnormalities	29	1	0	0	0	30
Genetic syndromes	5	0	0	0	0	5
Neurodevelopmental delay	4	1	0	0	0	5
Total	**437**	**33**	**5**	**1**	**0**	**476**

Table 4. Clinical findings in liveborn infants with respect to the NT thickness.

Disorder	n	NT (mm)
Heart defects:	8	
VSD	3	2.6/3.0/3.2
VSD, ASD and aortic coarctation	1	3.9
VSD, ASD and tricuspid valve anomaly	1	4.0
Hypoplastic left ventricle	1	3.4
Isolated valve anomaly	2	3.4/2.6
Other abnormalities:	30	
Hydronephrosis (isolated)	4	1.8/2.5/2.8/3.1
Hydronephrosis and ureteral stenosis	2	2.8/3.1
Vesicouretheral reflux	2	2.6/2.8
Cleft lip and/or cleft palate	4	1.5/2.1/3.1/3.1
Craniosynostosis	1	2.3
Hypoplasia of the corpus callosum	1	2.5
Hydrocephalus	1	3.2
Micrognathia	1	2.6
Hemangioma	2	1.8/1.9
Cystic adenomatoid malformation	1	2.4
Diaphragmatic hernia	1	3.2
Atresia of the duodenum	1	3.0
Unilateral renal agenesis	1	2.7

Disorder	n	NT (mm)
Cryptorchidism	2	3.2/4.4
Hypospadias	1	3.2
Polydactyly	1	2.3
Hip dysplasia	3	1.8/1.8/2.2
Talipes	1	2.9
Genetic syndromes and neurodevelopmental delay:	10	
Adrenogenital syndrome	1	3.0
Lipid metabolism disorder	1	1.9
Coeliac disease	1	1.6
Polycystic kidney disease	2	2.4/2.4
Unspecific genetic syndrome and neurodevelopmental delay	2	2.6/3.0
Neurodevelopmental delay	3	2.5/2.9/3.5

Table 5. Disorders described in forty-eight euploid infants.

3.4. Gender and preterm labor

The overall male: female ratio was 1.37:1. In the group of fetuses with NT thickness between 95th percentile to ≤ 3.4 mm the ratio was 1.27:1 and in the group with NT ≥ 3.5 mm 2.64:1.

The gender distribution of liveborn infants with respect to the abnormalities is presented in Table 6. Male gender was predominant among healthy infants and in the group with genetic syndromes neurodevelopmental delay.

Preterm delivery was registered in 41 cases (41/476; 8.6%). Thirty-one healthy babies (31/431; 9.5%) and 10 infants with abnormalities (10/48; 20.8%) were born preterm.

Infants	Males	Females
Healthy	253	175
Heart defect	1	7
Structural abnormalities	15	15
Genetic syndromes/ neurodevelopmental delay	8	2
Total	276	198

Table 6. Gender distribution of liveborn infants with respect to the abnormalities.

4. Discussion

We evaluated the pregnancy outcome of a subgroup of 512 fetuses with increased NT thickness and normal karyotype referring to 11,980 unselected pregnancies. According to the data of fetal loss, structural abnormalities, genetic disorders and neurodevelopmental delay, one out of 6 fetuses had an increased risk ≥1:300 of trisomy 21 calculated on the basis of maternal age, NT and fetal crown-rump length. The study confirms that 16.4% fetuses (84/512) were at increased risk of adverse pregnancy outcome.

The number of studies, which examined unselected pregnancy population with clear description of all adverse pregnancy outcomes, is limited [9]. Bilardo CM et al [14] noted that one out of five fetuses with increased NT had an adverse pregnancy outcome. Their study provides an overview of the selected pregnancy of 675 fetuses referred from other centers because of an increased NT measurement.

4.1. Fetal loss

In some studies it is not clear whether the fetuses with an unknown karyotype were included [17,18]. This is particularly important in the cases of fetal loss. We included only fetuses with known normal karyotypes. Karyotyping was provided in all cases of miscarriages, intrauterine deaths and terminations of pregnancies using amniocentesis or tissue samples obtained during surgical evacuation of the products of conception.

The increased NT thickness augments the risk of fetal loss. The allover fetal loss in our subgroup of fetuses was 7% (Table 2). We share the opinion that fetal loss in studies without a control group is very difficult to interpret [9,17-20]. The reported rates of spontaneous loss are 0.5-3.8% and the reported rates of termination of pregnancy are 2.3-16.9%.

Fifteen women terminated their pregnancies because of the fetal abnormalities (Table 3). But in 4 cases the pregnancy was terminated at the request of the parents because of an increased risk of trisomy 21, despite of the fact that no fetal malformation had been detected at the ultrasound examination. Westin M et al [9] describe similar experiences.

Our study shows similar weakness compared to the related studies, namely not all fetuses lost having undergone autopsy for ascertainment of fetal abnormalities, especially in the group of miscarriages [9,17-20].

4.2. Liveborn infants with abnormalities

The prevalence of structural abnormalities in our subgroup of newborns with increased NT was 8%. The percentage is higher than expected in general population (2-3%). A similar finding can be encountered in the studies without a control group (9.5-30.3%) [9].

Heart defects were confirmed in 8 out of 38 infants with structural abnormalities. The median NT thickness was significantly higher in fetuses with major heart defects compared to those with normal hearts [21-24]. In 8 infants with heart defects we found NT measurement between 3.4 and 4.4 mm. Although the measurement of NT thickness alone appears to be a moderately effective screening pool for the detection of heart abnormalities, its role in detection of specific congenital heart defects seems more promising [24]. When an increased NT is found, the fetus has to be screened for additional sonographic markers such as tricuspid regurgitation and abnormal ductus venosus Doppler flow profile. We share the opinion that in fetuses with an NT measurement ≥99th percentile, and/or in which tricuspid regurgitation and/or abnormal ductus venosus Doppler flow pattern is found, an earlier fetal echocardiograpy is indicated [23,24].

The second most common isolated structural abnormality was hydronephrosis followed by cleft lip and/or cleft palate (Table 5).

In 5 cases genetic syndromes were found. There were two cases of inherited polycystic kidney disease, and three "de novo" genetic syndromes. In comparison with other studies we detected no infants with neuromuscular disorders [13,14].

As Bilardo CM et al [14] pointed out, the most unpredictable aspect of increased NT is neurodevelopmental delay, which could be manifested unexpectedly, in the postnatal period. The reported incidence of neurodevelopmental delay in fetuses with or without recognizable genetic syndrome varies from 0 to 13% [14,25,26]. In our study 10.4% of newborns (5 out of 48) were diagnosed during the follow-up period of at least 18-months.

4.3. Gender and preterm labor

In our population of fetuses with increased NT thickness, male gender was predominant, especially in the group with NT ≥ 3.5 mm. The impact of male: female ratio on the degree of nuchal fluid accumulation has been reported with controversial results. Yaron et al [27] and Prefumo et al [28] did not find NT to be significantly related to gender, but Lam et al [29] and Timmerman et al [30] reported significantly larger NT in male fetuses. Also Spencer et al [31] found NT to be 3-4% smaller in both chromosomally normal and Down syndrome female fetuses.

5. Conclusion

Many couples enter any of the screening programs without an intricate understanding of the potential fetal and newborn complications. While it is reasonable for the future parents to consider normal karyotype as a "good" result, the healthcare professionals should counsel them that enlarged NT thickness is a strong marker for adverse pregnancy outcome, associated with miscarriage, intrauterine death, heart defects, numerous other structural abnormalities and genetic syndromes. Although the measurement of the nuchal translucency thickness was introduced over 15 years ago, we share the opinion that a general consensus on how to counsel parents of an euploid fetus with enlarged NT has not yet been achieved [13]. The larger studies with uniform protocols and long-term follow-up are needed to recommend the guidelines for objective parental counseling.

Author details

Ksenija Gersak[1], Darija M. Strah[2] and Maja Pohar-Perme[3]

1 Department of Obstetrics and Gynecology, University Medical Center Ljubljana, Slovenia

2 Diagnostic Centre Strah, Domzale, Slovenia

3 Institute for Biostatistics and Medical Informatics, Faculty of Medicine, University of Ljubljana, Slovenia

References

[1] Nicolaides KH. The 11-13+6 weeks scan. London: Fetal Medicine Foundation; 2004.

[2] Nicolaides KH, Azar G, Byrne D, et al. Fetal nuchal translucency: ultrasound screening for chromosomal defects in the first trimester of pregnancy. BMJ 1992;304(6831): 867-9.

[3] Nicolaides KH, Brizot ML, Snijders RJM. Fetal nuchal translucency: ultrasound screening for fetal trisomy in the first trimester of pregnancy. BJOG 1994;101:782-6.

[4] Pajkrt E, van Lith JMM, Mol BWJ, et al. Screening for Down's syndrome by fetal nuchal translucency measurement in a general obstetric population. Ultrasound Obstet Gynecol 1998;12:163–9.

[5] Economides DL, Whitlow BJ, Kadir R, et al. First trimester sonografic detection of chromosomal abnormalities in an unselected population. Br J Obstet Gynaecol 1998;105:58–62.

[6] Bindra R, Heath V, Liao A, et al. One stop assessment of risk for trisomy 21 at 11–14 weeks a prospective study of 15030 pregnancies. Ultrasound Obstet Gynecol 2002;20:219–25.

[7] Liu SS, Lee FK, Lee JL, et al. Pregnancy outcomes in unselected singleton pregnant women with an increased risk of first-trimester Down's syndrome. Acta Obstet Gynecol Scand 2004;83:1130–4.

[8] Rozenberg P, Bussières L, Chevret S, et al. Screening for Down syndrome using first-trimester combined screening followed by second-trimester ultrasound examination in an unselected population. Am J Obstet Gynecol 2006;195:1379–87.

[9] Westin M, Saltvedt S, Bergman G, et al. Is measurement of nuchal translucency thickness a useful screening tool for heart defects? A study of 16,383 fetuses. Ultrasound Obstet Gynecol 2006;27:632–9.

[10] Czuba B, Borowski D, Cnota W, et al. Ultrasonographic assessment of fetal nuchal translucency (NT) at 11th and 14th week of gestation-Polish multicentre study. Neuro Endocrinol Lett 2007;28:175–81.

[11] Kagan KO, Staboulidou I, Cruz J, et al. Two-stage first-trimester screening for trisomy 21 by ultrasound assessment and biochemical testing. Ultrasound Obstet Gynecol 2010;36:542–7.

[12] Gersak K, Pohar-Perme M, Strah DM. First trimester screening for trisomy 21 by maternal age, nuchal translucency and fetal nasal bone in unselected pregnancies. In: Day S, ed. Genetics and etiology of Down syndrome. Rijeka: Intech; 2011:301-312.

[13] Bilardo CM, Timmerman E, Pajkrt E, et al. Increased nuchal translucency in euploid fetuses-what should we be telling the parents? Prenat Diagn 2010;30:93-102.

[14] Bilardo CM, Müller MA, Pajkrt, E, et al. Increased nuchal translucency thickness and normal karyotype: time for parental reassurance. Ultrasound Obstet Gynecol 2007;30:11-8.

[15] Snijders RJM, Noble P, Sebire N, et al. UK multicentre project on assessment of risk for trisomy 21 by maternal age and fetal nuchal translucency thickness at 10 – 14 weeks of gestation. Lancet 1999;18:519–21.

[16] The Fetal Medicine Centre. Ultrasound scan procedures. http://www.fetalmedicine.com(accessed 1 July 2012).

[17] Maymon R, Jauniaux E, Cohen O, et al. Pregnancy outcome and infant follow-up of fetuses with abnormally increased first trimester nuchal translucency. Hum Reprod 2000;15:2023-7.

[18] Cheng CC, Bahado-Singh RO, Chen SC, et al. Pregnancy outcomes with increased nuchal translucency after routine Down syndrome screening. Int J Gynaecol Obstet 2004;84:5-9.

[19] Souka AP, Krampl E, Bakalis S, et al. Outcome of pregnancy in chromosomally normal fetuses with increased nuchal translucency in the first trimester. Ultrasound Obstet Gynecol 2001;18:9-17.

[20] Senat MV, De Keersmaecker B, Audibert F, et al. Pregnancy outcome in fetuses with increased nuchal translucency and normal karyotype. Prenat Diagn 2002;22:345-9.

[21] Ghi T, Huggon IC, Zosmer N, et al. Incidence of major structural cardiac defects associated with increased nuchal translucency but normal karyotype. Ultrasound Obstet Gynecol 2001;18:610-4.

[22] Müller MA, Bleker P, Bonsel GJ, et al. Nuchal translucency screening and anxiety levels in pregnancy and puerperium. Ultrasound Obstet Gynecol 2007;27:357-61.

[23] Vogel M, Sharland GK, McElhinney DB, et al. Prevalence of increased nuchal translucency in fetuses with congenital cardiac disease and a normal karyotype. Cardiol Young 2009;19:441-5.

[24] Clur SA, Ottenkamp J, Bilardo CM. The nuchal translucency and the fetal heart: a literature review. Prenat Diagn 2009;29:739-48.

[25] Maymon R, Herman A. The clinical evaluation and pregnancy outcome of euploid fetuses with increased nuchal translucency. Clin Genet 2004;66:426-36.

[26] Souka AP, Von Kaisenberg CS, Hyett JA, et al. Increased nuchal translucency with normal karyotype. Am J Obstet Gynecol 2005;192:1005-21.

[27] Yaron Y, Wolman I, Kupferminc MJ, et al. Effect of fetal gender on first trimester markers and on Down syndrome screening. Prenat Diagn 2001;21:1027-30.

[28] Prefumo F, Venturini PL, De Biasio P. Effect of fetal gender on first-trimester ductus-venosus blood flow. Ultrasound Obstet Gynecol 2003;22:268-70.

[29] Lam YH, Tang MH, Lee CP, et al. The effect of fetal gender on nuchal translucency at 10-14 weeks of gestation. Prenat Diagn 2001;21:627-9.

[30] Timmerman E, Pajkrt E, Bilardo CM. Male gender as a favorable prognostic factor in pregnancies with enlarged nuchal translucency. Ultrasound Obstet Gynecol 2009;34:373-8.

[31] Spencer K, Ong CY, Liao AW, et al. The influence of fetal sex in screening for trisomy 21 by fetal nuchal translucency, maternal serum free beta-hCG and PAPP-A at 10-14 weeks of gestation. Prenat Diagn 2000;20:673-5.

Chapter 3

Prenatal Screening and Diagnosis

Jaana Marttala

Additional information is available at the end of the chapter

http://dx.doi.org/10.5772/52861

1. Introduction

1.1. Maternal age

In recent years the prevalence of Down syndrome has been increasing. The increase in the prevalence might be partly explained by better compilation of statistics on Down syndrome today. Also, the mean maternal age at first delivery as well as the proportion of older mothers is increasing in all western countries and the risk of Down syndrome increases with advancing maternal age [1]. The proportion of mothers aged 35 years or older in France, Finland, Germany, Greece and United Kingdom were 15.8 %, 19.0 %, 17.0 %, 14.2 % and 17.2 % in 2001, respectively, in 2008 the proportions were 18.9 %, 18.2 %, 21.8 %, 20.9 % and 20.1 %, respectively (Eurostat). Screening for Down syndrome was first performed in 1970's using advanced maternal age or previous history of chromosomal abnormality. The prevalence of Down syndrome at term rises from 1/1527 at the maternal age of 20 years to 1/895 at age 30 and to 1/97 at age 40 [11]. Also the gestational age affects the prevalence of Down syndrome. The estimated rate of fetal loss in Down syndrome pregnancies is 43 % between gestational week 10 and term, 23 % between gestational week 15 and term and 12 % of births are stillbirths or result in a neonatal death [12]. Therefore, the risk of Down syndrome decreases as the pregnancy progresses. Table 1 presents the prevalence of Down syndrome pregnancies in different maternal age groups according to the gestational age.

Maternal age of 35 years or more used as a screening method can detect approximately 43-61 % of Down syndrome cases [13, 14]. However, the false positive rate (FPR) is high since the proportion of women aged 35 years or older is approximately 20 % in western countries. Chorionic villus sampling (CVS) and amniocentesis (AC) carry a 0.5-1.0 % risk of fetal loss [15]. Maternal age of 35 is an arbitrary threshold and there are better screening methods available today. The invasive test should not be offered only because of increased maternal age.

Maternal age (years)	Gestational age (weeks)						
	10	12	14	16	20	40	
20		1/983	1/1068	1/1140	1/1200	1/1295	1/1527
25		1/870	1/946	1/1009	1/1062	1/1147	1/1352
30		1/576	1/626	1/668	1/703	1/759	1/895
35		1/229	1/249	1/266	1/280	1/302	1/356
40		1/62	1/68	1/72	1/76	1/82	1/97
45		1/15	1/16	1/17	1/18	1/19	1/23

Table 1. The prevalence of Down syndrome according to maternal age and gestational age. (Modified from Snijders *et al.* 1999).

1.2. Second trimester screening

Abnormal levels of specific maternal serum markers were associated with Down syndrome in 1980's. Second trimester screening with maternal age and maternal serum markers was developed consisting of either double, triple or quadruple serum screening. Optimal window for second trimester serum screening is between 15 and 22 weeks of gestation. Double test includes maternal age, maternal serum free beta human chorionic gonadotropin (fβ-hCG) and alfafetoprotein (AFP). The additional serum markers are unconjugated oestriol (uE3) in triple screening and uE3 and inhibin-A in quadruple screening. The estimated FPRs for an 85 % detection rate (DR) for double, triple and quadruple screening are 13.1 %, 9.3-14 % and 6.2-7.3 %, respectively [9, 16]. For a 5 % FPR the DRs for double, triple and quadruple screening are approximately 59 %, 63 % and 72 %, respectively.

2. Screening for Down syndrome today

Screening for Down syndrome has moved from second trimester to first trimester during the last two decades. The most popular screening method today is combined first trimester screening where maternal serum biomarkers fβ-hCG and pregnancy associated plasma protein-A (PAPP-A) are used in combination with fetal nuchal translucency (NT) measurement, ultrasound dated gestational age and maternal age to calculate a woman's risk for Down syndrome using a computer based program. The serum markers and NT do not correlate with each other in chromosomally normal or abnormal fetuses [17]. Each screened woman has a priori risk which is based on her age and the gestational age. The risk calculation software program uses the Gaussian distributions of NT and serum values of normal and affected cases to calculate the LRs. These are described by their means of $\log_{10}$ MoMs, standard deviations and correlation coefficients between the markers. The screening test performs well if the Gaussian distributions of the markers in the normal and affected populations are separated. Alternatively, the screening test is impractical if the distributions overlap widely.

The median MoMs and standard deviations in the populations influence the degree of the overlap. A patient-specific risk for each screened woman is calculated by multiplying the a priori risk based on maternal age with the LR [18-21].

Maternal serum biochemistry reflects the degree of maturity of the placenta rather than directly measuring the presence or absence of Down syndrome. These markers have also limitations, such as the relatively narrow gestational window in which they can be used. In pregnancies that are affected by fetal chromosomal abnormalities the placental function is impaired and the levels of fβ-hCG and PAPP-A differ from normal pregnancies. The results of the maternal serum biochemistry are reported as multiples of the median (MoM) specific to the gestational week. MoM values are calculated by dividing a woman's marker level by the median level of that marker for the entire population at that gestational age in each laboratory. The use of MoM values therefore also allows the interpretation between the results from different laboratories in different countries. The expected levels of maternal serum markers are not only affected by maternal age and gestational age but also other factors like maternal weight, ethnic origin, the presence of insulin dependent diabetes mellitus, multiple pregnancy, smoking and vaginal bleeding. Screening program takes into account certain variables.

2.1. Screening markers

Human chorionic gonadotropin (hCG) was first purified from the pregnant women's urine. hCG is produced by the trophoblastic cells of the placenta from the 10th to 12th day after conception and it reaches its peak value in maternal circulation at 8 to 10 weeks of gestation. Then, a rapid decrease is seen and a plateau is reached at 20th week of gestation [22]. hCG was first used as a second trimester screening marker for Down syndrome. Later, it was shown that the free beta subunit of hCG (fβ-hCG) is an effective screening marker for Down syndrome in the first trimester of the pregnancy. In Down syndrome pregnancies maternal serum fβ-hCG levels are higher than in normal pregnancies during the first trimester of the pregnancy. The reported DRs for fβ-hCG alone are around 19-42 % for a 5 % FPR [9, 16]. The DR of fβ-hCG for Down syndrome is better at gestational week 13 than at gestational week 10 [9].

The association between abnormal levels of maternal serum pregnancy associated plasma protein-A (PAPP-A) and fetal aneuploidy was made in late 1980's and early 1990's [22, 23]. PAPP-A levels normally rise during pregnancy all the way to the delivery. PAPP-A is a metalloproteinase that cleaves insulin-growth factor binding protein-4 (IGFBP-4) which binds IGFs with high affinity thus preventing their interaction with the IGF-receptors that mediate cell growth and survival signals [24, 25]. IGFs are important in implantation, placental physiology and fetal growth [25]. Therefore, PAPP-A is believed to function as a growth factor of both fetus and placenta during the pregnancy. PAPP-A levels are lower in Down syndrome pregnancies during the first trimester of the pregnancy but the deviation from normal decreases with gestational age [20]. The DR for PAPP-A alone is approximately 52 % for a 5 % FPR [16].

Fetal NT in the first trimester of the pregnancy was described as the fluid-filled space under the skin behind the fetal neck in 1992 [7, 8]. NT is measured during first trimester ultrasound scan at gestational weeks 10-13. Ultrasound scan also offers accurate dating of the pregnancy, ascertainment of viable fetus or missed abortion, detection of multiple pregnancies, accurate dating of the pregnancy, identification of chorionicity and detection of some major fetal anomalies. NT measurement is not altered in multiple pregnancies or by assisted reproduction techniques. Large studies in low risk populations have shown the association between increased NT and chromosomal defects. The combination of maternal age and NT was reported to have a DR of 63.0-90.0 % for a FPR of 5.0-13.0 % [16, 26]. Therefore, NT measurement is the best single marker in screening for Down syndrome [16, 27].

The incidence of chromosomal defects is related to the thickness rather than the appearance of NT [28]. In initial studies, single millimeter cut-offs like 2.5 mm or 3.0 mm were used to define screen positivity but as it was learned that NT increases with CRL it was realized that it is important to take gestational age into account [29]. Later certain percentile cut-offs, like the fetal NT measurement equal to or above the 95th or 99th centile for CRL, were used. Today, most current screening programs advocate the use of gestational age based cut-offs for risk assessment of MoMs. However, some recent studies like a study of 36120 singleton pregnancies with complete first trimester NT and serum marker data have concluded that immediate invasive testing should be offered to all patients with NT measurement of 3 mm or greater since the addition of the first trimester serum markers do not seem to significantly reduce the final risk of fetal aneuploidy [30].

Also the risk of other adverse pregnancy outcomes increases with enlarging NT measurement. Between NT values of the 95th and 99th percentiles, the prevalence of major anomalies is 2.5 %. With NT measurement of 6.5 mm or larger, the risk is approximately 45 % [31]. The causes behind increased NT measurement are heterogenic which is in relation to the variety of adverse pregnancy outcomes that increased fetal NT has been associated with [32]. Congenital heart defect is the most common adverse pregnancy outcome that has been associated with increased NT [31]. The prevalence of congenital heart defects in children with Down syndrome is approximately 43 % [33]. Other suggested mechanisms include impaired or delayed development of lymphatic drainage [34], mediastinal compression and impedence to venous return caused by for example diaphragmatic hernia or skeletal dysplasias [35, 36], over-expression of certain collagen genes in trisomic fetuses [37], exomphalos, body stalk anomaly, fetal akinesia deformation sequence and genetic syndromes [38, 39].

2.2. Performance of the combined first trimester screening

Screening works better among a population where the incidence of the screened condition is high. Therefore, since the risk of Down syndrome increases with advancing maternal age, screening works better among the older women. Overall, more than half of the Down syndrome cases occur among the women aged 35 years or older [13, 14]. Reported screening perfomances are better in studies that have been conducted in high risk populations where the median maternal age is high and thereby the incidence of Down syndrome is also high. When the screened population reflects well the general low risk population and united screening strategy and high quality ultrasound machines are used, reliable screening results are drawn. Table 2 summarizes the performance of combined first trimester screening for trisomy 21 in large studies reported in the literature.

Study	Gestation	Sample size	Trisomy 21 (N)	Incidence of trisomy 21	Median age	Women at age of ≥ 35 (%)	Cut-off level	DR %	FPR %
Bindra *et al.* 2002 [40]	11 – 14	15030	82	1:175	34.0	47.1	1:300	90.2	5.0
Crossley *et al.* 2002 [41]	10 – 14	17229	45	1:383	29.9	15.4	1:250	82	5
Wald *et al.* 2003 [16]	10 – 13	39983	85	1:470	-	-	1:310	83	5
Wapner *et al.* 2003 [42]	10 – 14	8514	61	1:135	34.5	50.0	1:270	85.2	9.4
Malone *et al.* 2005 [9]	11 12 13	38167	117	1:326	30.1	21.6	1:300	87 85 82	5.0
Rozenberg *et al.* 2006 [43]	11 – 13	14934	51	1:293	30.9	-	1:250	79.6	2.7
Kagan *et al.* 2008 [44]	11 – 13	56771	395	1:143	35.4	-	1:200	89	4.6
Okun *et al.* 2008 [45]	11 – 13	14487	62	1:234	34.0	-	1:200	83.9	4.0
Borrell *et al.* 2009 [46]	11 12 13	7250	66	1:110	32.0	-	1:250	86 84 83	4.9 5.4 6.1
Kagan *et al.* 2009 [47]	11-13	19736	122	1:162	34.5	-	1:150	91.0	3.1
Leung *et al.* 2009 [48]	11 – 13	10363	38	1:272	32.0	27.4	1:300	91.2	5.4
Schaelike *et al.* 2009 [49]	11-13	10668	59	1:181	-	31.0	1:300	88.1	4.9
Wortelboer *et al.* 2009 [50]	10 – 14	20293	87	1:233	34.3	°/>36 yr 38.7	1:250	75.9	3.3
Salomon *et al.* 2010 [51]	11-13	21492	80	1:269	30.7	-	1:250	80.0	8.8
Wright *et al.* 2010 [52]	7-14	223361	886	1:252	31.9	-	1:100	90.0	3.0
Engels *et al.* 2011 [16]	9-14	26274 <36 17970 ≥36 8304	121 <36 52 ≥36 69	1:217 <36 1:346 ≥36 1:120	34.1	≥36 yr 31.6	1:200	95.2 <36 94.5 ≥36 95.8	6.6 <36 4.1 ≥36 13.0
Marttala *et al.* 2011 [53]	9 – 13	76949	188	1:409	29.3	19.3	1:250	81.9	4.3
Yeo *et al.* 2012 [54]	10-13	12585	31	1:406	-	-	1:300	87.1	5.1
Peuhkurinen *et al.* 2012 [55]	9-13	63945 <35 50941 ≥35 13004	<35 73 ≥35 115	<35 1:876 ≥35 1:113	<35 27.9 ≥35 37.8	16.9	1:250	<35 74.0 ≥35 87.0	<35 2.8 ≥35 11.9

Table 2. Performance of first trimester combined screening of Down syndrome in different studies.

Improving the screening means increase in the DR and decrease in the FPR and thus decrease in the number of invasive procedures needed to detect one case of Down syndrome and number of procedure related miscarriages. However, with current screening strategies, increase in DR means an increase also in the FPR. A decrease in invasive procedures is an important goal and therefore special attention should be given to decreasing the FPR.

As screening performance depends on maternal age the screening program takes into account maternal age [55]. DR and FPR increase with advancing maternal age. Worst screening performance is among the women aged 25-29 years [14, 43]. The overall screening performance may be an underestimation or overestimation on individual level depending on the screened woman's age. More focus on individual risk in counseling is needed. Among younger women, the possibility of a false negative screening result is higher and among older women the possibility of false positive screening result is higher. Possibly, lowering the screening cut-off level among women aged 35 or more could improve the balance between DR and FPR [14]. For example, in USA, improved prenatal screening tests and increased availability of screening for also the older women has declined the uptake of invasive testing over the past decade. Also the risk of procedure related miscarriage affects women's decision. The possibility for earlier screening during the first trimester has decreased the number of invasive tests more than the second trimester screening. Also a screening strategy that excludes maternal age, called advanced first trimester screening, might be an option among older women.

Most common factor for a false negative screening result is NT. Therefore, appropriate training and constant audit as well as possibly the certification of the competence should be required from the examiners performing ultrasound scans and NT measurements. Even more competence will be required if additional ultrasound markers like nasal bone will be included into the screening program. The quality of ultrasound machines is also important.

It is possible to provide pretest counseling, biochemical testing of the mother, and NT measurement at the same visit and post-test counseling on a combined risk estimate within a one-hour visit to a one-stop clinic [40]. However, screening performance differs according to the gestational age. The difference between fβ-hCG MoM values increases between unaffected and affected pregnancies as the pregnancy progresses. On the contrary, the difference in PAPP-A values decreases and PAPP-A is more effective screening marker than fβ-hCG. The maximum separation in PAPP-A levels is seen at 9-10 gestational weeks. Therefore, screening works better when PAPP-A is measured during 9-10 weeks of gestation rather than during gestational weeks 7-8 or 11-14. First trimester ultrasound scan is more accurate during the late first trimester. Therefore it would be rational to draw blood samples for the measurements of PAPP-A and fβ-hCG at gestational weeks 9-10 and have another visit at 12th gestational week for the ultrasound scan. Another option could be to measure PAPP-A at gestational weeks 9-10 and NT and fβ-hCG at 12th gestational week. This could improve DRs from 90 % to 92 % for a FPR of 3 % and from 93 % to 95 % for a FPR of 5 % [20, 47, 48, 50].

Also, fetal gender has been shown to affect the levels of maternal serum PAPP-A and fβ-hCG in Down syndrome pregnancies. The levels of fβ-hCG and PAPP-A were shown to be significantly increased and NT measurements significantly reduced in women carrying female fetuses compared to women carrying male fetuses [51]. In future, NIPD may replace contemporary prenatal diagnosis in those women who are at risk of fetal chromosomal abnormality after Down syndrome screening. However, at the moment, research should also focus on improving the sensitivity and specificity of the combined screening. This might happen by adding new biochemical and sonographic markers into screening.

2.3. Invasive testing

After a positive screening result, a diagnostic test is offered. Also women who are in increased risk for Down syndrome due to increased maternal age or have a family history of Down syndrome are offered invasive testing. CVS can be performed at 11-14 weeks of gestation and AC from 15 weeks of gestation. CVS and AC carry an approximately 0.5-1 % risk of miscarriage [15].

2.4. Other investigated screening markers

2.4.1. Additional ultrasound markers

Ductus venosus (DV) shunts approximately half of the well-oxygenated blood from the umbilical vein directly into the inferior vena cava thus bypassing the liver. The blood flow in the DV is normally forward and triphasic. The waveform of the blood flow has a peak during ventricular systole (S-wave) and diastole (D-wave), during the atrial contraction in late diastole there is a nadir (A-wave). Abnormal flow in the DV in the first trimester of the pregnancy has been associated with chromosomal abnormalities. The abnormal DV flow has been reported to detect approximately 65-75 % of the Down syndrome cases for a FPR of 5.0-21 % [56, 57]. Addition of DV assessment to combined screening can improve the DR from 89 % to 96 % with an increase in FPR from 2.3 % to 2.5 % [58].

Fetal tachycardia has been associated with Down syndrome. However, the results have been controversial and even when the association has been made the authors have not always suggested the use of fetal heart rate (FHR) in the screening program. Addition of FHR to combined screening improves the DR only marginally, from 89 % to 90 % for a FPR of 3.0 % [58].

Frontomaxillary facial (FMF) angle decreases normally with CRL from 85° at 45 mm to 75° at 84 mm [59]. The FMF angle measurements are above the 95th centile in approximately 69 % of Down syndrome fetuses and 5 % of euploid fetuses. Addition of FMF angle to combined screening can improve the DR from 90 % to 95 % for a FPR of 5.0 % [60].

Nasal bone (NB) has been found to be absent or hypoplastic in fetuses with Down syndrome. NB is classified as being absent in cases where NB appears as a thin line, or less echogenic than the overlying skin suggesting that the NB is not yet ossified. The DR for NB alone is approximately 73 % for a FPR of 0.5 % [83]. Addition of NB to combined screening can improve the DR from 89 % to 91 % for a FPR of 2.5 % [58].

Tricuspid regurgitation (TR) is defined by the Fetal Medicine Foundation as when the velocity of the flow exceeds 60 cm/s and occurs during at least half of the systole. In some studies, however, TR has been defined as when the flow exceeds 80 cm/s [62]. The DR for TR alone is approximately 59.4 % for a FPR of 8.8 % [63]. Addition of TR to combined screening can improve the DR from 75 % to 87 % for a FPR of 1.0 % [62]. Table 3 presents the reported DRs and FPRs for additional ultrasound markers alone and in combination with first trimester combined screening.

Ultrasound marker	Ultrasound marker + maternal age		Combined screening + ultrasound marker	
	Detection rate (%)	False positive rate (%)	Detection rate (%)	False positive rate (%)
Ductus venosus flow	65-75	5-21	96	2.5
Fetal heart rate	-	-	90	3
Frontomaxillary facial angle	69	5	95	5
Nasal bone	59.8-73	0.5-2.6	91 97	2.5 5
Tricuspid regurgitation	59.4	8.8	87 96	1 2.6

Table 3. Screening performance of the additional ultrasound markers used alone and in combination with combined first trimester screening markers.

There is no significant association between DV flow, FMF angle, NB or TR and the combined screening markers PAPP-A, fβ-hCG and NT [59, 64]. New sonographic markers may also be used in combination. Inclusion of the new sonographic markers in to screening requires appropriate training of the examiners and the imagining protocols need to be standardized.

2.4.2. Genetic sonogram

Genetic sonogram is an ultrasound examination performed during the second trimester of the pregnancy. During the genetic sonogram fetuses are evaluated for structural malformations and also searched for the sonographic markers of Down syndrome. Main markers include nuchal fold, short femur and humerus, pyelectasis, echogenic intracardiac focus, hyperechoic bowel and any major anomaly. Major abnormalities can be recognized approximately in 25 % of the Down syndrome pregnancies [65]. If there are one or more sonographic markers present, the baseline risk of Down syndrome increases. Similarly, the absence of markers conveys a reduction in the risk based on for example combined first trimester screening, previous chromosomal abnormality or advanced maternal age [66].

Besides major markers there are also minor, "soft", markers that can be evaluated during the scan. These include nuchal skinfold of 6 mm or more, choroid plexus cyst, enlarged cisterna magna over 10 mm, ventriculomegaly 10 mm or more, echogenic intracardiac focus, pericardial effusion, hydrops, two-vessel umbilical cord, polydactyly, clinodactyly, sandal gap, and club foot. The genetic sonogram has been reported to have a DR of 66.6 – 83.0 % for a 6.7 – 19.3 % FPR depending on the population. The screening performance is naturally lower in a low risk population [67, 68]. Combining the genetic sonogram into combined first trimester screening can improve the DR from 81 % to 90 % for a 5 % FPR [69].

If major defects are detected during the scan, fetal karyotyping is offered to determine the underlying cause and the risk of recurrence. Even if the condition, like diaphragmatic hernia, is treatable by a surgery, there might be a chromosomal abnormality behind it. Unlike major defects, minor defects are common and rarely associated with any other handicap than chromosomal abnormality. Therefore, detection of a minor defect should lead to a thorough search for other defects. The risk of a fetal anomaly should be individually evaluated since it increases with the number of minor defects detected. Second trimester ultrasound scan will likely have an important role also in the future in the detection of fetal Down syndrome and other chromosomal abnormalities.

2.4.3. *Other biochemical screening markers*

New biochemical screening markers are under investigation. A disintegrin and metalloprotease 12 (ADAM12) is a glycoprotein that is synthesized by placenta. Lowered levels of ADAM12 in maternal serum have been associated with Down syndrome and other chromosomal abnormalities such as trisomies 18 and 13 during the early first trimester of the pregnancy but its deviation from normality decreases as the pregnancy progresses [69-71]. ADAM12 is not a good screening marker for Down syndrome during gestational weeks 11-13 since its levels are not significantly different from normal. Although in other chromosomal abnormalities the levels differ significantly from normal, there is a significant association between ADAM12 and fβ-hCG and PAPP-A [95, 96]. Modeled DRs for ADAM12 in combination with first trimester combined screening markers are 97 % and 89 % for FPRs of 5 % and 1 % at gestational week 12 [70]. However, it seems that no additional benefit could be obtained be the inclusion of ADAM12 into the first trimester combined screening.

Inhibin A has been long used as a part of second trimester quadruple screening. High levels of inhibin A in Down syndrome pregnancies have also been found during the first trimester of the pregnancy. Using inhibin A with combined screening markers during the gestational weeks 9-11 can achieve an approximately 82.6 % DR for a 1.0 % FPR which is close to the performance of the integrated test [5].

Placental protein 13 (PP13) levels are not altered significantly in Down syndrome pregnancies but its levels are significantly decreased in trisomy 18 and 13, Turner syndrome and triploidy pregnancies [72, 73]. Placental growth factor (PlGF) levels in maternal serum have been reported to be decreased, increased or the same in Down syndrome pregnancies compared to unaffected pregnancies during the first and second trimester of the pregnancy. According to the literature, maternal serum PlGF is potentially useful in first trimester screening for fetal chromosomal abnormalities.

Using second trimester serum markers AFP, inhibin A and uE3 during the first trimester has also been studied. For the combination of PAPP-A, fβ-hCG, AFP and NT the estimated DR is 87.2 %, when AFP is replaced with uE3 the estimated DR is 87.9 % and for all the markers, 88.3 % for a 5 % FPR [20]. Inhibin A with combination of first trimester combined screening markers has been shown to achieve DRs of 81.4 % and 82.6 % at gestational weeks 7-8 and 9-11, respectively, for FPRs of 0.9 % and 1 % [5]. The studies on inhibin A have been controversial and some have found that inhibin A does not increase the screening performance in the first trimester [74].

Besides the biomarkers mentioned above, also other maternal serum proteins have been shown to be more abundant in control versus Down syndrome pregnancies in both first and second trimester of the pregnancy [75]. Large scale prospective studies in low risk populations evaluating the new maternal serum biomarkers need to be conducted before these markers could be implemented into the routine first trimester screening.

2.5. Integrated screening and contingent screening

In 1999 first trimester and second trimester screening were combined to create an integrated screening method which has been shown to achieve DRs around 85 %, 90 % and 94 % for FPRs of 1 %, 2 % and 5 %, respectively [76]. After first trimester combined screening is performed, no risk assessment is provided, instead, women return between gestational weeks 15 and 20 for measurements of serum quadruple markers. These screening methods are then combined with maternal age and an individual risk for Down syndrome is calculated. The advantage of integrated screening is its high sensitivity and specificity. However, first trimester screening results are withheld and the screening results are not available until the second trimester of the pregnancy. In the FaSTER trial, with a 5 % FPR, modeled DRs for integrated screening method were 96 %, 95 % and 94 % when the PAPP-A was measured during the gestational weeks 11, 12 or 13, respectively [9]. In the SURUSS study, integrated screening achieved a 93 % DR for a 5 % FPR. At an 85 % DR the FPR was 1.2 % [16].

Contingent screening policy was developed to reduce the number of NT measurements needed. This can be beneficial in the areas where there are no qualified personnel or high-quality ultrasound machines available or where distances are long. Firstly, first trimester serum sample is analyzed for the levels of PAPP-A and fβ-hCG. Secondly, women are divided into three groups, women in low, intermediate and high risk for chromosomal abnormalities according to the serum markers. Women in low risk are offered no further screening. Women in high risk are offered immediate invasive testing. NT screening is offered for those in intermediate risk and new risk calculation using first trimester serum markers and NT measurement is performed and invasive testing is offered for those in high risk. This method has been estimated to achieve DRs of 67.6 % and 88.6 % for FPRs of 2.3 % and 6.4 %, respectively [77, 78]. Contingent screening might put women in unequal positions as first trimester combined screening is known to achieve higher screening performances. Moreover, major structural abnormalities can be detected during the first trimester ultrasound scan [79, 80]. Also other variations of contingent screening including for example new sonographic markers have been developed.

3. Screening for Down syndrome in the future

3.1. Non-Invasive Prenatal Diagnosis (NIPD)

One of the hottest topics in prenatal medicine today is the noninvasive prenatal diagnosis (NIPD). Since 1997 many approaches have been made in the field of NIPD and today it is possible to determine fetal sex, fetal Rhesus D status and diagnose genetic disorders or carrier status for paternally inherited mutations [81]. Women in high risk of X-linked disorders like hemophilia can be offered noninvasive fetal sex determination. Y chromosome derived sequences can be found in maternal blood as early as eight weeks of gestation [82]. The detection of Y chromosome material indicates further investigations but if no evidence of detectable Y chromosome is found, unnecessary invasive testing with the risk of pregnancy loss, can be avoided. The costs of NIPD of fetal gender and invasive testing are similar [83, 84]. Y chromosome sequences can be detected with approximately 95.4 % sensitivity and 98.6 % specificity. Best test performance reported is for the real-time quantitative polymerase chain reaction (RTQ-PCR) after 20 weeks of gestation. Tests performed before seventh gestational week or using urine sample have been reported to be unreliable [85].

Detection of fetal rhesus D status can reduce the use of D immunoglobulin to prevent immune hemolytic disease of the newborn. The reported sensitivities and specificities for fetal Rhesus D sequence are greater than 95 % [86]. Reported false negative results are mainly due to a lack of fetal DNA in maternal blood sample due to too early gestation or insensitive methods. The presence of pseudogenes, mainly in African women, can lead to false positive results. However, current genotyping protocols in molecular diagnostic laboratories acknowledge the possibility of the pseudogene and do not amplify this region of the genome [87]. The first study evaluating the national clinical application of NIPD of fetal Rhesus D status conducted in Denmark, reported a sensitivity of 99.9 % and specificity of 96.5 % [88].

Fetal hemoglobin in maternal circulation was detected in 1956 indicating transplacental transmission of fetal erythrocytes [89]. Fetal cells were found in maternal blood during pregnancy in 1958 [90]. Nucleated red blood cells have a relatively short lifespan in maternal blood but other cells can reside in maternal blood for decades after delivery and therefore cause false positive or negative test results in subsequent pregnancies [87, 91]. Other problems besides the possibility of the presence of previous pregnancy include the rare number of fetal cells in maternal plasma, one cell per ml, and low efficiency of enrichment methods.

CffDNA, originating from the apoptotic trophoblasts derived from the embryo, was first detected in maternal circulation in 1997 [92, 93]. It has been shown that cffDNA is present in maternal circulation even before placental circulation has been established. It is present also in anembryonic gestations. Detected cffDNA sequences in maternal blood have been shown to reflect the placental genotype in cases of confined placental mosaicism [87]. Compared to intact fetal cells cffDNA has many advantages; it is almost a thousand times more present in maternal circulation than fetal cells, its mean half-life in maternal blood is approximately 16-30 minutes making it a marker of the current pregnancy [94, 95]. Even though the concentration of cffDNA in maternal blood is higher than that of the intact fetal cells, it is still low and it only comprises 3-6 % of the total cell-free DNA in maternal blood since the majority of cell-free DNA is of maternal origin. Also, half of the fetal genome is inherited from the mother and there are individual differences in the concentration of the total cffDNA [94, 96].

The newest strategy for noninvasive prenatal gene profiling is the maternal blood analysis of fetal mRNA. Discovery of fetal placenta-specific expressed mRNAs in the maternal serum and plasma was made in 2000 [97]. Fetal mRNA molecules have been shown to be easily detectable since they are very stable in maternal blood probably due to the association with particulate matters [99]. Numerous pregnancy-specific, fetal-specific mRNA transcripts that are independent from fetal gender and fetal genetic polymorphisms have been identified in maternal circulation [99, 100]. Studied noninvasive prenatal screening mRNA markers include for example placenta-specific 4 (PLAC4) which is cleared rapidly after delivery and has been reported to have a 90 % DR for a 3.5 % FPR for Down syndrome [100].

3.1.1. Current state of art in NIPD

Various methods for NIPD using cffNA in maternal circulation have been introduced. Massively parallel sequencing (MPS) of fetal DNA has high sensitivity and specificity for the detection of trisomy 21. The reported sensitivities range between 79.1 % and 100 % and specificities between 97.9 % and 100 %, respectively [101-104]. Similar sensitivities and specificities for trisomies 21 and 18 have been reported for targeted MPS method and for trisomy 21 with differential methylation and real-time multiplex ligation-dependent probe amplification (RT-MLPA). One study achieved a 100 % sensitivity and specificity for trisomy 21 by a targeted approach that was based on calculation of haplotype ratios from tandem single nucleotide polymorphisms (SNP) sequences on chromosome 21 combined with a quantitative DNA measurement technology [105].

The use of MPS as the screening strategy has been reported to achieve sensitivities of 91.9-100 % and 100 % with specificities of 98.9-100 % and 98.4-100 % for trisomy 18 and trisomy 13, respectively [106-108]. MPS combined with improved z-score test methodology, was reported to achieve 100 % DR with a 0 % FPR for Down syndrome, trisomy 18, trisomy 13, Turner syndrome and Klinefelter syndrome [109]. High troughput DNA sequencing has many advantages as the entire process can be automated and multiple samples be analyzed simultaneously so that thousands of sequencing reactions can occur in parallel as the test DNA is bound to a solid support such as an array.

One method called the RNA-SNP approach measures the ratio of alleles for a SNP in placenta-derived mRNA molecules in maternal plasma [100]. PLAC4 mRNA has been used for this method [110]. The RNA-SNP method detects the deviated RNA-SNP allelic ratio on PLAC4 mRNA which is caused by the imbalance in chromosome 21 dosage. The RNA-SNP strategy is only suitable to women with a fetus heterozygous for the studied SNP in the PLAC4 gene. Method can be based on a mass spectrometry (MS) method or digital-PCR which enhances the precision [100, 111]. Digital-PCR method is more costly but it can be used in analysis of plasma samples with low concentration of PLAC4 mRNA such in early pregnancy samples.

Another method used is the measurement of the total concentration of PLAC4 mRNA in maternal plasma is increased in Down syndrome pregnancies because of the extra gene copy in the placenta [112]. The mRNA quantification method can be used for pregnancies with homozygous fetuses. However, it is not yet known if there are other factors such as increased apoptosis in aneuploid placentas that might contribute to the increase of circulating PLAC4 mRNA in maternal plasma. The diagnostic accuracies of RNA-SNP approach, using blood samples from women carrying heterozygous fetuses for the PLAC4 mRNA, on the MS and digital-PCR platforms have identical sensitivities and specificities of 90-100 % and 89.7-96.5 %, respectively [100, 112].

Also gene sequences present in neonatal and maternal whole blood have been studied [81, 87]. In amniotic fluid, abundant amounts of both cffRNA and cffDNA can be found and the present cell-free nucleic acids (cffNA) are nearly exclusively of fetal origin. Also, the cffNA appears to originate from fetal tissues that are either in direct contact with the amniotic fluid or drain into the amniotic fluid and there seems to be no NA derived from the placenta. Intial studies on the molecular pathophysiology in the living fetus suggest that the majority of dysregulated gene espression in aneuploid fetuses occurs in genes present in other chromosomes than the one involved in the chromosomal abnormality. Another finding is the oxidative stress in fetuses affected by Down syndrome which may result in the mental retardation and Alzheimer's disease [87]. After birth, analysis of cffNA from neonatal saliva can be used to monitor neonatal health and development. This offers comprehensive, real-time information regarding many organs and tissues which could allow the monitoring of premature neonates in terms of health, disease and development [113].

The reported data indicates that highly accurate NIPD of chromosomal abnormalities by maternal blood sample is achievable during the first trimester of the pregnancy. However, the gestational window of NIPD is still to be researched. Although studies have reported high sensitivities and specificities, approximately 1 % FPRs have been reported. Therefore, at the moment, invasive testing is still required after positive test result and the method might be more incisively regarded as an "advanced screening test" rather than a diagnostic test and pregnancy termination should not be offered only based on a positive NIPD test. However, it has been estimated that 98 % of the invasive procedures could be avoided if AC or CVS were based on the MPS test results [101]. Most studies to date have been small and conducted in high risk women. Large-scale objective clinical trials are needed to evaluate the sensitivity and specificity of NIPD in low risk general populations. The future costs of NIPD can be only estimated and are dependent on the relative costs of NIPD, Down syndrome screening and number of invasive tests that are performed.

NIPD of fetal Rhesus D genotype has been widely validated in Europe but it is slower been undertaken in United States of America. It is anticipated that besides fetal sex determination and Rhesus D detection, over the next few years also the NIPD of fetal aneuploidy will be possible and NIPD will be refined to include also other trisomies than trisomy 21. However, it may take longer to develop proper techniques to detect other pathogenic rearrangements. Ultrasound scan during the early pregnancy will be necessary even if NIPD would become a routine screening method. Increased levels of cffNA in maternal blood have been associated, besides chromosomal abnormalities, with various pathological conditions like pre-eclampsia, hemolytic anemia, elevated liver enzymes, low platelets syndrome and placental abnormalities like placenta accrete [87, 114].

3.1.2. Ethics in NIPD

NIPD has many benefits as definitive diagnoses can be made earlier in the pregnancy when termination of an affected pregnancy is safer, parental anxiety is reduced and costs are decreased. As testing becomes safer the uptake will probably increase and thus additional health and economic benefits can be reached. However, NIPD also raises many ethical issues. Counseling needs to be informative so that women could make the decision fully aware of the consequences of possible findings. At the moment, counseling is offered for every woman but only those who have received a positive screening result are offered more detailed information about Down syndrome as they are offered invasive testing. The nature of NIPD, however, is closer to invasive diagnosis than screening. Therefore, all women should be comprehensively counseled before the testing. This probably requires much more genetic counselors than are currently available.

In recent years, private sector has been funding research around NIPD. This might lead to expensive testing. Until now, Down syndrome screening has had a minimal effect on birth incidence of genetic disorders. As testing becomes safer and more accurate than before more affected pregnancies may be found and possibly terminated. This might affect the public attitudes towards affected individuals and their families. Women might feel more pressured by the society to test and terminate affected pregnancies. Also commercial and insurance sectors might perceive economic benefits in decreasing the prevalence of disorders. As the technology develops, also less severe disorders, late-onset disorders, nonmedical traits and predispositions can be detected prenatally. Codes of practice should be developed as well as regulatory recommendations made [158]. In United States of America, several professional organizations have stated that noninvasive fetal gender determination should only be offered for medical indications. However, via the internet the test is available directly to the consumers and the technology might also be used for fetal sex selection.

Women seem to feel positive about the new improvements in the screening field. However, they find it hard to fully realize the new choices and consequences that will follow with NIPD [115]. Among the healthcare providers there seems to be a lack of knowledge or conviction about using NIPD. Healthcare providers hold genetic counseling and professional society approval important and they are more willing to offer cffDNA testing for chromosomal abnormalities and single-gene disorders than determination of sex and behavioral or late-onset conditions. Standards of care and professional guidelines are necessary.

4. Other implications for combined Down syndrome screening method

Using the algorithm for Down syndrome, combined screening detects approximately 55.6 % of trisomy 18 cases, 36.4 % of trisomy 13 cases and 60 % of other aneuploidies for a 4.3 %

FPR. When specific algorithm for trisomy 18 is used, the DR for trisomy 18 is reported to be 74.0 - 88 % with a slight increase of 0.1 % in the FPR. Using the specific algorithm for trisomy 13 improves the DR for trisomy 13 to approximately 54.5 - 73 % for an additional 0.1 % increase in the FPR [116, 117].

Adverse pregnancy outcomes like pregnancy loss, hypertension, preeclampsia, eclampsia, preterm delivery, small for gestational age newborns and fetal death cannot yet be predicted in the early pregnancy. Closer surveillance and possible new treatments could be studied on women in high risk to avoid the adverse pregnancy outcomes in the future. As well as increased NT measurements, also abnormal levels of maternal serum biochemical markers have been associated with pregnancy complications.

5. Ethical aspects of the first trimester screening

Participating in the screening for chromosomal abnormalities and the diagnostic testing is voluntary. Women have an opportunity to retrieve screening at any point. It is essential that women make an informed decision when they decide to participate in the screening. When a positive screening result is received, detailed and objective counseling should be offered about the condition at issue and about the procedure and its risks. Health professionals' personal opinions should not affect the woman's decision. However, it is known that the many issues like the age, level of medical knowledge, opinion about the screening test, specialty and attitudes towards the patients affect the counseling. Due to the complexity of the screening, women need to assimilate a lot of information which might not always be successful. If the possibility of a chromosomal abnormality is introduced for the first time when the screening is offered, worry can be caused. The possibility to terminate the pregnancy after a chromosomal abnormality is detected raises many ethical issues about the right of the disabled to be born regardless of their disability. Screening is also thought to be insulting towards people with a chromosomal or a structural anomaly. Screening does not produce diagnoses, only risks for chromosomal abnormalities. The limitations of the screening should be told for the women participating in the screening. One redeeming feature of the screening is that it provides a great deal of knowledge about chromosomal and structural abnormalities equally for every screened woman.

6. Screening in multiple pregnancies and in ART pregnancies

Screening in multiple pregnancies is more difficult than in singleton pregnancies. Firstly, maternal serum biochemistry is less effective in multiple pregnancies since placental analytes from normal fetus/fetuses can mask abnormal levels in the affected fetus. Moreover, abnormal levels of maternal serum biochemical markers cannot distinguish which fetus is the affected one [118]. Secondly, second trimester ultrasound examination is more challenging because of the limitations due to the positions of the fetuses and interposition of fetal parts.

Nuchal translucency measurement together with maternal age, however, has been shown to be an effective screening method in multiple pregnancies. The DR is comparable to that in singleton pregnancies for a slightly higher FPR. Also, determination of fetus-specific risk is possible with this technique. The limitation of ultrasound in twins is that they can be influenced by hemodynamic imbalance between the twins' circulation. Other possible screening markers in multiple pregnancies are DV flow and NB [119-121].

Screening in pregnancies conceived using assisted reproductive technologies (ART) has been studied by different research groups and contradictory results have been reported. In some studies fβ-hCG and NT have been enlarged in ART pregnancies and PAPP-A levels decreased, while others have reported no significant differences in these markers. It seems that decreased PAPP-A levels in ART pregnancies is the most discriminating factor leading to increased FPR in these pregnancies. However, some have reported no significant difference in FPR in ART pregnancies compared with spontaneous pregnancies [191].

7. Cost-effectiveness of the screening and international differences in screening strategies

The demands for the prenatal screening performance are high. Also, the cost-effectiveness of the screening should be good. There are some estimations about the screening costs in different countries but overall, the cost and patient acceptability of the alternative policies of screening tests depend on the existing infrastructure of antenatal care, which varies between different countries and centers. Screening and diagnostic tests for chromosomal abnormalities have been developed and been available for several decades and the research for new strategies is ongoing. National committees review available evidence and national screening statistics and each country adopts testing modalities in its own way. In dissimilar healthcare systems guidelines for best practice evolve different ways. There are differences in what tests are offered, insurance coverage, counseling and the national legal situation for terminating an affected pregnancy. Global knowledge about testing practices gets more and more important for the counselors as people immigrate between the countries and into different cultures. In Europe, almost 90 % of couples who receive a prenatal diagnosis of Down syndrome decide to terminate the pregnancy. However, the legal situation concerning pregnancy termination differs between countries [123]. Most couples that feel that they would continue the pregnancy even though the fetus would be diagnosed with a chromosomal abnormality do not participate in the screening program [124]. There are significant differences in screening modalities between for example United Kingdom and the United States of America despite many similarities between the countries [125]. The introduction of prenatal screening has, however, led to a reduction in live-births of Down syndrome cases internationally.

http://dx.doi.org/10.5772/52861

Author details

Jaana Marttala

Department of Obstetrics and Gynecology, Oulu, Finland

References

[1] Hook EB (1981) Rates of chromosome abnormalities at different maternal ages. Obstet Gynecol 58(3): 282-285.

[2] Merkatz IR, Nitowsky HM, Macri JN, Johnson WE. An association between low maternal serum alpha-fetoprotein and fetal chromosomal abnormalities. Am J Obstet Gynecol. 1984; 148: 886-94.

[3] Bogart MH, Pandian MR, Jones OW. Abnormal maternal serum chorionic gonadotropin levels in pregnancies with fetal chromosome abnormalities. Prenat Diagn. 1987; 7: 623-30.

[4] Canick JA, Knight GJ, Palomaki GE, Haddow JE, Cuckle HS, Wald NJ. Low second trimester maternal serum unconjugated oestriol in pregnancies with down's syndrome. Br J Obstet Gynaecol. 1988; 95: 330-3.

[5] Christiansen M, Norgaard-Pedersen B. Inhibin A is a maternal serum marker for down's syndrome early in the first trimester. Clin Genet. 2005; 68: 35-9.

[6] Haddow JE, Palomaki GE, Knight GJ, Williams J, Pulkkinen A, Canick JA, et al. Prenatal screening for down's syndrome with use of maternal serum markers. N Engl J Med. 1992; 327: 588-93.

[7] Nicolaides KH, Azar G, Byrne D, Mansur C, Marks K. Fetal nuchal translucency: Ultrasound screening for chromosomal defects in first trimester of pregnancy. BMJ. 1992; 304: 867-9.

[8] Ville Y, Lalondrelle C, Doumerc S, Daffos F, Frydman R, Oury JF, et al. First-trimester diagnosis of nuchal anomalies: Significance and fetal outcome. Ultrasound Obstet Gynecol. 1992; 2: 314-6.

[9] Malone FD, Canick JA, Ball RH, Nyberg DA, Comstock CH, Bukowski R, et al. First- and Second-Trimester Evaluation of Risk (FASTER) Research Consortium. First-trimester or second-trimester screening, or both, for down's syndrome. N Engl J Med. 2005; 353: 2001-11.

[10] de Graaf IM, Tijmstra T, Bleker OP, van Lith JM. Womens' preference in down syndrome screening. Prenat Diagn. 2002; 22: 624-9.

[11] Snijders RJ, Sundberg K, Holzgreve W, Henry G, Nicolaides KH. Maternal age- and gestation-specific risk for trisomy 21. Ultrasound Obstet Gynecol. 1999; 13: 167-70.

[12] Morris JK, Wald NJ, Watt HC. Fetal loss in down syndrome pregnancies. Prenat Diagn. 1999; 19: 142-5.

[13] Marttala J, Yliniemi O, Gissler M, Nieminen P, Ryynanen M. Prevalence of down's syndrome in a pregnant population in finland. Acta Obstet Gynecol Scand. 2010; 89: 715-7.

[14] Engels MA, Heijboer AC, Blankenstein MA, van Vugt JM. Performance of first-trimester combined test for down syndrome in different maternal age groups: Reason for adjustments in screening policy? Prenat Diagn. 2011; 31: 1241-5.

[15] Tabor A, Alfirevic Z. Update on procedure-related risks for prenatal diagnosis techniques. Fetal Diagn Ther. 2010; 27: 1-7.

[16] Wald NJ, Rodeck C, Hackshaw AK, Walters J, Chitty L, Mackinson AM. First and second trimester antenatal screening for down's syndrome: The results of the serum, urine and ultrasound screening study (SURUSS). J Med Screen. 2003; 10: 56-104.

[17] Brizot ML, Snijders RJ, Butler J, Bersinger NA, Nicolaides KH. Maternal serum hCG and fetal nuchal translucency thickness for the prediction of fetal trisomies in the first trimester of pregnancy. Br J Obstet Gynaecol. 1995; 102: 127-32.

[18] Reynolds TM, Penney MD. The mathematical basis of multivariate risk screening: With special reference to screening for down's syndrome associated pregnancy. Ann Clin Biochem. 1990; 27: 452-8.

[19] Wald NJ, Hackshaw AK. Combining ultrasound and biochemistry in first-trimester screening for down's syndrome. Prenat Diagn. 1997; 17: 821-9.

[20] Cuckle HS, van Lith JM. Appropriate biochemical parameters in first-trimester screening for down syndrome. Prenat Diagn. 1999; 19: 505-12.

[21] Tsukerman GL, Gusina NB, Cuckle HS. Maternal serum screening for down syndrome in the first trimester: Experience from belarus. Prenat Diagn. 1999; 19: 499-504.

[22] Talmadge K, Boorstein WR, Fiddes JC. The human genome contains seven genes for the beta-subunit of chorionic gonadotropin but only one gene for the beta-subunit of luteinizing hormone. DNA. 1983; 2: 281-9.

[23] Brambati B, Macintosh MC, Teisner B, Maguiness S, Shrimanker K, Lanzani A, et al. Low maternal serum levels of pregnancy associated plasma protein A (PAPP-A) in the first trimester in association with abnormal fetal karyotype. Br J Obstet Gynaecol. 1993; 100: 324-6.

[24] Lawrence JB, Oxvig C, Overgaard MT, Sottrup-Jensen L, Gleich GJ, Hays LG, et al. The insulin-like growth factor (IGF)-dependent IGF binding protein-4 protease se-

creted by human fibroblasts is pregnancy-associated plasma protein-A. Proc Natl Acad Sci U S A. 1999; 96: 3149-53.

[25] Baker J, Liu JP, Robertson EJ, Efstratiadis A. Role of insulin-like growth factors in embryonic and postnatal growth. Cell. 1993; 75: 73-82.

[26] Malone FD, D'Alton ME, Society for Maternal-Fetal M. First-trimester sonographic screening for down syndrome. Obstet Gynecol. 2003; 102: 1066-79.

[27] Marttala J, Kaijomaa M, Ranta J, Dahlbacka A, Nieminen P, Tekay A, et al. False-negative results in routine combined first-trimester screening for down syndrome in finland. Am J Perinatol. 2012; 29: 211-6.

[28] Snijders RJ, Noble P, Sebire N, Souka A, Nicolaides KH. UK multicentre project on assessment of risk of trisomy 21 by maternal age and fetal nuchal-translucency thickness at 10-14 weeks of gestation. fetal medicine foundation first trimester screening group. Lancet. 1998; 352: 343-6.

[29] Braithwaite JM, Morris RW, Economides DL. Nuchal translucency measurements: Frequency distribution and changes with gestation in a general population. Br J Obstet Gynaecol. 1996; 103: 1201-4.

[30] Comstock CH, Malone FD, Ball RH, Nyberg DA, Saade GR, Berkowitz RL, et al. Is there a nuchal translucency millimeter measurement above which there is no added benefit from first trimester serum screening? Am J Obstet Gynecol. 2006; 195: 843-7.

[31] Bilardo CM, Muller MA, Pajkrt E, Clur SA, van Zalen MM, Bijlsma EK. Increased nuchal translucency thickness and normal karyotype: Time for parental reassurance. Ultrasound Obstet Gynecol. 2007; 30: 11-8.

[32] Souka AP, Von Kaisenberg CS, Hyett JA, Sonek JD, Nicolaides KH. Increased nuchal translucency with normal karyotype. Am J Obstet Gynecol. 2005; 192: 1005-21.

[33] Weijerman ME, van Furth AM, van der Mooren MD, van Weissenbruch MM, Rammeloo L, Broers CJ, et al. Prevalence of congenital heart defects and persistent pulmonary hypertension of the neonate with down syndrome. Eur J Pediatr. 2010; 169: 1195-9.

[34] Haak MC, Bartelings MM, Jackson DG, Webb S, van Vugt JM, Gittenberger-de Groot AC. Increased nuchal translucency is associated with jugular lymphatic distension. Hum Reprod. 2002; 17: 1086-92.

[35] Sepulveda W, Wong AE, Casasbuenas A, Solari A, Alcalde JL. Congenital diaphragmatic hernia in a first-trimester ultrasound aneuploidy screening program. Prenat Diagn. 2008; 28: 531-4.

[36] Ngo C, Viot G, Aubry MC, Tsatsaris V, Grange G, Cabrol D, et al. First-trimester ultrasound diagnosis of skeletal dysplasia associated with increased nuchal translucency thickness. Ultrasound Obstet Gynecol. 2007; 30: 221-6.

[37] von Kaisenberg CS, Krenn V, Ludwig M, Nicolaides KH, Brand-Saberi B. Morphological classification of nuchal skin in human fetuses with trisomy 21, 18, and 13 at 12-18 weeks and in a trisomy 16 mouse. Anat Embryol (Berl). 1998; 197: 105-24.

[38] Daskalakis G, Sebire NJ, Jurkovic D, Snijders RJ, Nicolaides KH. Body stalk anomaly at 10-14 weeks of gestation. Ultrasound Obstet Gynecol. 1997; 10: 416-8.

[39] Souka AP, Snijders RJ, Novakov A, Soares W, Nicolaides KH. Defects and syndromes in chromosomally normal fetuses with increased nuchal translucency thickness at 10-14 weeks of gestation. Ultrasound Obstet Gynecol. 1998; 11: 391-400.

[40] Bindra R, Heath V, Liao A, Spencer K, Nicolaides KH. One-stop clinic for assessment of risk for trisomy 21 at 11-14 weeks: A prospective study of 15 030 pregnancies. Ultrasound Obstet Gynecol. 2002; 20: 219-25.

[41] Crossley JA, Aitken DA, Cameron AD, McBride E, Connor JM. Combined ultrasound and biochemical screening for down's syndrome in the first trimester: A scottish multicentre study. BJOG. 2002; 109: 667-76.

[42] Wapner R. Thom E. Simpson JL. Pergament E. Silver R. Filkins K. Platt L. Mahoney M. Johnson A. Hogge WA. Wilson RD. Mohide P. Hershey D. Krantz D. Zachary J. Snijders R. Greene N. Sabbagha R. MacGregor S. Hill L. Gagnon A. Hallahan T. Jackson L. First Trimester Maternal Serum Biochemistry and Fetal Nuchal Translucency Screening (BUN) Study Group. First-trimester screening for trisomies 21 and 18. N Engl J Med. 2003; 349: 1405-13.

[43] Rozenberg P, Bussieres L, Chevret S, Bernard JP, Malagrida L, Cuckle H, et al. Screening for down syndrome using first-trimester combined screening followed by second-trimester ultrasound examination in an unselected population. Am J Obstet Gynecol. 2006; 195: 1379-87.

[44] Kagan KO, Wright D, Baker A, Sahota D, Nicolaides KH. Screening for trisomy 21 by maternal age, fetal nuchal translucency thickness, free beta-human chorionic gonadotropin and pregnancy-associated plasma protein-A. Ultrasound Obstet Gynecol. 2008; 31: 618-24.

[45] Okun N, Summers AM, Hoffman B, Huang T, Winsor E, Chitayat D, et al. Prospective experience with integrated prenatal screening and first trimester combined screening for trisomy 21 in a large canadian urban center. Prenat Diagn. 2008; 28: 987-92.

[46] Borrell A, Borobio V, Bestwick JP, Wald NJ. Ductus venosus pulsatility index as an antenatal screening marker for down's syndrome: Use with the combined and integrated tests. J Med Screen. 2009; 16: 112-8.

[47] Kagan KO, Etchegaray A, Zhou Y, Wright D, Nicolaides KH. Prospective validation of first-trimester combined screening for trisomy 21. Ultrasound Obstet Gynecol. 2009; 34: 14-8.

[48] Leung TY, Chan LW, Law LW, Sahota DS, Fung TY, Leung TN, et al. First trimester combined screening for trisomy 21 in hong kong: Outcome of the first 10,000 cases. J Matern Fetal Neonatal Med. 2009; 22: 300-4.

[49] Schaelike M, Kossakiewicz M, Kossakiewicz A, Schild RL. Examination of a first-trimester down syndrome screening concept on a mix of 11,107 high- and low-risk patients at a private center for prenatal medicine in germany. Eur J Obstet Gynecol Reprod Biol. 2009; 144: 140-5.

[50] Wortelboer EJ, Koster MP, Stoutenbeek P, Elvers LH, Loeber JG, Visser GH, et al. First-trimester down syndrome screening performance in the dutch population; how to achieve further improvement? Prenat Diagn. 2009; 29: 588-92.

[51] Salomon LJ, Chevret S, Bussieres L, Ville Y, Rozenberg P. Down syndrome screening using first-trimester combined tests and contingent use of femur length at routine anomaly scan. Prenat Diagn. 2010; 30: 783-9.

[52] Wright D, Spencer K, Kagan KK, Torring N, Petersen OB, Christou A, et al. First-trimester combined screening for trisomy 21 at 7-14 weeks' gestation. Ultrasound Obstet Gynecol. 2010; 36: 404-11.

[53] Marttala J, Ranta JK, Kaijomaa M, Nieminen P, Laitinen P, Kokkonen H, et al. More invasive procedures are done to detect each case of down's syndrome in younger women. Acta Obstet Gynecol Scand. 2011; 90: 642-7.

[54] Yeo GS, Lai FM, Wei X, Lata P, Tan DT, Yong MH, et al. Validation of first trimester screening for trisomy 21 in singapore with reference to performance of nasal bone. Fetal Diagn Ther. 2012.

[55] Peuhkurinen S, Laitinen P, Ryynanen M, Marttala J. First trimester down syndrome screening is less effective and the number of invasive procedures is increased in women younger than 35 years of age. J Eval Clin Pract. 2012.

[56] Maiz N, Staboulidou I, Leal AM, Minekawa R, Nicolaides KH. Ductus venosus doppler at 11 to 13 weeks of gestation in the prediction of outcome in twin pregnancies. Obstet Gynecol. 2009; 113: 860-5.

[57] Maiz N, Valencia C, Kagan KO, Wright D, Nicolaides KH. Ductus venosus doppler in screening for trisomies 21, 18 and 13 and turner syndrome at 11-13 weeks of gestation. Ultrasound Obstet Gynecol. 2009; 33: 512-7.

[58] Kagan KO, Staboulidou I, Cruz J, Wright D, Nicolaides KH. Two-stage first-trimester screening for trisomy 21 by ultrasound assessment and biochemical testing. Ultrasound Obstet Gynecol. 2010; 36: 542-7.

[59] Borenstein M, Persico N, Kaihura C, Sonek J, Nicolaides KH. Frontomaxillary facial angle in chromosomally normal fetuses at 11 + 0 to 13 + 6 weeks. Ultrasound Obstet Gynecol. 2007; 30: 737-41.

[60] Borenstein M, Persico N, Kagan KO, Gazzoni A, Nicolaides KH. Frontomaxillary facial angle in screening for trisomy 21 at 11 + 0 to 13 + 6 weeks. Ultrasound Obstet Gynecol. 2008; 32: 5-11.

[61] Cicero S, Curcio P, Papageorghiou A, Sonek J, Nicolaides K. Absence of nasal bone in fetuses with trisomy 21 at 11-14 weeks of gestation: An observational study. Lancet. 2001; 358: 1665-7.

[62] Falcon O, Faiola S, Huggon I, Allan L, Nicolaides KH. Fetal tricuspid regurgitation at the 11 + 0 to 13 + 6-week scan: Association with chromosomal defects and reproducibility of the method. Ultrasound Obstet Gynecol. 2006; 27: 609-12.

[63] Huggon IC, DeFigueiredo DB, Allan LD. Tricuspid regurgitation in the diagnosis of chromosomal anomalies in the fetus at 11-14 weeks of gestation. Heart. 2003; 89: 1071-3.

[64] Cicero S, Bindra R, Rembouskos G, Spencer K, Nicolaides KH. Integrated ultrasound and biochemical screening for trisomy 21 using fetal nuchal translucency, absent fetal nasal bone, free beta-hCG and PAPP-A at 11 to 14 weeks. Prenat Diagn. 2003; 23: 306-10.

[65] Bromley B, Lieberman E, Shipp TD, Benacerraf BR. The genetic sonogram: A method of risk assessment for down syndrome in the second trimester. J Ultrasound Med. 2002; 21: 1087,96; quiz 1097-8.

[66] Benacerraf BR. The role of the second trimester genetic sonogram in screening for fetal down syndrome. Semin Perinatol. 2005; 29: 386-94.

[67] Benn PA, Kaminsky LM, Ying J, Borgida AF, Egan JF. Combined second-trimester biochemical and ultrasound screening for down syndrome. Obstet Gynecol. 2002; 100: 1168-76.

[68] Aagaard-Tillery KM, Malone FD, Nyberg DA, Porter TF, Cuckle HS, Fuchs K, et al. Role of second-trimester genetic sonography after down syndrome screening. Obstet Gynecol. 2009; 114: 1189-96.

[69] Laigaard J, Spencer K, Christiansen M, Cowans NJ, Larsen SO, Pedersen BN, et al. ADAM 12 as a first-trimester maternal serum marker in screening for down syndrome. Prenat Diagn. 2006; 26: 973-9.

[70] Laigaard J, Cuckle H, Wewer UM, Christiansen M. Maternal serum ADAM12 levels in down and edwards' syndrome pregnancies at 9-12 weeks' gestation. Prenat Diagn. 2006; 26: 689-91.

[71] Valinen Y, Peuhkurinen S, Jarvela IY, Laitinen P, Ryynanen M. Maternal serum ADAM12 levels correlate with PAPP-A levels during the first trimester. Gynecol Obstet Invest. 2010; 70: 60-3.

[72] Koster MP, Wortelboer EJ, Cuckle HS, Stoutenbeek P, Visser GH, Schielen PC. Placental protein 13 as a first trimester screening marker for aneuploidy. Prenat Diagn. 2009; 29: 1237-41.

[73] Akolekar R, Perez Penco JM, Skyfta E, Rodriguez Calvo J, Nicolaides KH. Maternal serum placental protein 13 at eleven to thirteen weeks in chromosomally abnormal pregnancies. Fetal Diagn Ther. 2010; 27: 72-7.

[74] Spencer K, Liao AW, Ong CY, Geerts L, Nicolaides KH. First trimester maternal serum placenta growth factor (PIGF)concentrations in pregnancies with fetal trisomy 21 or trisomy 18. Prenat Diagn. 2001; 21: 718-22.

[75] Nagalla SR, Canick JA, Jacob T, Schneider KA, Reddy AP, Thomas A, et al. Proteomic analysis of maternal serum in down syndrome: Identification of novel protein biomarkers. J Proteome Res. 2007; 6: 1245-57.

[76] Saller DN,Jr, Canick JA. Current methods of prenatal screening for down syndrome and other fetal abnormalities. Clin Obstet Gynecol. 2008; 51: 24-36.

[77] Christiansen M, Olesen Larsen S. An increase in cost-effectiveness of first trimester maternal screening programmes for fetal chromosome anomalies is obtained by contingent testing. Prenat Diagn. 2002; 22: 482-6.

[78] Vadiveloo T, Crossley JA, Aitken DA. First-trimester contingent screening for down syndrome can reduce the number of nuchal translucency measurements required. Prenat Diagn. 2009; 29: 79-82.

[79] Souka AP, Pilalis A, Kavalakis I, Antsaklis P, Papantoniou N, Mesogitis S, et al. Screening for major structural abnormalities at the 11- to 14-week ultrasound scan. Am J Obstet Gynecol. 2006; 194: 393-6.

[80] Oztekin O, Oztekin D, Tinar S, Adibelli Z. Ultrasonographic diagnosis of fetal structural abnormalities in prenatal screening at 11-14 weeks. Diagn Interv Radiol. 2009; 15: 221-5.

[81] Maron JL, Bianchi DW. Prenatal diagnosis using cell-free nucleic acids in maternal body fluids: A decade of progress. Am J Med Genet C Semin Med Genet. 2007; 145C: 5-17.

[82] Bustamante-Aragones A, Rodriguez de Alba M, Gonzalez-Gonzalez C, Trujillo-Tiebas MJ, Diego-Alvarez D, Vallespin E, et al. Foetal sex determination in maternal blood from the seventh week of gestation and its role in diagnosing haemophilia in the foetuses of female carriers. Haemophilia. 2008; 14: 593-8.

[83] Hill M, Finning K, Martin P, Hogg J, Meaney C, Norbury G, et al. Non-invasive prenatal determination of fetal sex: Translating research into clinical practice. Clin Genet. 2011; 80: 68-75.

[84] Hill M, Taffinder S, Chitty LS, Morris S. Incremental cost of non-invasive prenatal diagnosis versus invasive prenatal diagnosis of fetal sex in england. Prenat Diagn. 2011; 31: 267-73.

[85] Devaney SA, Palomaki GE, Scott JA, Bianchi DW. Noninvasive fetal sex determination using cell-free fetal DNA: A systematic review and meta-analysis. JAMA. 2011; 306: 627-36.

[86] Macher HC, Noguerol P, Medrano-Campillo P, Garrido-Marquez MR, Rubio-Calvo A, Carmona-Gonzalez M, et al. Standardization non-invasive fetal RHD and SRY determination into clinical routine using a new multiplex RT-PCR assay for fetal cell-free DNA in pregnant women plasma: Results in clinical benefits and cost saving. Clin Chim Acta. 2012; 413: 490-4.

[87] Bianchi DW, Maron JL, Johnson KL. Insights into fetal and neonatal development through analysis of cell-free RNA in body fluids. Early Hum Dev. 2010; 86: 747-52.

[88] Clausen FB, Christiansen M, Steffensen R, Jorgensen S, Nielsen C, Jakobsen MA, et al. Report of the first nationally implemented clinical routine screening for fetal RHD in D- pregnant women to ascertain the requirement for antenatal RhD prophylaxis. Transfusion. 2012; 52: 752-8.

[89] Bromberg YM, Salzberger M, Abrahamov A. Transplacental transmission of fetal erythrocytes with demonstration of fetal hemoglobin in maternal circulation. Obstet Gynecol. 1956; 7: 672-4.

[90] Weiner W, Child RM, Garvie JM, Peek WH. Foetal cells in the maternal circulation during pregnancy. Br Med J. 1958; 2: 770-1.

[91] Lurie S, Mamet Y. Red blood cell survival and kinetics during pregnancy. Eur J Obstet Gynecol Reprod Biol. 2000; 93: 185-92.

[92] Lo YMD, Corbetta N, Chamberlain PF, Rai V, Sargent IL, Redman CW, et al. Presence of fetal DNA in maternal plasma and serum. The Lancet. 1997; 350: 485-7.

[93] Alberry M, Maddocks D, Jones M, Abdel Hadi M, Abdel-Fattah S, Avent N, et al. Free fetal DNA in maternal plasma in anembryonic pregnancies: Confirmation that the origin is the trophoblast. Prenat Diagn. 2007; 27: 415-8.

[94] Lo YM, Tein MS, Lau TK, Haines CJ, Leung TN, Poon PM, et al. Quantitative analysis of fetal DNA in maternal plasma and serum: Implications for noninvasive prenatal diagnosis. Am J Hum Genet. 1998; 62: 768-75.

[95] Lo YM, Lau TK, Zhang J, Leung TN, Chang AM, Hjelm NM, et al. Increased fetal DNA concentrations in the plasma of pregnant women carrying fetuses with trisomy 21. Clin Chem. 1999; 45: 1747-51.

[96] Wright CF, Burton H. The use of cell-free fetal nucleic acids in maternal blood for non-invasive prenatal diagnosis. Hum Reprod Update. 2009; 15: 139-51.

[97] Poon LL, Leung TN, Lau TK, Lo YM. Presence of fetal RNA in maternal plasma. Clin Chem. 2000; 46: 1832-4.

[98] Ng EK, Tsui NB, Lam NY, Chiu RW, Yu SC, Wong SC, et al. Presence of filterable and nonfilterable mRNA in the plasma of cancer patients and healthy individuals. Clin Chem. 2002; 48: 1212-7.

[99] Farina A, Chan CW, Chiu RW, Tsui NB, Carinci P, Concu M, et al. Circulating corticotropin-releasing hormone mRNA in maternal plasma: Relationship with gestational age and severity of preeclampsia. Clin Chem. 2004; 50: 1851-4.

[100] Lo YM, Tsui NB, Chiu RW, Lau TK, Leung TN, Heung MM, et al. Plasma placental RNA allelic ratio permits noninvasive prenatal chromosomal aneuploidy detection. Nat Med. 2007; 13: 218-23.

[101] Chiu RW, Akolekar R, Zheng YW, Leung TY, Sun H, Chan KC, et al. Non-invasive prenatal assessment of trisomy 21 by multiplexed maternal plasma DNA sequencing: Large scale validity study. BMJ. 2011; 342: c7401.

[102] Chiu RW, Chan KC, Gao Y, Lau VY, Zheng W, Leung TY, et al. Noninvasive prenatal diagnosis of fetal chromosomal aneuploidy by massively parallel genomic sequencing of DNA in maternal plasma. Proc Natl Acad Sci U S A. 2008; 105: 20458-63.

[103] Ehrich M, Deciu C, Zwiefelhofer T, Tynan JA, Cagasan L, Tim R, et al. Noninvasive detection of fetal trisomy 21 by sequencing of DNA in maternal blood: A study in a clinical setting. Am J Obstet Gynecol. 2011; 204: 205.e1,205.11.

[104] Palomaki GE, Kloza EM, Lambert-Messerlian GM, Haddow JE, Neveux LM, Ehrich M, et al. DNA sequencing of maternal plasma to detect down syndrome: An international clinical validation study. Genet Med. 2011; 13: 913-20.

[105] Ghanta S, Mitchell ME, Ames M, Hidestrand M, Simpson P, Goetsch M, et al. Non-invasive prenatal detection of trisomy 21 using tandem single nucleotide polymorphisms. PLoS One. 2010; 5: e13184.

[106] Fan HC, Blumenfeld YJ, Chitkara U, Hudgins L, Quake SR. Noninvasive diagnosis of fetal aneuploidy by shotgun sequencing DNA from maternal blood. Proc Natl Acad Sci U S A. 2008; 105: 16266-71.

[107] Sehnert AJ, Rhees B, Comstock D, de Feo E, Heilek G, Burke J, et al. Optimal detection of fetal chromosomal abnormalities by massively parallel DNA sequencing of cell-free fetal DNA from maternal blood. Clin Chem. 2011; 57: 1042-9.

[108] Chen EZ, Chiu RW, Sun H, Akolekar R, Chan KC, Leung TY, et al. Noninvasive prenatal diagnosis of fetal trisomy 18 and trisomy 13 by maternal plasma DNA sequencing. PLoS One. 2011; 6: e21791.

[109] Lau TK, Chen F, Pan X, Pooh RK, Jiang F, Li Y, et al. Noninvasive prenatal diagnosis of common fetal chromosomal aneuploidies by maternal plasma DNA sequencing. J Matern Fetal Neonatal Med. 2012.

[110] Kido S, Sakuragi N, Bronner MP, Sayegh R, Berger R, Patterson D, et al. D21S418E identifies a cAMP-regulated gene located on chromosome 21q22.3 that is expressed in placental syncytiotrophoblast and choriocarcinoma cells. Genomics. 1993; 17: 256-9.

[111] Lo YM, Lun FM, Chan KC, Tsui NB, Chong KC, Lau TK, et al. Digital PCR for the molecular detection of fetal chromosomal aneuploidy. Proc Natl Acad Sci U S A. 2007; 104: 13116-21.

[112] Tsui NB, Akolekar R, Chiu RW, Chow KC, Leung TY, Lau TK, et al. Synergy of total PLAC4 RNA concentration and measurement of the RNA single-nucleotide polymorphism allelic ratio for the noninvasive prenatal detection of trisomy 21. Clin Chem. 2010; 56: 73-81.

[113] Maron JL, Johnson KL, Rocke DM, Cohen MG, Liley AJ, Bianchi DW. Neonatal salivary analysis reveals global developmental gene expression changes in the premature infant. Clin Chem. 2010; 56: 409-16.

[114] Benn PA, Chapman AR. Practical and ethical considerations of noninvasive prenatal diagnosis. JAMA. 2009; 301: 2154-6.

[115] Kooij L, Tymstra T, Berg P. The attitude of women toward current and future possibilities of diagnostic testing in maternal blood using fetal DNA. Prenat Diagn. 2009; 29: 164-8.

[116] Marttala J, Peuhkurinen S, Ranta JK, Laitinen P, Kokkonen HL, Honkasalo T, et al. Screening and outcome of chromosomal abnormalities other than trisomy 21 in northern finland. Acta Obstet Gynecol Scand. 2011; 90: 885-9.

[117] Ekelund CK, Petersen OB, Skibsted L, Kjaergaard S, Vogel I, Tabor A, et al. First trimester screening for trisomy 21 in denmark: Implications on detection and birth rates of trisomy 18 and trisomy 13. Ultrasound Obstet Gynecol. 2011; 38: 140-4.

[118] Matias A, Montenegro N, Blickstein I. Down syndrome screening in multiple pregnancies. Obstet Gynecol Clin North Am. 2005; 32: 81,96, ix.

[119] Sebire NJ, Snijders RJ, Hughes K, Sepulveda W, Nicolaides KH. Screening for trisomy 21 in twin pregnancies by maternal age and fetal nuchal translucency thickness at 10-14 weeks of gestation. Br J Obstet Gynaecol. 1996; 103: 999-1003.

[120] Matias A, Ramalho C, Montenegro N. Search for hemodynamic compromise at 11-14 weeks in monochorionic twin pregnancy: Is abnormal flow in the ductus venosus predictive of twin-twin transfusion syndrome? J Matern Fetal Neonatal Med. 2005; 18: 79-86.

[121] Sepulveda W, Wong AE, Dezerega V. First-trimester ultrasonographic screening for trisomy 21 using fetal nuchal translucency and nasal bone. Obstet Gynecol. 2007; 109: 1040-5.

[122] Kirkegaard I, Henriksen TB, Torring N, Uldbjerg N. PAPP-A and free beta-hCG measured prior to 10 weeks is associated with preterm delivery and small-for-gestational-age infants. Prenat Diagn. 2011; 31: 171-5.

[123] Boyd PA, Devigan C, Khoshnood B, Loane M, Garne E, Dolk H, et al. Survey of prenatal screening policies in europe for structural malformations and chromosome anomalies, and their impact on detection and termination rates for neural tube defects and down's syndrome. BJOG. 2008; 115: 689-96.

[124] Kobelka C, Mattman A, Langlois S. An evaluation of the decision-making process regarding amniocentesis following a screen-positive maternal serum screen result. Prenat Diagn. 2009; 29: 514-9.

[125] Tapon D. Prenatal testing for down syndrome: Comparison of screening practices in the UK and USA. J Genet Couns. 2010; 19: 112-30.

Section 2

Diseases in Children with Down Syndrome

Chapter 4

Control of Dental Biofilm and Oral Health Maintenance in Patients with Down Syndrome

Ana Paula Teitelbaum and Gislaine Denise Czlusniak

Additional information is available at the end of the chapter

http://dx.doi.org/10.5772/53348

1. Introduction

The greatest prophylaxis challenge in dentistry is the control of dental biofilm and consequently, avoiding dental caries and gingival inflammation [1]. This control is generally carried out through mechanical and / or chemical methods. Although the mechanical methods (toothbrush and dental floss) are considered efficient, they are not sufficiently so in certain cases [2], [3].

Individuals with Down syndrome (DS) present various oral diseases, such as the presence of pseudoprognatismo, hard palate and lower ogival shape; pseudomacroglossia due to hypotonia tongue; high prevalence and susceptibility to periodontal problems due to error in the autoregulatory mechanism immune, and poor occlusal relationship, with a predominance of anterior crossbite and / or later. The position of the tongue protruded, produces abnormal strength in the lower anterior teeth, which normally are in a position to cross-bite. These factors favor the onset of severe periodontitis, leading to early loss of teeth. However, there is a lower incidence of dental caries, which has been attributed mainly to the increase in buffer capacity of saliva [4].

Some dental anomalies can be observed, as the presence of hypodontia or oligodontia, tooth conoids, microteeth, hypocalcification enamel, fusion and twinning can also be an increase in the size of the clinical crown of molars and the inclination of the occlusal surface to the lingual, making access to restorative procedures. Furthermore, the rash and exfoliation of the primary teeth and eruption of the permanent are delayed, and there is a high prevalence of bruxism [4], and these alterations interfere with the quality of toothbrushing.

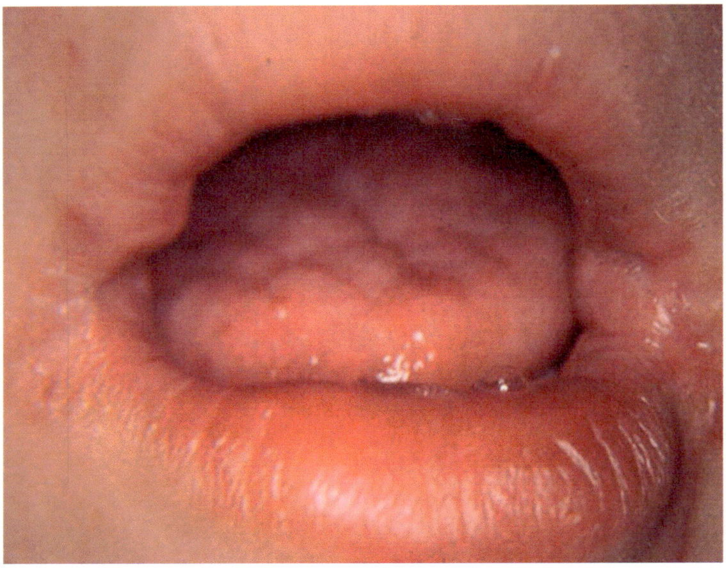

Figure 1. Pseudomacroglossia due to hypotonia tongue

There is agreement among many authors on the existence of factors predisposing to periodontal disease in patients with Down syndrome. Although poor oral hygiene, poor nutrition and local irritants may exacerbate this problem, they can not be regarded as its main cause. The greater predisposition to periodontal disease has been attributed to characteristics of patients with chromosomal abnormalities of trisomy [5]·It is therefore essential to establish strategies to p revent periodontal disease in these individuals.

Second Cornejo et al. [6] (1996), which conducted a study in 86 individuals with DS living in Argentina, aged between 3 and 19 years, the presence of the changes described above puts them at a disadvantage in relation to oral health, compared with noncarriers.

Besides the inherent disadvantage to the individual, access to dental care is also difficult for these people. Allison et al. [7] (2000), in a study conducted in France, compared the levels of care received dental services and oral hygiene habits among children with DS and their siblings. According to parents and / or guardians, the group with DS had difficulty finding access to dental services and oral care compared to their phenotypically normal siblings. In Brazil, studying the prevalence of dental caries in primary and permanent teeth of children with DS in Sao Jose dos Campos (SP), Moraes et al. [8] (2002) found that the values of ceo and CPO-D were similar to those identified by the Municipal Health Department, in a survey of dental caries in children from public schools. However, the authors found a frequency of 9.25% and 4.76% decayed teeth restored among the children examined, against the values of 3.98% and 5.88%, respectively, obtained by the Municipal Health.

All these mentioned aspects can be inferred that it would be essential to adopt appropriate measures aimed at controlling biofilm among the DS patients, to prevent the installation of dental caries and gingival inflammation, because the microorganisms in the biofilm and act decisively etiologic agents in the origin and development of caries and periodontal also (König et al. [9] 2002). In 1965, Löe et al. [10] demonstrated the direct relationship between the biofilm and the development of gingivitis in humans, concluding that the removal of biofilm employing brushing and flossing, could result in reversal in health (Löe et al. [10] 1965, Theilade et al. [11] 1966). For this reason, control of the biofilm has an important role in the prevention, treatment and maintenance of periodontal health.

2. Mechanical control of dental biofilm

The mechanical control is to remove biofilm employing proper technique of brushing, combined with a dentifrice and auxiliary materials such as wire or dental tape (Owens et al. [12] 1997).

The ability to remove dental biofilm by the use of different types of brushes is basically the same. There is no ideal brush, and your choice should be guided by the needs of each individual patient and clinical observations of the professional. However, there are characteristics that facilitate the oral hygiene procedures, as the presence of small head multitufuladas, soft bristle, rounded second study by Panzeri et al. [13] (1993).

The toothbrushing is an effective procedure for the maintenance of proper oral hygiene. However, to get a good cleaning of the oral cavity, in addition to toothbrushes, other factors must be considered such as time, frequency, brushing technique, manual skills and motivation of patients (Halla [14] 1982).

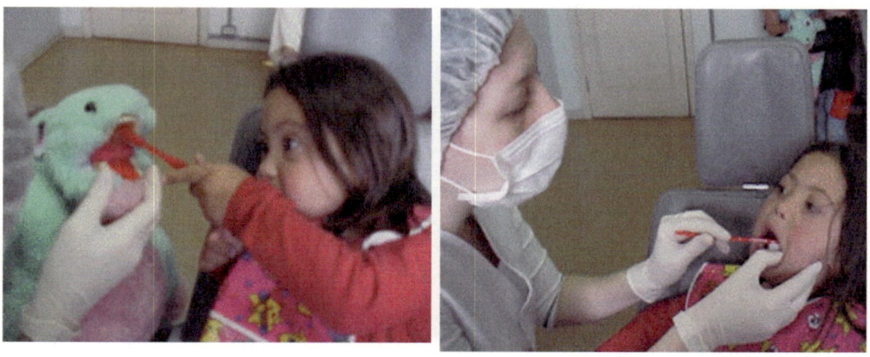

Figure 2. Motivation of patients and toothbrushing

Several authors report that, although brushing is the most widespread and universally suitable for the mechanical removal of the plate are not known techniques ideal nor brushes which, by itself, may promote a perfect cleaning. All this technical device should be associated with constant motivation [12],[15]-[16].

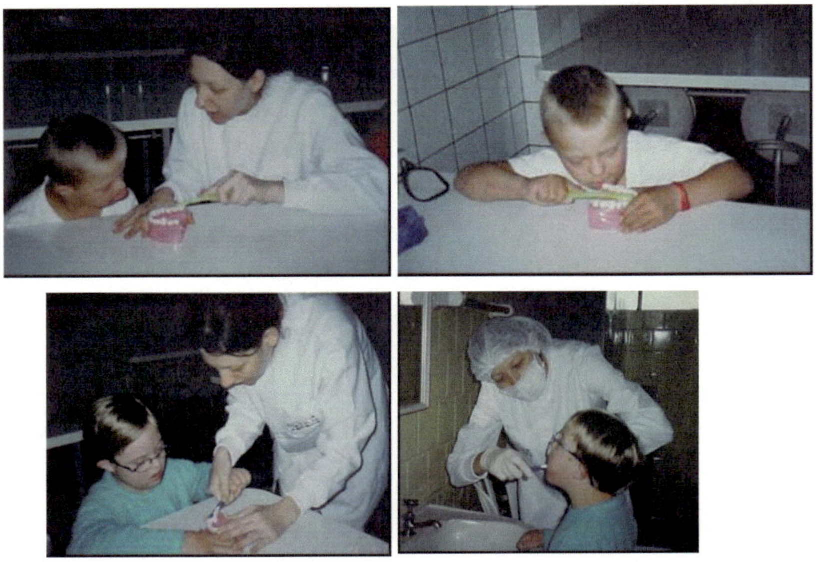

Figure 3. Toothbrushing technique and manual skills

The control of dental biofilm is a preventive action that involves a number of aspects, such as health education, which is achieved through constant guidance and motivation for people on oral hygiene (Bijella [17]1999).

The manual dexterity and, many times, the motivation, are indispensable factors for efficient oral hygiene through mechanical means in patients with Down syndrome [18]-[22]. Thus, the key to success in promoting and maintaining a satisfactory oral health in these patients is the application of a rigorous program of oral hygiene constant [23].

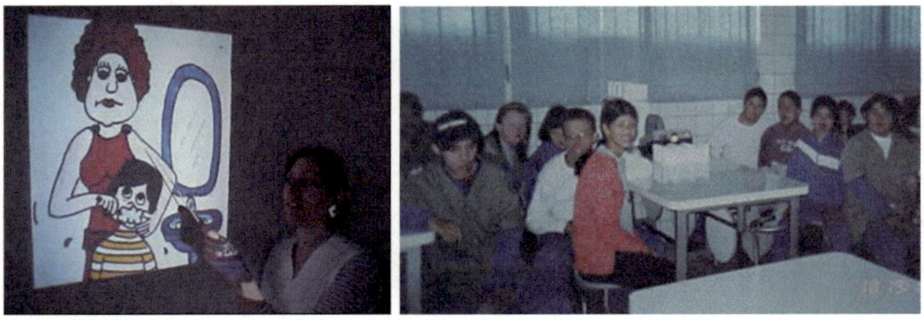

Figure 4. Lecture to motivate the control of biofilm

Mental disability is another aspect to be considered as difficult to awareness of the importance of oral health, difficulty in learning the techniques of brushing and lack of concentration at the time of toothbrushing [24],[25]. This difficulty leads these patients to have high levels of plaque-dependent oral diseases, especially periodontal changes [6]. It is therefore essential to establish strategies to prevent periodontal disease in these individuals.

http://dx.doi.org/10.5772/53348

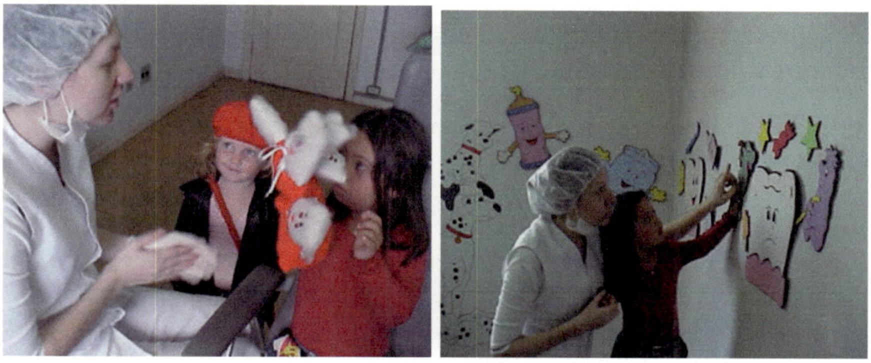

Figure 5. Constant guidance and motivation

Second Nielsen [26] (1990), the type and degree of disability are also important factors, since the greater the degree of mental deficiency the worse the level of hygiene.

3. Dentifrices with disclosing agent dental biofilm

The obstacles inherent to children with Down syndrome and the difficulties faced by parents and / or people in charge for toothbrushing, lead the professional in dentistry to look for a substance capable of aiding and stimulating these patients in the mechanical control of the dental biofilm. Studies suggest the use of disclosing agents, such as erythrosine, to remove dental biofilm more easily. For this reason, the presence of a disclosing agent in the formulation of the dentifrice could aid in the removal of the dental biofilm [27].

Are disclosing the chemicals used for staining bacteria, which show the colonies, invisible or barely visible, that adhere to tooth surfaces, making them visible, thus supporting the maintenance of oral hygiene while facilitating their removal (Bellini et al. [27]1974). Among the forms of application of disclosing the most commonly used in dentistry are tablets or solutions (Medeiros [28]1991).

The proven merit of disclosing meant that its use became a source of motivation (Toassi, Petry [29]2002), are indicated as excellent aids in determining the state of oral hygiene. Shown to be valuable as a teaching tool in education, not only by convincing the population for the presence of dental biofilm, as well as raising awareness about the need for its removal (Cristiano, Bignelli [30]1995).

Second Bouquet [31] (1971) and Gillings [32] (1977), the disclosing must provide ease of application and handling, good flavor, not blushing residually plastic restorations or tooth cracks, do not stain the mucosal lip, cheek and gum, to be of contrasting color facilitate the differentiation from the marginal gingiva and does not cause tissue irritation.

There are a variety of disclosing the market, among them are methylene blue, eosin, erythrosin, fluorescein sodium, neutral red and proflavine monosulfate. According to the work of

Silva et al. [33] (2002), among all the solutions mentioned, eosin, erythrosine and neutral red showed the greatest ability to blush, ease of removal and absence of antimicrobial activity, are essential requirements in studies evaluating methods of hygiene and guidance patient.

Erythrosine a dye consisting of the disodium salt of 3 ', 6' - dihydroxy - 2 ', 4', 5 ', 7' - tetraiodospiro [isobenzenofurano -1 (3H), 9 - [9H] xateno] - 3 - one and may contain up to 4.0% Fluoresceins a lesser degree of iodination, and chloride and / or sodium sulfate and water of crystallization. Must contain at least 85% calculated as total dye $C_{20}H_6I_4O_5Na_2$. Presented as physical characteristics: fine powder, red or brown odorless, soluble in water and hidroscópio giving red solution should not exhibit fluorescent room light, also soluble in ethanol, glycerin and propylene glycol. Practically insoluble in ether, mineral oil and fats (Standing Committee Review of the Brazilian Pharmacopoeia [34] 1996).

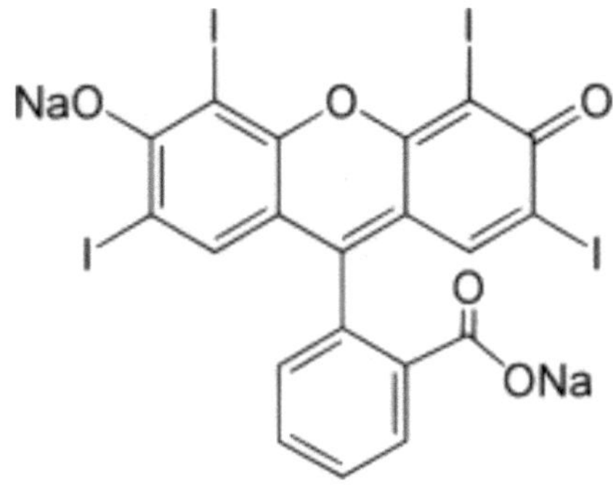

Figure 6. Structural formula erythrosine

The use of a dentifrice containing the color erythrosine as agent for removal of dental biofilm during toothbrushing is an excellent resource to stimulate the patient in your dental hygiene (Quintanilla, Bastos [35]1988), because the presence of this dye to facilitate parents and individuals / or guardians to view the plaque, especially in places where there is greater difficulty of removal during brushing (Duarte et al. [36]1990).

The use of toothpaste containing erythrosine, Dentplaque ®, was approved by the ADA, and is used as part of a program to promote oral health, being distributed by the Ministry of Health in 1999, the Health Secretariat of São Paul, including the Regional Health of Piracicaba, Piracicaba encompassing than 25 cities in the region (Silva et al. [37] 2004).

According to research Quintanilla et al. [38] (1989) where they studied the clinical behavior of the dentifrice added erythrosine Dentplaque ® 0.5% by comparing the new proposal to existing, as the common dentifrice and dental plaque disclosing in tablet form coadjuntor dentifrice common comparing the percentage of plaque remaining and the time taken to perform each of the three proposals in nine females with mean age of 21.33 years, and all with private have never experienced the use of a plaque disclosing. Individuals selected for the sample received no instruction on brushing technique, since the aim was to assess whether humans would be able to remove plaque evident on the surfaces of the teeth, according to the manual skills of each participant. The time was recorded in seconds since the beginning of each experiment (opening the packages), to its end. To evaluate the remaining plate, disclosure was made with basic fuchsin after each experiment, and recorded the number of stained surfaces, indicating the remaining plaque. The authors found that the average time of tooth brushing with toothpaste containing erythrosine has become more than double when compared to an ordinary toothpaste. Regarding the plaque index, the authors observed that the impregnation of the dye this is most efficient method III (Dentplaque ®), because the dye is rubbed on the plaque while toothbrushing, when compared to other (MI - toothbrushing with dentifrice common; M II - use of disclosing tablets plaque and toothbrushing with dentifrice common).

However, Rodrigues et al. [39] (1994) found different result. Undertook a study on the effectiveness of the dentifrices containing erythrosine Dentplaque ® in the stimulation process to dental hygiene for 45 male children, aged 6-12 years living in an orphanage in the city of Rio de Janeiro. These children were divided randomly into three groups of 15 patients maintained the same dietary habits. Initially, all received instructions on oral hygiene and toothbrushing technique, through lectures and posters illustrative devices. Were given tuition every 30 days during the 90 days of the survey. The brushing technique recommended in this study was to headphones, and recommended its implementation soon after meals. The control group made use of the brush with your regular dentifrice, the second group made use of a disclosing in tablet form before each brushing, and use your usual toothpaste, and the third group used a dentifrice containing erythrosine for toothbrushing routine. These children were supervised daily by an official of the orphanage properly oriented. In the initial evaluation, all were subjected to three more evaluations, with a 30-day interval between them being given the simplified oral hygiene index of Greene & Vermillion. The authors concluded that there were no statistical differences in relation to reducing the level of dental plaque in the three groups, but it was observed that the dentifrice was the easiest way of disclosure, and inserts a method of assimilation more difficult for children aged 6-12 years.

The same result of the work of Rodrigues et al. [39] (1994) found in Silva et al. [97] (2004), with 62 students at a public school in the city of Piracicaba, aged between 12 and 14 years. Participants were divided into groups: dentifrice with erythrosine Dentplaque ® (Group I) and the use of disclosing tablets (Group II). The plaque reduction was observed in all groups did not show statistically significant differences between them. However, the authors noted that factors that had limited the completion of this study, as the amount of sample, the low amount of plaque revealed by the index and the small amount of plaque shown by the students may have influenced the results, covering the response of the methods. In addition, the fact that some individuals participated in this study only the initial assessment, refusing to participate in the final evaluation, the amount of the sample was reduced to 18 participants.

In this context, the use of a dentifrice with erythrosine, as an agent for plaque removal should encourage the completion of a thorough toothbrushing, presumably more closely individual (Silva et al. [40] 2003).

4. Chemical control of dental biofilm

Studies have shown that mechanical control produces significant reductions in gingivitis in people with special needs. However, many patients with Down syndrome, besides being unable to cooperate, do not have sufficient manual dexterity to do toothbrushing or to use dental floss. Consequently, the use of chemical and / or antimicrobial agents as aids in plaque control can be indicated for these individuals. Considering the fact that toothbrushing with dentifrice is the most common tool for good oral hygiene, adding chlorhexidine to dentifrices could be seen as a practical means of improving the quality of oral hygiene [2, 41-47].

The chemicals and / or antimicrobial agents are often used in dental plaque reduction and can be used in conjunction with the mechanical control in preserving health and treatment of gingivitis, in some patients (Mandel [48] 1994), especially those that have little manual dexterity to the realization of toothbrushing (Fischman [49] 1979).

The attributes required for a chemical agent can play its effectiveness in controlling supragingival biofilm was postulated by Loesche [50] (1976). According to the author, the chemical agent to be effective against microorganisms responsible for inflammation and must have substantivity, ie, the intraoral retention capacity, to achieve a contact time sufficient to act on the microorganisms existing, and to maintain inhibition dental biofilm formation by a longer period. Furthermore, the product must be stable at room temperature for a considerable time and safe for human use.

Other features should also be observed for a chemical agent to be considered effective, such as lack of toxicity, not to be allergenic, have clinical evidence of significant reductions of plaque and gingivitis, be selective and have specificity to act on pathogenic microbiota, provide a pleasant taste have to be affordable and easy to use (Van Der Ouderra [51] 1991).

Chemical control of biofilm can be made to prophylactic or therapeutic. In the first case, the goal would be that there were an imbalance in the microbiota, when mechanical methods are ineffective. In the therapeutic sense with respect to individuals who already have changes in order to achieve the predominant bacteria-related diseases, aiming at restoring the microbiota and its harmony with the host (Marsh [52] 1992).

In 1954, Davies et al. [53] synthesized in the laboratory substance large bacterial action against Gram + and Gram -, and fungi. From this time, the chlorhexidine is now used as a general disinfectant for the treatment of various infections.

It was marketed in the 60s, by Imperial Chemical Industries (England), and one of the first applications of chlorhexidine in dentistry to control biofilm was performed by Schiott and Löe [54] (1970). The authors recommend the use of 10 mL of chlorhexidine digluconate 0.2% twice a day for one minute in order to prevent the accumulation of plaque and gingivitis subsequent. Since then, this compound has been considered the most effective agent in the chemical control dental biofilm (Souza, Abreu [55] 2003).

http://dx.doi.org/10.5772/53348

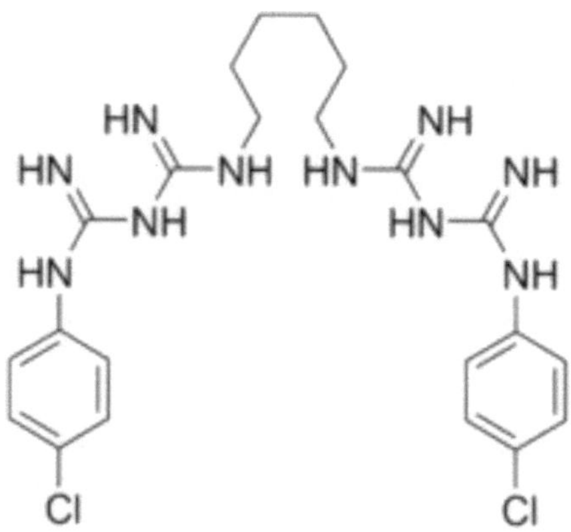

Figure 7. Structural formula chlorhexidine

Chlorhexidine is a cationic agent, a bis-guanidine non-toxic molecule is a symmetrical, with two rings and two 4-chlorophenyl groups ethane pentânicos connected by a central hexamethylene chain. Is prepared in the form of various salts, and gluconate, the digluconate or chlorhexidine acetate in its composition (Vinholis et al. [56] 1996). The chlorhexidine digluconate salt is one of the most widely used in the preparation of therapeutic formulations, because of its greater solubility in water and physiological pH, dissociates releasing the active component (Bonacorsi et al. [57] 2000).

The main site of action of chlorhexidine, both in prokaryotes and in eukaryotic cells is the cytoplasmic membrane. The mechanism of action of chlorhexidine begins with a call in the bacterial cell wall, when the adsorption of positive charges in the molecule of the substance to the surface of the negative charges increases the permeability of the bacterial cell walls of microorganism and allows the agent to penetrate the cytoplasmic occurring disruption of cell membrane leakage of intracellular components and low molecular weight, as potassium ions. At this stage the bacteriostatic effect is considered and reversible. While in high concentrations, lead to enzyme inhibition (ATPase), extravasation of macromolecules (nucleotides) and clotting components of the cytoplasm, due to the interaction of chlorhexidine with cytoplasmic proteins and nucleic acid, thus reaching the stage of bactericidal and irreversible (Bonacorsi et al. [57] 2000).

The chlorhexidine is usually effective against Gram positive and Gram-negative bacteria, fungi, yeasts and Candida albicans. It has broad spectrum antibacterial, high substantivity, is safe and effective (Quagliato [58] 1991).

Second Vinholis et al. [56] (1996), there are three mechanisms for chlorhexidine inhibition of biofilm:

Chlorhexidine is connected by means of electrostatic forces to the groups of acidic proteins such as phosphates, sulphates and carboxyl ions found in saliva and mouth tissues, there avoiding the formation of the acquired pellicle.

The ability of bacteria to bind to the tooth can be reduced by the absorption of chlorhexidine to the capsule of extracellular polysaccharides.

Chlorhexidine can compete with Ca + + ions. The mechanism is probably due to a direct competition between ions and / or availability of the drug and the carboxylic groups in the oral tissues. Can also inhibit the formation of bridges between the Ca + bacteria and surfaces, and the bacteria together. Due to its cationic properties, chlorhexidine can bind to the hydroxyapatite of enamel, and the acquired pellicle salivary proteins (Gjermo 59 1989).

5. Dentifrices with chlorhexidine

The chemical agent chlorhexidine as deputy in the control of dental biofilm is useful in situations where oral hygiene is inefficient, is compromised or is impossible to be realized. This antimicrobial agent is particularly suited to individuals who, because of physical or mental limitations, they are incapable, in whole or in part, the appropriate mechanical removal of plaque, were considered patients with special needs (Al-Tannir, Goodman [60] 1994).

That the dentifrices are used in conjunction with toothbrushing, causes the addition of chlorhexidine greater deserves attention, since it does not represent changes to the patient, as is routine in the same. Importantly, most studies of dentifrices containing chlorhexidine has been made with experimental formulations (Sathler, Fischer [61] 1996).

Experimental studies have shown that dentifrices with 0.5% chlorhexidine were less effective than rinsing mouthwash with 0.2% chlorhexidine (Addy et al. [62] 1989, Jenkins et al. [63] 1990). In a study by Gjermo and Rolla [64] (1970), the use of dentifrices with 0.6% chlorhexidine and 0.8% applied in trays on the teeth to avoid interference from the mechanical action of toothbrushing, showed a reduction in the rate of plate, and these results were consistent with those obtained with mouthwash.

Second Jenkins et al. [42] (1993), introduction of 1% chlorhexidine dentifrices promoted to an improvement in gingival index and plaque index, similar to those experienced in rinsing with 0.2% chlorhexidine. The authors also state that the association of fluoride with chlorhexidine dentifrices does not inhibit chlorhexidine.

The use of chlorhexidine dentifrice is a controversial subject. Some research on the short-term clinical effect of reducing plaque and gingival show the effectiveness of this substance (Torres 65 2000). This was proved in the study of Storhaug 46 (1977), which evaluated the use of toothpaste containing 0.8% chlorhexidine in 27 patients with special needs, from 4 to 12 years in a clinic held by the government of Norway. These patients were selected to test the effects of toothbrushing performed with the plaque index, gingival index, according to the criteria proposed by Löe and Silness. Patients were then divided into two groups: 17 children were using toothpaste containing chlorhexidine (GI) and 10 children used a placebo dentifrice (GII). After 6 weeks of study, there was significant reduction in plaque index of the group that used chlorhexidine compared with the control group and gingival index, no significant differences for the group that used chlorhexidine. However, clinically, the acute signs of inflammation are gone. The author stated that the conventional techniques of oral hygiene can be difficult to implement for this group of patients and chlorhexidine, in its various forms of application, an agent is extremely useful for maintaining oral health of patients with special needs.

Russell and Bay [44] (1981) observed that the use of toothpaste the basis of 1% chlorhexidine in daily brushing of children with epilepsy and mental retardation, reflected in a significant improvement in plaque and gingival index in this group of patients.

Dolles and Gjermo [41] (1980) evaluated the effect of three dentifrices in reducing dental caries and gingivitis (DI - dentifrice containing chlorhexidine (2%), IBD - with fluoride toothpaste (0.1% NaF) and DIII - chlorhexidine dentifrice with the two % and fluorine (0.1% NaF) for two years. Ninety-one students from 13 to 15 years of age participated in the research. the group using the dentifrice with fluoride and chlorhexidine showed a lower rate of dental caries, although the gingival conditions improved in the three groups, showing no statistical differences.

In a study of experimental gingivitis, Jenkins et al. 42 (1993), found that a dentifrice formulation of 1% chlorhexidine and 1000 ppm F (NaF) produced statistically significant reductions in plaque and gingivitis, compared with the placebo dentifrice. Subsequently, Yates et al. 47 1993, proposed to assess the clinical effects of chlorhexidine dentifrice 1%, with or without the 1000ppmF (NaF) previously tested by Jenkins et al. 42 1993. This study aimed to evaluate the control of plaque and gingivitis using: a) dentifrice containing 1% chlorhexidine called single asset, b) 1% of dentifrice containing fluoride clorexidina/1000ppm called active double c) negative control for six months. The sample consisted of two hundred ninety-seven individuals aged between 18 and 61 years. The periodontal parameters used were the plaque index, gingival bleeding and staining that were recorded at the beginning, six, 0,24 weeks, along with the index calculation was also recorded in the sixth, twelfth and twenty-fourth week. After prophylaxis performed at baseline, the subjects used the assigned dentifrice twice a day for one minute, without any other additional information on oral hygiene were given, just the direction we should use enough toothpaste to cover the head of the toothbrush. It was not permitted to use any other adjunctive oral hygiene product. At the end of the study all subjects were examined by a hygienist and extrinsic staining, supragingival plaque and calculus were removed. The results showed reduction of plaque index and bleeding in all groups, but a significant improvement occurred in the chlorhexidine group. In contrast to these results, staining and calculus indices were more significant in the test groups compared with the control group. The authors concluded that the side effects of chlorhexidine are acceptable, the dentifrice containing chlorhexidine can be recommended for the same clinical applications than the other products based on chlorhexidine. The compatibility of fluoride with chlorhexidine in one of the products could be effective in preventing tooth decay, and fluoride dentifrice containing chlorhexidine and could provide benefits to gingival health than preventive and therapeutic applications in clinical dentistry.

The action of a dentifrice containing 1% chlorhexidine in reducing dental plaque and gingival bleeding in 156 children over a period of twelve weeks, residents in Ga-Rankuwa (Pretoria, South Africa), aged between 12 and 14 years were evaluated by Gugushe et al. [2] (1994). The children were divided into three groups, which used conventional dentifrice (group A - 51 subjects), placebo dentifrice (group B - 49 individuals) and chlorhexidine dentifrice (group C - 56 individuals). Before starting the experiment, they were instructed on oral hygiene, had their records of plaque index, gingival taken and received professional dental prophylaxis. The record of the indices was repeated in the sixth and twelfth weeks. All patients were instructed to make tooth brushing morning and night. In the presence of plaque, it was observed that the rate decreased in all groups, with reductions substantially equal groups A and B and further reduction to the group C In relation to the gingival index, a reduction very similar in all groups (approximately 4%) without significant differences. However, the dentifrice with 1% chlorhexidine was more effective in controlling dental plaque as compared with the conventional dentifrice and placebo.

In a clinical study by Sanz et al. [45] (1994), the experimental dentifrice containing chlorhexidine 0.4% and 0.345 mg of zinc, contributed significantly to the improvement of oral hygiene, both in relation to the plaque and gingivitis and bleeding, resulting in fewer spots than those found in the group who used mouthwash with chlorhexidine 0.12%. The investigators concluded that the tested dentifrice can be viewed as a promising alternative for the use of substances effective in reducing plaque and gingivitis, and offer minimal side effects.

In respect the effect on the microflora of the mouth, the dentifrices to 1% chlorhexidine and tested for a period of 6 months, promoted reduction of aerobic microorganisms and anerróbicos (Maynard et al. [66] 1993).

Considering the fact that toothbrushing with dentifrice is the most common habits of oral hygiene (Owens et al. [12] 1997), this practice can be seen as a plausible way for the introduction of chemicals to improve the oral health (Yates et al. [47] 1993).

According to Newman [67] (1986), the introduction of antimicrobial agents in dentifrices aims to improve the effectiveness of toothbrushing, promoting a positive effect in reducing biofilm.

Thus, Teltelbaum et al. [68,69] (2009, 2010) conducted a study with patients with SD, where he developed a dentifrice containing these two substances, chlorhexidine and erythrosine and evaluated the mechanical and chemical control of dental biofilm. The mechanical and chemical control of dental biofilm in patients with Down syndrome, of using different experimental dentifrices in forty institutionalized children between ages 7 and 13 years in the mixed dentition in an experimental cross-over, blind clinical trial where we used the following protocols: fluoridated dentifrice (protocol G1); fluoridated dentifrice + chlorhexidine (protocol G2); fluoridated dentifrice + chlorhexidine + plaquedisclosing agent (protocol G3); and fluoridated dentifrice + plaque-disclosing agent (protocol G4). Each experimental stage lasted 10 days with a 15-day washout. The evaluated parameters were plaque index and gingival bleeding and initial clinical conditions between each stage were similar. The dentifrices containing plaque-disclosing agent, irrespective of their association with chlorhexidine, produced a greater reduction in the final plaque index. As for gingival bleeding, the dentifrice containing erythrosine and the one containing chlorhexidine produced similar results. The dentifrice containing an association of chlorhexidine and erythrosine gave the best results. Thus, with the methodology employed, it was possible to conclude that the combination of drugs (chlorhexidine, fluorine and erythrosine) within one dentifrice can be useful in controlling dental biofilm and in the reduction of gingival bleeding [68,69].

Author details

Ana Paula Teitelbaum[1] and Gislaine Denise Czlusniak[1]

1 Department of Dentistry, Ponta Grossa Dental School, Center for Higher Education of Campos Gerais (CESCAGE), Ponta Grossa, Paraná, Brazil

2 Department of Dentistry, School of Dentistry, Ponta Grossa State University, Ponta Grossa, Paraná, Brazil

References

[1] Sekino S, Ramberg P, Uzel NG, Socransky S, Lindhe J. Effect of various chlorhexidine regimens on salivary bacteria and de novo plaque formation. J Clin Periodontol 2003;30:919–25.

[2] Gugushe TS, de Wet FA, Rojas-Silva O. Efficacy of an experimental dentifrice formulation on primary school children in Ga-Rankuwa, Pretoria. J Dent Assoc S Afr 1994;49:209–12.

[3] Owens J, Addy M, Faulkner J, Lockwood C, Adair R. A short-term clinical study design to investigate the chemical plaque inhibitory properties of mouthrinses when used as adjuncts to toothpastes: applied to chlorhexidine. J Clin Periodontol 1997;24:732–7.

[4] Sabbagh-Haddad A, Ciamponi AL, Guaré RO. Pacientes especiais. In Guedes-Pinto AC. Odontopediatria. São Paulo: Santos; 2003. p. 893-931.

[5] Reuland-Bosma W, Dijk J. Periodontal disease in Down's syndrome: a review. J Clin Periodontol. 1986; 13(1);64-73.

[6] Cornejo LS, Zak GA, Dorronsoro de Cattoni ST, Calamari SE, Azcurra AI, Battellino LJ. S. Bucodental health condition in patients with Down syndrome of Cordoba City, Argentina. Acta Odontol Latinoam. 1996; 9(2):65-79.

[7] Alisson PJ, Hennequin M, Faulks D. Dental care access among individuals with Down syndrome in France. Spec Care Dent. 2000; 20(1):28-34.

[8] Moraes MEL, Bastos MS, Moraes LC,Rocha JC. Prevalência de cárie pelo índice CPO-D em portadores de síndrome de Down. Pós-Grad Rev Odontol. 2002; 5(2): 64-73.

[9] König J, Storcks V, Kocher T, Bössmann K, Plagmann HC. Anti-plaque effect of tempered 0,2% chlorhexidine rinse: an in vivo study. J Clin Periodontol. 2002; 29(3): 207-10.

[10] Löe H, Theilade E, Jensen SB. Experimental gingivitis in man. J Periodontol. 1965; 36:177-87.

[11] Theilade E, Wright WH, Jensen SB, Löe H. Experimental gingivitis in man II. A longitudinal clinical and bacteriological investigation. J Periodontal Res. 1966; 1: 1-13.

[12] Owens J, Addy M, Faulkner J, Lockwood C, Adair R. A short-term clinical study desing to investigate the chemical plaque inhibitory properties of mounthrinses when used as adjuncts to toothpastes: applied to chlorexidine. J Clin Periodontol. 1997; 24(10):732-7.

[13] Panzeri H, Lara EHG, Zaniquelli O, Schiavetto F. Avaliação de algumas características das escovas dentais do mercado nacional. Rev ABO Nac. 1993; 1(1):23-9.

[14] Halla DA. Propósito das escovas dentárias. Rev Paul Odontol. 1982; 4(2):42-7.

[15] Pannuti CM, Saraiva MC, Ferraro A, Falsi D, Cai S, Lotufo, RF. Efficacy of a 0,5% chlorhexidine gel on the control of gingivitis in brazilian mentally handicapped patients. J Clin Periodontol. 2003; 30:573-6.

[16] Palomo F, Wantland L, Sanchez A, DeVizio W, Carter W, Baines E.The MFTB. The importance of oral health education in prevention programs for children. J Bras Odontol Odontopediatr Baby.1999; 2(6): 127-31.

[17] Bijella MFTB. A importância da educação em saúde bucal nos programas preventivos para crianças. J Bras Odontopediatr Odontol Bebê. 1999; 2(6): 127-31.

[18] Seagriff-Curtin P, Pugliese S, Romer M. Dental considerations for individuals with Down syndrome. N Y State Dent J 2006;72:33–5.

[19] Boyd D, Quick A, Murray C. The Down syndrome patient in dental practice, Part II: clinical considerations. N Z Dent J 2004;100:4–9.

[20] Surabian SR. Developmental disabilities and understanding the needs of patients with mental retardation and Down syndrome. J Calif Dent Assoc 2001;29:415–23.

[21] Shyama M, Al-Mutawa SA, Honkala S, Honkala E. Supervised toothbrushing and oral health education program in Kuwait for children and young adults with Down syndrome. Spec Care Dentist 2003;23:94–9.

[22] Shapira J, Stabholz A. A comprehensive 30-month preventive dental health program in a pre-adolescent population with Down's syndrome: a longitudinal study. Spec Care Dentist 1996;16:33–7.

[23] Tensini DA, Fenton SJ. Oral heath needs of persons with physical or mental disabilities. Dent Clin North Am. 1994; 38(3):483-98.

[24] Brown RH. Dental treatment of the mongoloid child. ASDC J Dent Child. 1965; 32:73-81.

[25] Scully C. Down's syndrome: aspects of dental care. J Dent. 1976; 4(4):167-74.

[26] Nielsen LA. Plaque and gingivitis in children with cerebral palsy relation to CP-diagnosism, mental and motor handicap. Tandlaegernes Tidsskr. 1990; 5(11):316-20.

[27] Bellini HT, Anerud A, Moustafa MH. Disclosing wafers in an oral hygiene instruction program. Odontol Revy 1974;25:247–53.

[28] Medeiros UV. Aspectos gerais no controle da placa bacteriana -controle da placa bacteriana em saúde pública. Rev Assoc Paul Cir Dent. 1991; 45(3):479-83.

[29] Toassi RFC, Petry PC. Motivação no controle do biofilme dental e sangramento gengival em escolares. Rev Saude Publica. 2002; 36(5):634-7.

[30] Cristiano, OS, Bignelli P. Contribuição ao Estudo de Reveladores de Placa Bacteriana Dental. [Monografia]. Ribeirão Preto: Faculdade de Odontologia da USP;1995.

[31] Bouquet P. Stains and dental plaque detection with clinical reports. Rev Fr Odontostomatol. 1971; 18(10):1239-61.

[32] Guillings ED. Recent developments in dental plaque disclosants. Austr Dent J. 1977; 22(4): 260-6.

[33] Silva CHL, Paranhos HFO, Ito IY. Evidenciadores de biofilme em prótese total: avaliação clínica e antimicrobiana. Pesqui Odontol Bras. 2002; 16(3):270-5.

[34] Comissão Permanente de Revisão da Farmacopéia Brasileira. Farmacopéia Brasileira. 4 ed. São Paulo: Atheneu;1996.

[35] Quintanilha LELP, Bastos JRM. Dentifrício como revelador de placa. RGO. 1988; 36(4):296.

[36] Duarte CA, Lascala NT, Muenchi A. Estudo clínico da influência dos evidenciadores de placa bacteriana na motivação de pacientes à higiene bucal sob supervisão e orientação direta. Rev Odontol Univ São Paulo. 1990 ; 4(4): 278-83.

[37] Silva D D, Gonçalo CS, Sousa MLR, Wada RS. Aggregation of plaque disclosing agent in a dentifrice. J Appl Oral Sci. 2004; 12(2):154-8.

[38] Quintanilha LELP, Lima ALP, Siqueira ES, Carvalho RA. Evidenciador de placa bacteriana veiculado por dentifrício. Odontol Hoje. 1989; 18:499-508.

[39] Rodrigues RMJ, Cruz RA, Campos VA. Eficiência de um dentifrício contendo eritrosina no processo de estimulação à higiene dental de crianças. RBO. 1994; 51(1):11-6.

[40] Silva DD, Sousa MLR, Gomes VE, Cury JA. Estabilidade do flúor e da embalagem de um dentifrício evidenciador de placa bacteriana. Rev Odonto Cienc. 2003; 18(39):8-12.

[41] Dolles OK, Gjermo P. Caries increment and gingival status during 2 years' use of chlorhexidine- and fluoride-containing dentifrices. Scand J Dent Res 1980;88:22–7.

[42] Jenkins S, Addy M, Newcombe R. The effects of a chlorhexidine toothpaste on the development of plaque, gingivitis and tooth staining. J Clin Periodontol 1993;20:59–62.

[43] Pieper K, Dirks B, Kessler P. Caries, oral hygiene and periodontal disease in handicapped adults. Community Dent Oral Epidemiol 1986;14:28–30.

[44] Russell BG, Bay LM. Systemic effects of oral use of chlorhexidine gel in multihandicapped epileptic children. Scand J Dent Res 1981;89:264–9.

[45] Sanz M, Vallcorba N, Fabregues S, Muller I, Herkstroter F. The effect of a dentifrice containing chlorhexidine and zinc on plaque, gingivitis, calculus and tooth staining. J Clin Periodontol 1994;21:431–7.

[46] Storhaug K. Hibitane in oral disease in handicapped patients. J Clin Periodontol 1977;4:102–7.

[47] Yates R, Jenkins S, Newcombe R, Wade W, Moran J, Addy M. A 6-month home usage trial of a 1% chlorhexidine toothpaste (1). Effects on plaque, gingivitis, calculus and toothstaining. J Clin Periodontol 1993;20:130–8.

[48] Mandel ID. Antimicrobial mouthrinses: overview and update. J Am Dent Assoc. 1994; 125:2-10.

[49] Fischman SL. Design of studies to evaluate plaque control agents. J Dent Res. 1979; 58(12):2389-95.

[50] Loesche W. Chemotherapy of dental plaque infections. Oral Sci Rev. 1976; 9: 65-107.

[51] Van Der Ouderaa FG. Anti – plaque agents. Rational and prospects for prevention of gengivites and periodontol disease. J Clin Periodontol. 1991; 18(6):447-54.

[52] Marsh PD. Microbiological aspects of the chemical control of plaque and gengivitis. J Dent Res. 1992; 71(7):1431-8.

[53] Davies GE, Francis J, Martin AR, Rose Fl, Swain G. 1:6-di 4-chlorophenyldiguanidohexane (hibitane) laboratory investigation of a new antibacterial agent of high potency. Br J Pharmacol Chemother. 1954; 9(2): 192-6.

[54] Löe H, Schiott CR. The effect of mouthrinses and topical application of chlorhexidine on the development of dental plaque and gingivitis in man. J Periodontal. 1970; 5(2): 79-83.

[55] Souza RR, Abreu MHNG. Análise crítica da indicação da clorexidina no controle da placa bacteriana e doença periodontal. Arq Odontol. 2003; 39(3): 175-81.

[56] Vinholis AHC, Marcantonio RAG, Marcantonio E. Mecanismo de ação da clorexidina. Rev Periodontia. 1996; 5(3):281-3.

[57] Bonacorsi C, Devienne KF, Raddi MSG. Citotoxidade in vitro de soluções de digluconato de clorexidina preparadas em farmácias de manipulação. Rev Bras Cienc Farm. 2000; 21(1):125-32.

http://dx.doi.org/10.5772/53348

[58] Quagliato CE. Clorexidina – a mais conhecida substância antimicrobiana. Odonto-Cad Doc. 1991; 1(4):104-6.

[59] Gjermo P. Chlorhexidine and related compounds. J Dent Res. 1989(special issue); 68:1602-8.

[60] Al-Tannir M, Goodman HS. A review of chlorhexidine and its use in special populations. Spec Care Dentist. 1994; 14(3):116-22.

[61] Sathler LWL, Fischer RG. O efeito anti-placa do triclosan contido em dentifrícios. Rev Periodont. 1996; 5(3):267-72.

[62] Addy M, Jenkins S, Newcombe R Comparison of two commercially available chlorhrexidine mouthrinses I. Staing and antimicrobial effects in vitro. Clin Prev Dent. 1989; 11(4):10-4.

[63] Jenkins S, Addy M, Newcombe R. The effects of 0.5% chlorhexidine and 0.2% triclosan containing toothpastes on salivary bacterial counts. J Clin Periodontol. 1990;17(2): 85-9.

[64] Gjermo P, Rolla G. Plaque innibition by antibacterial dentifrices. Scand J Dent Res. 1970; 78(4):464-70.

[65] Torres MCM. Utilização da clorexidina em seus diversos veículos. RBO. 2000; 57(3): 174-80.

[66] Maynard JH, Jenkins SM, Moran J, Addy M, Newcombe R, Wade WG. A 6-mounth home usage trial of a 1% chlorhexidine toothpaste II. Effects on the oral microflora. J Clin Periodontol. 1993; 20(3):207-11.

[67] Newman HN. Modes of application of antiplaque chemicals. J Clin Periodontol. 1986; 13(10):965-74.

[68] Teitelbaum AP, Popchapski MT, Jansen JL, Sabbagh-Haddad A,.Santos FA, Czlusniak GC. Evaluation of the mechanical and chemical control of dental biofilm in patients with Down syndrome. Community Dentistry and Oral Epidemiology 2009;37; 463-7.

[69] Teitelbaum AP, Pinto MHB, Czlusniak GD, Sabbagh-Haddad A,.Santos FA. Action of experimental dentifrices on oral health of children with down syndrome. IJD. International Journal of Dentistry 2010; 9;128-35.

Chapter 5

How to Design an Exercise Program TO Reduce Inflammation in Obese People With Down Syndrome

Francisco J. Ordonez, Gabriel Fornieles,
Alejandra Camacho, Miguel A. Rosety,
Antonio J Diaz, Ignacio Rosety, Natalia Garcia and
Manuel Rosety-Rodriguez

Additional information is available at the end of the chapter

http://dx.doi.org/10.5772/ 52984

1. Introduction

Obesity in people with Down syndrome: a big problem.

Over the last decade, a significant increase in the life expectancy of people with Down syndrome (DS) has been observed. The higher life expectancy has caused a higher incidence of morbidity as they age [1]. Many of these disorders have been associated to obesity that is a major health problem in people with intellectual disabilities. Not only for its prevalence but also for its negative impact on their health status and quality of life.

In a more detailed way, it is widely accepted that obesity is a serious problem that is overwhelmingly prevalent in the general population. However, the magnitude of this problem is even worse in people with intellectual disability in general and Down syndrome in particular. A cross-sectional study with adult clients (n=470) of three Dutch intellectual disability care providing organizations and found that healthy behavior was low, with 98.9% of the participants having an unhealthy diet and 68.3% a lack of exercise [2]. In a more detailed way, women and people with Down syndrome were significantly more at risk of being obese [3].

Obesity and overweight are independent risk factors for chronic disease and have been shown to make a significant contribution to the reduced life expectancy of adults with intellectual disability. Further, the increased visceral fat in females with DS might indicate a higher risk of metabolic syndrome in this group [4].

Accordingly, recent studies have concluded that more attention needs to be paid to the rising fat mass percentages seen in individuals with Down syndrome in order to minimize negative, long-term health consequences [5,6].

In reviewing the current evidence, the effectiveness of interventions was judged on both the extent of and the maintenance of weight reduction.

It is widely accepted promoting appropriate levels of physical activity remains an important component for both weight loss and management and should have its place as a lifestyle and behavioral change in people with Down syndrome [7,8,9].

However, the interventions that have been conducted has achieved a degree of success in promoting weight reduction in the short term. There is less evidence about whether intervention programs can maintain weight loss effectively in the long term. In fact, current guidelines highlight the interventions that lead to modest, maintainable weight lose for people with intellectual disability will have significant benefits on both health and welfare.

The latter authors also concluded that much of the research on obesity in adults with Down syndrome has design weaknesses, including small sample sizes and a lack of controlled studies [10].

Association between obesity and low-grade systemic inflammation

Accumulating evidence derived from both clinical and experimental studies highlight obesity may be viewed as a chronic low-grade inflammatory disease as well as a metabolic disease [11,12]. Therefore, it is widely accepted adipose tissue is not merely a fat storage depot. In contrast, endocrine and paracrine aspects of adipose tissue have become an active research area in the last years.

Recent studies have reported that parenchymal and stromal cells (fibroblats, endothelial cells and immune cells) in adipose tissue change dramatically in number and cell type during the course of obesity, which is referred to as "adipose tissue remodeling." In this regard, recent evidence suggests that the intimate crosstalk between mature adypocytes and stromal cells in adipose tissue plays a critical role in the dysregulation of adipocytokine production [13].

These findings were of particular interest since adults with intellectual disabilities experience high rates of obesity. Although Down syndrome has been traditionally considered an atheroma free model [14] recent studies have also reported individuals with intellectual disability suffer from low-graded systemic inflammation that has been proposed as a pathogenic mechanism of several disorders [15]. Previous studies showing increased levels of soluble intercellular adhesion molecule (sICAM-3) and soluble vascular cell adhesion molecule (sVCAM-1) in plasma, also suggested the presence of a moderate dysfunction of endothelial cells in subjects with Down syndrome [16].

Similarly, plasmatic concentrations of IL-6, IL-18 and CRP (C-reactive protein) levels were highly correlated with measures of total and visceral adiposity in obese adults with Prader-Willi Syndrome (PWS) [17]. The reported excessive visceral adiposity in subjects with PWS may be associated with decreased production and lower circulating levels of adiponectin

[18]. These data are of particular interest since increased low-grade inflammation is associated with increased arterial stiffness, a recognized marker for increased cardiovascular risk in people with Prader-Willi syndrome [19].

Importantly, some frequently diagnosed comorbidities could affect systemic inflammation in people with intellectual disability. In fact, obstructive sleep apnea, is a syndrome that has itself been linked to increased low-grade inflammation both in general population [20] and people with Prader-Willi syndrome [19].

Adipokines and acute phase proteins are important mediators of adverse effects (insulin resistance) so that the normalization of their levels has been reported as a therapeutic target in subjects at high cardiovascular risks [21,22].

Contradictory data have been reported about the effect of statins on adiponectin plasma levels. In this respect, atorvastatin (10-80 mg/day) increased adiponectin plasma levels in subjects at high cardiovascular risk. Further, adiponectin concentrations were positively correlated with high-density lipoprotein-cholesterol both before and after atorvastatin treatment [23]. Similar results were found using simvastatin (40mg/day) suggesting a novel anti-inflammatory effect of this drug [24].

Fortunately several studies have reported both endurance and resistance training programs at low/moderate intensity may reduce proinflammatory adipokines both at early life stages and elderly in obese people without intellectual disability [25]. However, to the best of our knowledge, there is a lack of information in people, especially women, with intellectual disabilities. Accordingly additional studies based on specific training programs that are adaptable to the needs of individuals with intellectual disability are strongly required [26].

In addition, it would be of interest to reduce the length of training programs previously published. In fact, it is expected shorter training programs may facilitate their follow-up, reducing drop-out rates.

Regular exercise in Down Syndrome

The benefits of physical activity are universal for general population, including those with disabilities [14, 27].

In fact, the participation of people with disabilities in sports and recreational activities promotes social inclusion, minimizes deconditioning, optimizes physical functioning, and enhances overall welfare [14,28]. Further sports participation enhances the psychological well-being of people with disabilities through the provision of opportunities to form friendships, express creativity, increase self-esteem, develop a self-identity, and foster meaning and purpose in life [29].

Physical consequences of inactivity for persons with disabilities include among others: reduced cardiovascular fitness, osteoporosis and impaired circulation. In addition, the psychosocial implications of inactivity include decreased self-esteem, decreased social acceptance, and ultimately, greater dependence on others for daily living [14].

Despite the benefits associated to regular exercise, subjects with disabilities are still, to a large extent, more restricted in their participation than their peers without disabilities. They may experience negative societal stereotypes and low performance expectations, rendering them with limited opportunities for participation in physical activities [30].

In this regard, people with Down syndrome are especially at risk because of physical and health impairments, as well as perceived and real barriers to participation in exercise [31].

In a more detailed way, it is accepted that persons with Down syndrome exhibit low peak aerobic capacities and maximal heart rates when compared with healthy non-disabled peers. These findings may be explained by a lower walking economy that is mainly related to their inability to adapt efficiently to positive variations in walking speed [32]. Furthermore, they present a different catecholamine response to exercise [33]. Accordingly, intervention programs based on regular exercise should be designed by taking into account their chronotropic incompetence. On the contrary, sessions theoretically designed at moderate intensity for the general population become exhausting for participants with Down syndrome, leading to undesired results and increased withdrawal rates.

However, it is important to note that environmental and family factors seem to be more significant determinants of participation than characteristics of the subjects themselves. In fact, families who engage in physical activities themselves tend to promote similar participation for their relatives with disabilities. Conversely, inactive role models, competing demands and time pressures, unsafe environments, lack of adequate facilities, insufficient funds, and inadequate access to quality daily physical education seem to be more prevalent among populations with special needs. The establishment of short-term goals, emphasizing variety and enjoyment, and positive reinforcement through documented progress toward goals can help spark and sustain the motivation for participation [14, 27,34].

In summary, misconceptions and attitudinal barriers at the level of the individual, the family, and the community need to be addressed to integrate people with disabilities into recreational and sports activities [14].

Another point of interest is that physical activity comes with an inherent risk for injury. For people with intellectual disability, previous studies have reported their injury risk may be complicated by preexisting disability [26]. Accordingly it is important for caregivers, educators and others to identify strategies to minimize risks of illness and injury related to participation through activity adaptations and safety precautions.

Fortunately, little or no sport-related injuries are reported in the literature during intervention programs based on regular exercise [32,35,36]. It may be explained, at least in part, due to the preparticipation physical examination (PPPE) and the design of specific training programs that are adaptable to the needs of individuals with intellectual disability. This is of particular interest since injuries and discomfort may lead to participants to interrupt their training program, increasing withdrawal rates and sedentary lifestyle [37].

2. Body

Problem statement

Accumulating evidence derived from both clinical and experimental studies highlight the association of visceral obesity with a proinflammatory status in general population [11,12]. Recent studies have also reported individuals with intellectual disability suffer from low-grade systemic inflammation that has been proposed as a pathogenic mechanism of several disorders [15]. The adipokines are important mediators of these adverse effects so that the normalization of their levels has been reported as a therapeutic target [21].

Fortunately several studies have reported both endurance and resistance training programs at low/moderate intensity may reduce proinflammatory adipokines both at early life stages and elderly in obese people without intellectual disability [25]. However, to the best of our knowledge, there is a lack of information in people, especially women, with intellectual disabilities.

Accordingly, this study was designed to assess the influence of a 10-week aerobic training program on plasmatic levels of adipokines in obese women with Down syndrome.

Application area

Healthcare costs are continuously increasing because of the increasing life expectancy among people with disabilities [1]. This is a strong argument for strengthening the role of preventive strategies, such as exercise, with the aim to reduce future costs.

However, researchers suggest that people with an intellectual disability undertake less physical activity than the general population and many rely, to some extent, on others to help them to access activities [34,38].

Currently, a wide variety of sporting activities are accessible to people with disabilities, and guidelines are available to assist caregivers, volunteers, educators and healthcare-providers in recommending activities appropriate for those people with specific conditions. These training programs should be not only effective but safe since previous studies have reported their sport-related injury risk may be complicated by preexisting disability.

Research course & method used

A 10-week aerobic training program was designed by a multidisciplinary team to reduce plasmatic adipokines in obese women with Down syndrome. In order to achieve this goal, twenty obese adult women with Down syndrome volunteered for the present interventional study. They had an intelligence quotient (IQ) range of 50–69, determined by Stanford-Binet Scale, being diagnosed as having mild intellectual disability. Eleven of them were randomly assigned to perform a 10-week aerobic training program, 3 sessions/ week, consisting of warming-up followed by a main part in a treadmill (30-40 min [increasing 2 minutes and half each two weeks]) at a work intensity of 55-65% of peak heart rate (increasing a 2.5% each two weeks) and a cooling-down period. Control group included

9 age, sex and BMI matched women with Down syndrome. Fat mass percentage and fat distribution were measured.

Plasmatic levels of TNF-α, IL-6 and leptin were assessed by commercial ELISA kits (Immunotech, MA, USA). High-sensitive C-Reactive Protein (hs-CRP) in plasma was assessed by nephelometric methods on a BN-II analyzer (Dade-Behring Diagnostics, Marburg, Germany). Fat mass percentage was assessed by bioelectrical impedance analysis BIA (Tanita TBF521). To determine waist to hip ratio, waist and hip circumferences were measured with an anthropometric tape (Holtain Ltd). Furthermore, each participant underwent a maximal continuous treadmill graded exercised test. All outcomes at individual level were assessed firstly at baseline and secondly 72-h after the end of the intervention. Written informed consent was obtained from all their parents or legal representatives. Further this protocol was approved by an Institutional Ethics Committee.

The results were expressed as a mean (SD). The statistical analysis of the data was performed using Student's *t*-test for paired data. Pearson´s correlation coefficient (r) was used to identify potential associations among tested parameters. The significance of the changes observed was ascertained to be p<0.05.

Results

When compared to baseline results, plasmatic levels of TNF-α (11.7±2.6 vs. 10.2±2.3 pg/ml; p=0.022), IL-6 (8.0±1.7 vs. 6.6±1.4 pg/ml; p=0.014) and leptin (54.2±6.7 vs. 45.7±6.1 ng/ml; p=0.026) were significantly reduced in interventional group. Similarly, C-reactive protein level was significantly decreased after being exercised (0.62±0.11 vs. 0.53± 0.09mg/dl;p=0.009). Regarding anthropometric measurements, both fat mass percentage (38.9±4.6 vs. 35.0±4.2%; p=0.041) and WHR (1.12±0.006 vs. 1.00±0.005 cm; p=0.038) were also reduced. We also found significant associations between WHR and IL-6 (r=0.51; p<0.001). VO_2max was also increased in exercised at the end of the experience (20.2±5.8 vs. 23.7±6.3 ml/kg/min; p=0.0007) suggesting an improvement of their physical fitness.

In contrast, control group showed no changes in any of the tested parameters.

Further research and Discussion

The main finding of this study was that aerobic training reduced significantly plasmatic levels of adipokines (TNF-α, IL-6 and leptin) as well as C-reactive protein (CRP) in adult women with Down syndrome. Similar results regarding anti-inflammatory effect of a 16-week aerobic training program have been reported in young women without intellectual disability [39]. Furthermore, a 6-month aerobic training program (four times/week, 45-60 min/session) reduced plasmatic levels of TNF in adults with type 2 diabetes [40].

Another challenge of this study was to identify significant associations between plasmatic adipokines and indices of obesity in order to provide an easier, quicker, cheaper and no-invasive assessment of the outcomes. The strongest correlation was found between IL-6 and waist-to-hip ratio (WHR). Our findings not only confirmed adipokines correlated with indirect body fat mass measures in obese women without intellectual disability [41,42]. It also provided the evidence that abdominal fat was significantly correlated to plasmatic levels of CRP.

To the best of our knowledge this is the first study conducted exclusively in premenopausal women with intellectual disability, in attempt to keep our sample homogeneous. To date, many studies focused on the influence of regular exercise in people with intellectual disability have recruited mixed (males and females) groups in order to increase their sample size to strengthen research designs and increase generalization of study findings [43,44,45]. A few studies have been conducted in males [35,36,46].

However, less attention has been paid to women in spite of the higher prevalence of obesity in the latter [4]. This finding may contribute to explain women with DS are observed to have a shorter life expectancy than men with DS [47]. A major strength of the present study was that we discarded gender mismatching, which itself influences total adiposity and fat distribution.

Further, it should be emphasized that our sample size was similar to the largest ones reported in previous exercise intervention research on persons with trisomy 21[35,36,43,44]. This is of particular interest since studying subjects with intellectual disabilities is associated with many challenges that restrict the number of participants investigated.

The present protocol lasted just 10 weeks, so that it may be considered more feasible and practical for participants and guidance. In order to promote sustainability of these healthy programs based on exercise, it is essential targeting not only participants but also their parents, caregivers, educators, etc. However the latter have received little attention so that future studies designed as cluster-randomized interventions are highly required [38].

As was hypothesized, peak VO2max was also significantly increased after being exercised for 10 weeks. These results are lower than that of male adults with Down syndrome.[46] In this respect, it is widely known that persons with Down syndrome exhibit low peak aerobic capacities and maximal heart rates when compared with healthy non-disabled peers. This finding may be explained by a lower walking economy that is mainly related to their inability to adapt efficiently to positive variations in walking speed.[32] Furthermore, they present a different catecholamine response to exercise.[33] Accordingly, intervention programs based on regular exercise should be designed by taking into account their chronotropic incompetence. On the contrary, sessions theoretically designed at moderate intensity for the general population become exhausting for participants with Down syndrome, leading to undesired results and increased withdrawal rates.

Finally, despite the high prevalence of obesity in people with Down syndrome, it should be pointed out it may be even more prevalent in several genetic syndromes such as Prader-Willy syndrome, Bardet-Biedl syndrome, Cohen syndrome etc. Accordingly further studies on these populations are also required [10].

3. Conclusion

In summary, it was concluded a 10-week aerobic training program reduced plasmatic levels of adipokines and acute phase proteins in adult obese women with Down syndrome. Therefore, additional long-term, well-conducted studies are required to determine whether correction of this low-grade proinflammatory status improves clinical outcomes of people with trisomy 21.

Authors gratefully acknowledge financial support (Exp Nº211/10) by Women´s Institute (Ministry of Health and Consumer Affairs, Spanish Government)

Author details

Francisco J. Ordonez[1], Gabriel Fornieles[2], Alejandra Camacho[3], Miguel A. Rosety[1], Antonio J Diaz[2], Ignacio Rosety[1], Natalia Garcia[4] and Manuel Rosety-Rodriguez[2*]

*Address all correspondence to: manuel.rosetyrodriguez@uca.es

1 Human Anatomy Department. School of Sports Medicine, Spain

2 Medicine Department. School of Sports Medicine, Spain

3 Juan Ramon Jimenez Hospital, Spain

4 Pathology Department. School of Medicine, Spain

References

[1] Tenenbaum, A., Chavkin, M., Wexler, I. D., Korem, M., & Merrick, J. (2012). Morbidity and hospitalizations of adults with Down syndrome. *Research in Developmental Disabilities*, 33, 435-41.

[2] de Winter, C. F., Magilsen, K. W., van Alfen, J. C., Penning, C., & Evenhuis, H. M. (2009). Prevalence of cardiovascular risk factors in older people with intellectual disability. *American Journal on Intellectual and Developmental Disabilities*, 114, 427-36.

[3] De Winter, C. F., Bastiaanse, L. P., Hilgenkamp, T. I., Evenhuis, H. M., & Echteld, M. A. (2012). Overweight and obesity in older people with intellectual disability. *Research in Developmental Disabilities*, 33, 398-405.

[4] González-Agüero, A., Ara, I., Moreno, L. A., Vicente-Rodríguez, G., & Casajús, J. A. (2011). Fat and lean masses in youths with Down syndrome: gender differences. *Research in Developmental Disabilities*, 32, 1685-93.

[5] Bhaumik, S., Watson, J. M., Thorp, C. F., Tyrer, F., & Mc Grother, C. W. (2008). Body mass index in adults with intellectual disability: distribution, associations and service implications: a population-based prevalence study. *Journal of Intellectual Disability Research*, 52, 287-98.

[6] Sohler, N., Lubetkin, E., Levy, J., Soghomonian, C., & Rimmerman, A. (2009). Factors associated with obesity and coronary heart disease in people with intellectual disabilities. *Social Work in Health Care*, 48, 76-89.

[7] Elmahgoub, S. M., Lambers, S., Stegen, S., Van Laethem, C., Cambier, D., & Calders, P. (2009). The influence of combined exercise training on indices of obesity, physical fitness and lipid profile in overweight and obese adolescents with mental retardation. *Journal of Strength and Conditioning Research*, 168, 1327-33.

[8] Melville, CA, Boyle, S., Miller, S., Macmillan, S., Penpraze, V., Pert, C., Spanos, D., Matthews, L., Robinson, N., Murray, H., & Hankey, C. R. (2011). An open study of the effectiveness of a multi-component weight-loss intervention for adults with intellectual disabilities and obesity. *British Journal of Nutrition*, 105, 1553-62.

[9] Ordonez, F. J., Rosety, M., & Rosety-Rodriguez, M. (2006). Influence of 12-week exercise training on fat mass percentage in adolescents with Down syndrome. *Medicine and Science Monitor*, 12, CR416-9.

[10] Hamilton, S., Hankey, C. R., Miller, S., Boyle, S., & Melville, CA. (2007). A review of weight loss interventions for adults with intellectual disabilities. *Obesity Review*, 8, 339-45.

[11] Inadera, H. (2008). The usefulness of circulating adipokine levels for the assessment of obesity-related health problems. *International Journal of Medical Sciences*, 5, 248-262.

[12] Popko, K., Gorska, E., Stelmaszczyk-Emmel, A., Plywaczewski, R., Stoklosa, A., Gorecka, D., Pyrzak, B., & Demkow, U. (2010). Proinflammatory cytokines Il-6 and TNF-α and the development of inflammation in obese subjects. *European Journal of Medical Research*, 15, 120-122.

[13] Suganami, T., Tanaka, M., & Ogawa, Y. (2012). Adipose tissue inflammation and ectopic lipid accumulation. Endocrinology Journal Aug 9. [Epub ahead of print]

[14] Murdoch, J. C., Rodger, J. C., Rao, S. S., Fletcher, C. D., & Dunnigan, M. G. (1977). Down's syndrome: an atheroma-free model? *British Medical Journal*, 2, 226-8.

[15] De Winter, C. F., Magilsen, K. W., van Alfen, J. C., Willemsen, S. P., & Evenhuis, H. M. (2011). Metabolic syndrome in 25% of older people with intellectual disability. *Family Practice*, 28, 141-4.

[16] Licastro, F., Chiappelli, M., Porcellini, E., Trabucchi, M., Marocchi, A., & Corsi, MM. (2006). Altered vessel signalling molecules in subjects with Downs syndrome. *International Journal of Immunopathology and Pharmacology*, 19, 181-5.

[17] Caixàs, A., Giménez-Palop, O., Broch, M., Vilardell, C., Megía, A., Simón, I., Giménez-Pérez, G., Mauricio, D., Vendrell, J., Richart, C., & González-Clemente, J. M.

(2008). Adult subjects with Prader-Willi syndrome show more low-grade systemic inflammation than matched obese subjects. *Journal of Endocrinological Investigation*, 31, 169-75.

[18] Kennedy, L., Bittel, D. C., Kibiryeva, N., Kalra, S. P., Torto, R., & Butler, M. G. (2006). Circulating adiponectin levels, body composition and obesity-related variables in Prader-Willi syndrome: comparison with obese subjects. *International Journal of Obesity*, 30, 382-7.

[19] Viardot, A., Sze, L., Purtell, L., Sainsbury, A., Loughnan, G., Smith, E., Herzog, H., Steinbeck, K., & Campbell, L. V. (2010). Prader-Willi syndrome is associated with activation of the innate immune system independently of central adiposity and insulin resistance. *The Journal of clinical endocrinology and metabolism*, 95, 3392-9.

[20] Minoguchi, K., Yokoe, T., Tazaki, T., Minoguchi, H., Tanaka, A., Oda, N., Okada, S., Ohta, S., Naito, H., & Adachi, M. (2005). Increased carotid intima-media thickness and serum inflammatory markers in obstructive sleep apnea. *American Journal of Respiratory and Critical Care Medicine*, 172, 625-630.

[21] Athyros, V. G., Tziomalos, K., Karagiannis, A., Anagnostis, P., & Mikhailidis, D. P. (2010). Should adipokines be considered in the choice of the treatment of obesity-related health problems? *Current Drug Targets*, 11, 122-35.

[22] Szotowska, M., Czerwienska, B., Adamczak, M., Chudek, J., & Wiecek, A. (2012). Effect of low-dose atorvastatin on plasma concentrations of adipokines in patients with metabolic syndrome. *Kidney and Blood Pressure Research*, 35, 226-32.

[23] Blanco-Colio, L. M., Martín-Ventura, J. L., Gómez-Guerrero, C., Masramon, X., de Teresa, E., Farsang, C., Gaw, A., Gensini, G., Leiter, L. A., Langer, A., & Egido, J. (2008). Adiponectin plasma levels are increased by atorvastatin treatment in subjects at high cardiovascular risk. *European Journal of Pharmacology*, 586, 259-65.

[24] Lazich, I., Sarafidis, P., de Guzman, E., Patel, A., Oliva, R., & Bakris, G. (2012). Effects of combining simvastatin with rosiglitazone on inflammation, oxidant stress and ambulatory blood pressure in patients with the metabolic syndrome: the SIROCO study. *Diabetes and Obesity Metabolism*, 14, 181-6.

[25] Rubin, D. A., & Hackney, A. C. (2010). Inflammatory cytokines and metabolic risk factors during growth and maturation: influence of physical activity. *Medicine and Sport Science*, 55, 43-55.

[26] Ramirez, M., Yang, J., Bourque, L., Javien, J., Kashani, S., Limbos, M. A., & Peek-Asa, C. (2009). Sports injuries to high school athletes with disabilities. *Pediatrics*, 123, 690-6.

[27] Durstine, J. L., Painter, P., Franklin, BA, Morgan, D., Pitetti, K. H., & Roberts, S. O. (2000). Physical activity for the chronically ill and disabled. *Sports Medicine*, 30, 207-219.

[28] Grandisson, M., Tétreault, S., & Freeman, A. R. (2012). Enabling integration in sports for adolescents with intellectual disabilities. *Journal of Applied Research in Intellectual Disabilities*, 25, 217-30.

[29] Weiss, J., Diamond, T., Demark, J., & Lovald, B. (2003). Involvement in Special Olympics and its relations to self-concept and actual competency in participants with developmental disabilities. *Research in Developmental Disabilities*, 24, 281-305.

[30] King, G., Law, M., King, S., Rosenbaum, P., Kertoy, M. K., & Young, N. L. (2003). A conceptual model of the factors affecting the recreation and leisure participation of children with disabilities. *Physical and Occupational Therapy in Pediatrics*, 23, 63-90.

[31] Terblanche, E., & Boer, P. H. (2012). The functional fitness capacity of adults with Down syndrome in South Africa. Journal of Intellectual Disability Research Jul 10. [Epub ahead of print]

[32] Mendonca, G. V., Pereira, F. D., Morato, P. P., & Fernhall, B. (2010). Walking economy of adults with Down syndrome. *International Journal of Sports Medicine*, 31, 10-15.

[33] Fernhall, B., Baynard, T., Collier, S. R., et al. (2009). Catecholamine response to maximal exercise in persons with Down syndrome. *American Journal of Cardiology*, 103, 724-726.

[34] Martin, E., Mc Kenzie, K., Newman, E., Bowden, K., & Morris, P. G. (2011). Care staff intentions to support adults with an intellectual disability to engage in physical activity: an application of the Theory of Planned Behaviour. *Research in Developmental Disabilities*, 32, 2535-41.

[35] Ordonez, F. J., Rosety, I., Rosety, M. A., Camacho-Molina, A., Fornieles, G., Rosety, M., & Rosety-Rodriguez, M. (2012). Aerobic training at moderate intensity reduced protein oxidation in adolescents with Down syndrome. *Scandinavian Journal of Medicine and Sciences in Sports*, 22, 91-94.

[36] Rosety-Rodriguez, M., Rosety, I., Fornieles-Gonzalez, G., Diaz, A., Rosety, M., & Ordonez, F. J. (2010). A 12-week aerobic training programme reduced plasmatic allantoin in adolescents with Down syndrome. *British Journal of Sports Medicine*, 44, 685-687.

[37] Mahy, J., Shields, N., Taylor, N. F., & Dodd, K. J. (2010). Identifying facilitators and barriers to physical activity for adults with Down syndrome. *Journal of Intellectual Disability Research*, 54, 795-805.

[38] Elinder, L. S., Bergström, H., & Hagberg, J. (2010). Promoting a healthy diet and physical activity in adults with intellectual disabilities living in community residences: design and evaluation of a cluster-randomized intervention. *BMC Public Health*, 10, 761.

[39] Arikawa, A. Y., Thomas, W., Schmitz, K. H., & Kurzer, MS. (2011). Sixteen weeks of exercise reduces C-reactive protein levels in young women. *Medicine and Sciences in Sports and Exercise*, 43, 1002-9.

[40] Kadoglou, N. P., Iliadis, F., Angelopoulou, N., Perrea, D., Ampatzidis, G., Liapis, C. D., & Alevizos, M. (2007). The anti-inflammatory effects of exercise training in patients with type 2 diabetes mellitus. *European Journal of Cardiovascular Prevention and Rehabilitation*, 14, 837-43.

[41] Ackermann, D., Jones, J., Barona, J., Calle, M. C., Kim, J. E., La Pia, B., Volek, J. S., Mc Intosh, M., Kalynych, C., Najm, W., Lerman, R. H., & Fernandez, M. L. (2011). Waist circumference is positively correlated with markers of inflammation and negatively with adiponectin in women with metabolic syndrome. *Nutrition Research*, 31, 197-204.

[42] Bahceci, M., Gokalp, D., Bahceci, S., Tuzcu, A., Atmaca, S., & Arikan, S. (2007). The correlation between adiposity and adiponectin, tumor necrosis factor alpha, interleukin-6 and high sensitivity C-reactive protein levels. Is adipocyte size associated with inflammation in adults? *Journal of Endocrinological Investigation*, 30, 210-214.

[43] González-Agüero, A., Vicente-Rodríguez, G., Gómez-Cabello, A., Ara, I., Moreno, L. A., & Casajús, J. A. (2012 A). A 21-week bone deposition promoting exercise programme increases bone mass in young people with Down syndrome. *Dev Med Child Neurol*, 54, 552-6.

[44] Cowley, P. M., Ploutz-Snyder, L. L., Baynard, T., Heffernan, K. S., Jae, S. Y., Hsu, S., Lee, M., Pitetti, K. H., Reiman, M. P., & Fernhall, B. (2011). The effect of progressive resistance training on leg strength, aerobic capacity and functional tasks of daily living in persons with Down syndrome. *Disability and Rehabilitation*, 33, 2229-2236.

[45] Mendonca, G. V., Pereira, F. D., & Fernhall, B. (2011). Effects of combined aerobic and resistance exercise training in adults with and without Down syndrome. *Archives of Physical Medicine and Rehabilitation*, 92, 37-45.

[46] Mendonca, G. V., & Pereira, F. D. (2009). Influence of long-term exercise training on submaximal and peak aerobic capacity and locomotor economy in adult males with Down's syndrome. *Med Sci Monit*, 15, 33-39.

[47] Tyrer, F., Smith, L. K., & Mc Grother, C. W. (2007). Mortality in adults with moderate to profound intellectual disability: a population-based study. *Journal of Intellectual Disability Research*, 51, 520-7.

Chapter 6

Heart Diseases in Down Syndrome

A. K. M. Mamunur Rashid

Additional information is available at the end of the chapter

http://dx.doi.org/10.5772/46009

1. Introduction

Down syndrome (trisomy 21) is the common disorder among chromosomal anomalies. Trisomy 21 remains the commonest with its incidence 1:650 – 1: 1000 live births (Hassold TA and Sherman S 2000). The clinical manifestations of Down syndrome (DS) are numerous and can present in any body system. The most significant include intellectual impairment, short stature, heart disease, digestive disorders and orthopedic abnormalities (Ramakrishnan V, 2011).

Cardiac malformations present at birth are an important component of pediatric cardiovascular disease and contribute a major percentage of clinically significant birth defects with an estimated prevalence of 4 to 5 per 1000 live births. It is estimated that 4 to 10 live born infants per 1000 have cardiac malformation, 40% of which are diagnosed in the first year of life.(Hoffman J I, 1990 ; Moller J H et al, 1993). Congenital heart defect are the most common of all birth defects, which is found to affect nearly 1% of newborns, and their frequency in spontaneously aborted pregnancies is estimated to be tenfold higher (Behrman RE et al., 2000). In the year 2000, prevalence of CHD in the pediatric population was estimated at approximately 623000 (320000 with single lesion, 165000 with moderately complex disease, and 138000 with highly complex CHD). (Hoffman J I et al, 2004) Among the CHD the incidence of ventricular septal defect (VSD) has been demonstrated to be high as 5% in 2 independent cohorts of 5000 serial newborns, 5000 serial premature infants. (Roguin N et al., 1995; Du Z D et al., 1996)

The causes for CHD can be categorized in to three major groups such as chromosomal, single gene disorder (10-15%) and multiple factors (85-90%). (Payne M et al., 1995)

Its association of congenital heart disease is well known. Among all cases of congenital heart diseases, 4%-10% are associated with Down syndrome, and 40%-60% of Down syndrome patients present congenital heart disease. Cardiac malformation in DS is the principal cause of mortality in the first two years of life. (Rodriguez LH, 1984; Stoll C, et al., 1998) This congenital heart disease contributes significantly to the morbidity and mortality of children with Down syndrome, who may develop congestive heart failure, pulmonary vascular disease, pneumonia, or failure to thrive. In the first few days life symptoms or signs may be absent or minimal despite the presence of significant congenital heart disease. The characteristic heart defects seen in Down syndrome derives from the abnormal development of endocardial cushions and results in a spectrum of defects involving the atrioventricular septum and valves. Accounting for approximately 63% of all DS-CHD, their lesion varies in severity from persistent of the common atrioventricular canal and membranous ventricular septal defects to ostiumprimum patency with valvular anomalies. (Cooney T P et al., 1982; Anderson R H, 1991) The specificity of atriventricularseptal defects for trisomy 21 is emphasized by the observation that individuals with Down syndrome account for 70% of all atriventricularseptal defects. (Ferencz C et al.,1997) This is followed by patent ductus arteriosus and atrial septal defects. Other forms of complex heart disease can occur including overriding aorta and Tetralogy of fallot. (Berr C and Borghi E, 1990) The hypothesis suggests the existence of a gene or gene clusters on chromosome 21 which is involved in cell adhesion and likely plays an important role in valvuloseptal morphogenesis, but when over expressed, result in the defects of Down syndrome – congenital heart disease. (Barlow G M et al., 2001)

2. Etiology and genetics

Down syndrome which is normally caused by trisomy 21 is a major cause of congenital heart disease and provides an important model with which to link individual to the pathways controlling heart development. The characteristic heart defect seen in Down syndrome derives from the abnormal development of the endocardial cushions and results in a spectrum of defects involving atrioventricular septum and valves. Accounting for approximately 63% of all DS-CHD,(Van PR et al., 1996) these lesions vary in severity from persistence of the common atrioventricular canal and membranous ventricular septal defects to Ostium primum patency with valvular anomalies. (Cooney TP et al., 1982; Anderson RH, 1991) Independent and intersecting approaches to identifying the gene(s) for DS-CHD have included mapping genes known to be involved in cardiac development (none of which localized to chromosome 21) and studying rare individuals with CHD and partial duplications of chromosome 21. There are number of genetic tests that can assist the clinician in diagnosing genetic alterations in the child with CHD. These include cytogenetic technique, fluorescence in situ hybridization (FISH), and DNA mutation analysis.(Pierpont ME et al., 2007) The studies initially suggested that subsets of the DS phenotype were associated with three copies of chromosome band 21q22.2-22.3(Rahmani Z et al., 1989; McCormick MK et al., 1989; Korenberg JR et al., 1990) and later, that DS-CHD was caused by the over expression of genes in the region including D21S55 through the telomere.(Korenberg JR etal., 1992; Delabar JM et al.,1993; Korenberg JR et al., 1994) Another work focused on the identification of a transcriptional map of DS-CHD region using a 3.5 Mb contiguous clone array covering the interval from D21S55 through

MX1/2.(Hubert RS et al., 1997) Recent study speculate that the over expression of Down syndrome cell adhesion molecule may have the potential to perturb epithelial-mesenchymal transformation and/or the migration and proliferation of mesenchymal cells, and possibly thus contribute to the increased intercellular adhesion seen in DS cushion fibroblasts and abnormal cushion development seen in DS-CHD. The DSCAM gene constitutes a large part of the DS-CHD region, spanning more than 840Kb of the region between D21S3 and (PFKL) as determined from BAC contigs (Yamakawa K et al., 1998) and genomic sequence analysis.(Hattori M et al., 2000) The study for DS-CHD suggests that the candidate region for DS-CHD may be narrowed to D21S3 (Defined by VSD), through PFKL (defined by TOF), comprising 5.5 Mb. This represents significant reduction of the previously described candidate region, which spanned 10.5 Mb from D21S55 to the telomere. (Korenberg JR et al., 1992; Korenberg JR et al., 1994) This study supports the hypothesis that trisomy for a gene in the DS-CHD candidate region is essential for the production of DS-CHD including TOF and VSD, trisomy for additional genes located in the telomere and other regions likely contributes the phenotypic variability of DS-CHD. (Barlow GM et al., 2001)

3. Type of heart defects in children with Down syndrome

- Atrioventricular septal defects (AVSDs)- These are the most common in children with Down syndrome.
- Atrial Septal Defects (ASDs)
- Patent Ductus arteriosus (PDA)
- Tetralogy of Fallot (TOF)

In a study by TRJ Tubman & et al. among 34 babies of Down syndrome had congenital heart disease detected by echocardiography (13 had atrioventricularseptal defects, seven secendum atrial septal defects, six solitary patent ductusarteriosus, five isolated ventricular septal defects, and three combinations of heart defects.)(Tubman TRJ et al., 1991)

Another study showed the association between CHD and DS in atrioventricularseptal defect 56 (35%), ventricular septal defect 48 (30%),ASD 14 (8.7%), TOF 8(5%), PDA 18 (11.2%) and other heart defects 20(12.5%). (Ramakrishnan, V. 2011)

4. Presentations

4.1. Atroventricular Septal Defects (AVSDs)

These heart defects are marked by a hole in the wall between the top chambers (atria) and bottom chambers (ventricles) and one common valve between the two atria. In some cases, there might not be a hole between the bottom chambers. Or the valves may be joined together, but either or both might leak.

Because of the high pressure in the left ventricle which is needed to pump the blood around the body, blood is forced through the holes in the central heart wall (septum) when the ventricles contracts. This increases the pressure in the right ventricles. This increased pressure (pulmonary hypertension) results in excess blood flow to the lung.

Some of the early symptoms seen are difficulty in eating, weight gain, fast irregular breathing and a degree of cyanosis (blueness) particularly noticeable around the mouth, fingers and toes. Clinical examination may show an enlarged heart and liver, and a diagnosis of heart failure may be given. This term, not all children will exhibit symptoms early in life, and those that do will not always show all of these features.

4.2. Ventricular Septal Defects (VSDs)

In this defect there is a hole between the bottom clambers (pumping chambers or ventricles). Because of the higher pressure in the left side of the heart this allows oxygenated blood to flow through the hole from the left to the right side of the heart and back to the lungs in addition to the normal flow. The amount of blood flow from the left to right ventricle depends on the size of the hole and on the pressure between the ventricles. In other words, the higher the rate of flow means more strain on the heart. The abnormal blood flow is responsible for the murmur that may be heard.

Generally patients with a small VSD will not exhibit symptoms (they are asymptomatic) and the problem may only be found when a murmur is detected upon routine examination. Patients with a moderate VSD may breathe quickly, exhibit poor weight gain and be slower at eating. These children are also much more prone to chest infection. This tends to be more pronounced when the hole is large.

4.3. Atrial Septal Defects (ASDs)

In this defect there is a hole between the top chambers (receiving chambers or atria). Because of the higher pressure in the left side of the heart, oxygenated blood flows through the hole from the left to the right side, and back to the lungs, in addition to the normal flow.

There are three types of atrial septal defects; the most common is when there is a hole in the middle of the central heart wall. Holes in the lower part of the septum, called primum defect (partial atrioventricularseptal defect), are often associated with a problem of the mitral valve that often results in a leak. Less common are sinus venosus defects or holes in the top of the septum. These are associated with an abnormality of the right upper lung vein.

Generally patients with an ASD defect will exhibit no symptoms and the problem is only found when a routine clinical examination detects a heart murmur. Occasionally children with this problem will exhibit poor weight gain and a failure to thrive, and if there is mitral valve leakage there may be early symptoms of breathlessness.

4.4. Patent Ductus Anteriosus (PDA)

This defect is the continuance of a direct connection between the aorta and the lung (pulmonary) artery, which normally closes shortly after birth. A baby in the womb is supplied oxygen by the placenta via the umbilical cord. The baby's lungs are not expanded and require only a small amount blood for them to grow. The ductus is a blood vessel that allows blood to bypass the baby's lungs.

If the ductus has partially closed and only a narrow connection remains, the baby won't show symptoms. If the connection is larger, the baby may be breathless and tired and show poor weight gain.

4.5. Tetralogy of fallot

A small percentage of babies with Down syndrome have this complex heart condition which combines the most common defect associated with Down syndrome, AVSD, with Tetralogy of fallot.

This anomaly includes four different heart problems:

- A hole between the top chambers and a hole between the bottom chambers
- Combined mitral and tricuspid valves (common atrioventricular valve)
- Narrowed pulmonary artery (from heart to lungs) or the area under or above the valve, or all three
- Thickening of the right bottom chamber (ventricle)

The combination of these defects early in life almost seems to balance out such that the child may be rather blue, but not too breathless. There can, of course, be too much blueness or too much breathlessness, depending on the severity of the different conditions.

In Tetralogy of fallot (TOF), often caynosis is not present at birth but increasing hypertrophy of the right ventricular infundibulum and cyanosis occur usually in the later part of infancy. But cyanosis is present since birth if Tetralogy of Fallot is accompanied with Down Syndrome. This may be due to increased hypertrophy of the right ventricular infundibulum in patient of TOF with DS at birth. (AKMM Rashid et al., 2009)

5. Case

A case of eleven months boy was admitted in a hospital with the complaints of bluish discoloration of lip and finger since birth and low grade fever, cough for seven days. Bluish discoloration aggravates during crying. He was born to an elderly mother and was completely immunized. There was no such illness in the family. On examination the child was cyanosed, heart rate 130/m, weight 7.5 kg. He had got mongoloid face with flat occiput, depressed nasal bridge, upward slanting of eyes, medial epicanthic fold. There was gap between the first and second toes with clinodactyly. On examination of the precordium there was left parasternal heave, pansystolic murmur was present in the lower sternal border. There was motor developmental delay. The boy was clinically diagnosed with congenital cyanotic heart disease with Down syndrome. On investigation his hemoglobin was 78%, Total leucocyte count 14700/cum, Neutrophil 82%, X – Ray chest had the feature of boot shaped cardiac shadow. ECG showed right ventricular hypertrophy. Karyotyping showed trisomy 21. Tetralogy of fallot was detected by Echocardiogram. Finally the child was diagnosed as Down Syndrome with Tetralogy of Fallot. (AKMM Rashid et al., 2009)

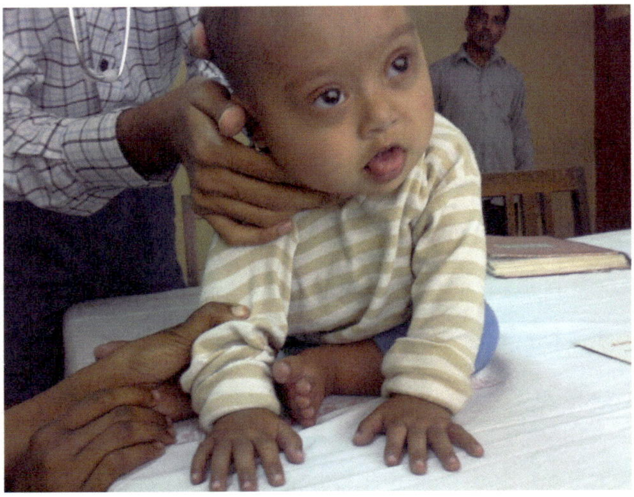

Figure 1. Patient with Down syndrome.

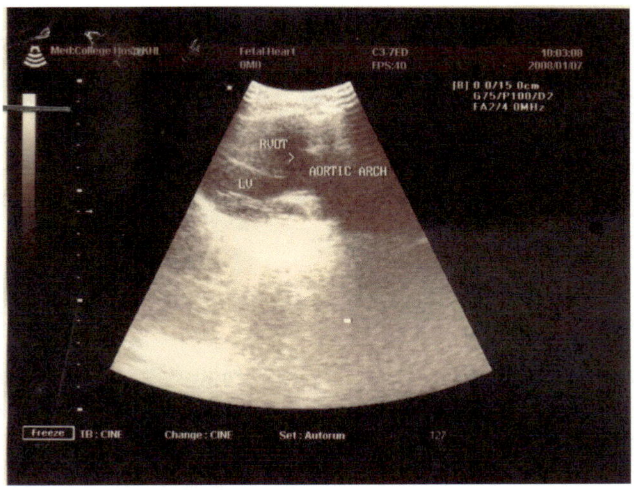

Figure 2. Echocardiogram showing Tetralogy of Fallot.

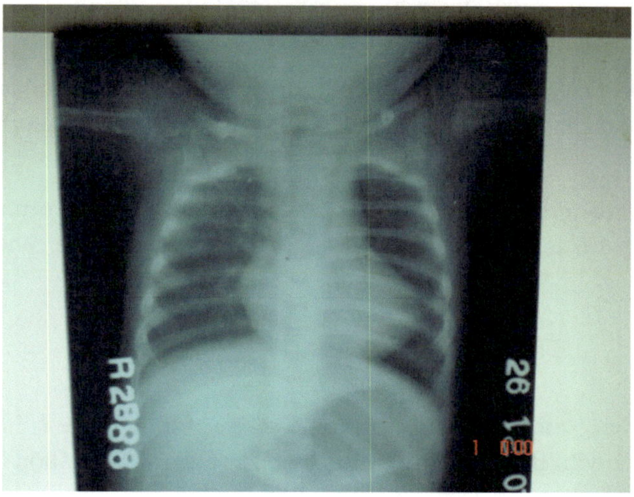

Figure 3. X-ray chest showing : boot shaped heart.

6. Other heart related problems in Down syndrome

In addition to the heart defects associated with Down syndrome, high blood pressure in the lungs (pulmonary hypertension) is more common in people with Down syndrome. This high blood pressure may be a result of malformation of the lung tissue, but the exact cause is not known. High blood pressure may limit the amount of blood flow to the lungs and therefore decrease the likelihood of symptoms of congestive heart failure seen in babies with complete AV canals or large ventricular septal defects.

7. Diagnosis

All babies that have been diagnosed with Down syndrome should have a cardiology evaluation because of the high incidence of associated congenital heart defects. A good history and physical examination should be performed in all Down syndrome children to rule out any obvious heart defect. Early diagnosis of congenital heart disease particularly of large left to right shunts, could enable a paediatrician to follow the baby carefully, to start medical treatment with diuretics and digoxin at an earlier stage and possibly to plan for earlier surgical intervention should this be indicated. Babies should be seen as early in life as possible, preferably in the first six months of life before pulmonary vascular disease can develop.

Electocardiogram can be very helpful in making the diagnosis of AV canal defect, even in the absence of physical findings.(Shashi V et al., 2002)

Echocardiography has to be performed routinely early in life in Down syndrome can detect congenital heart disease that might otherwise be missed. Early detection may help prevent complications such as pulmonary vascular disease that may adversely affect the outcome of cardiac surgery.

Occasionally a repeat electrocardiogram, chest x-ray, or echocardiogram is performed to further evaluate clinical changes. These tests are likely to be repeated before surgical repair is recommended.

Rarely, a cardiac catheterization is required for complete evaluation prior to corrective surgery especially in patients where elevated pressures in the lungs are a concern.

8. Treatment

Children with Down syndrome and symptoms of congestive heart failure can be initially managed medically with the use of diuretics, blood pressure medications to allow the heart to eject more blood out to the body rather than out to the lungs; and/or digoxin, a medication and to improve the pumping ability of the heart.

If the baby is having difficulty with feeding and weight gain, nasogastric tube feeding with calorie formula or fortified breast milk can be used to help with growth.

These are all temporary solutions to allow the baby to grow while deciding if and when surgery is indicated. If the baby has no signs of heart failure or is controlled well with medications, the decisions for surgical closure can be delayed. The decision must be individualized to each child's physical state as well as the family's concerns. The majority of cases of AVSD usually require surgical intervention; this generally takes place within the first six months of life.

Many VSD, will close spontaneously or get much smaller, so, it is normal practice to leave a child with a small or moderate VSD and monitor their progress before deciding to operate. Surgery may be needed if there is failure to thrive despite medication, or concern about pulmonary hypertension. If a large VSD is present, surgery is almost always recommended.

Small holes in ASD which allows little blood flow from left to right generally causes no problems. If they are located in the middle portion of the central heart wall, they may even close on their own. However, moderate and large holes do not close, and the extra work over the years places a strain of the right side of the heart causing an enlargement of both pumping chambers. Therefore, Surgery is recommended in the first few years of life or larger holes, before excessive strain has been placed on the heart.

If the ductus open for more than three months, it is unlikely to close on its own and surgical closure is imperative.

The types of surgery in TOF depend on the severity of the AVSD or the Fallots. Usually the children are quite blue and require a BT shunt to increase the amount of blue going to the lungs. Then another operation is performed later- usually at 1-2 years of age- so, that the holes can be closed, the valves repaired and the way out to the lung artery widened. (Cincinnati Children's hospital medical Center, 2006)

9. Long-term outlook

Over all, survival beyond one year of age is 85 percent in all children with Down syndrome. Over 50 percent of individuals with Down syndrome live to be greater than 50 years of age.

Congenital heart disease is the most common causes of death in early childhood. However, as of the late 1980s, 70 percent of children with Down syndrome and congenital heart disease lived beyond their first birth day with improved medical and surgical care, these numbers continue to improve. (Cincinnati Children's hospital medical Center, 2009)

Abbreviation

ASD – Atrial Septal Defect

AVSD- Atrioventricular Septal Defect

BAC- Beta-site APP –Cleaving

CHD- Congenital Heart Disease

DSCAM- Down syndrome cell adhesion molecule

DS- Down syndrome

MX- Myxovirus resistance

PDA- Patent Ductus Arteriosus

PFKL- Phosphofructo-kinase liver types

TOF- Tetralogy of fallot

VSD-Ventricular Septal defect

BT- Blalock Taussig

Author details

A. K. M. Mamunur Rashid

Dept. of Pediatrics, Khulna Medical College, Khulna, Bangladesh

References

[1] AKM Mamunur Rashid, Biswajit Basu, Md. Mizanur Rahman. Tetralogy of Fallot in Down syndrome (Trisomy 21)- An uncommon association. Pak J Med Sci, 2009 vol. 25, no.4, 698-700.

[2] Anderson RH. Simplifying the understanding of congenital malformations of the heart. Int J Cardiol 1991; 32: 131-42.

[3] Barlow G M., Xiao-Ning Chen, Zheng Y. Shi, Gary E Lyons, David M. Kurnit, Livija Celle, Nancy B. Spinner, Elaine Zackai, Mark J. Pettenati, Alexander J. Van Riper, Michael J. Vekemans, Corey H. Mjaatvedt, Julie R Korenberg. Genetics in Medicine March/April 2001-Vol.3, No.2, 91-101.

[4] Behrman RE, Kliegman RM and Jenson HB. From congenital heart disease. Philadelphia: Harcourt Asia Pvt. Ltd. Nelson Textbook of Pediatrics. 2000; 16 1362-63.

[5] Berr C and Borghi E. Risk of Down syndrome in relatives of trisomy 21 children. A case-control study. Ann Genet 1990;33:137-40.

[6] Cooney TP, Thurlbeck WM. Pulmonary hypoplasia in Down's syndrome. N Engl J Med 1982; 307: 1170-73.

[7] Cincinnati Children's hospital medical Center. Heart- Related Syndrome (Trisomy 21). 2006 :1-4. www.cincinnatichildrens.org/health/heart-encyclopedia/anomalies/pda

[8] Cincinnati Children's hospital medical Center. Down Syndrome (Trisomy 21). 2009:1-4. www.cincinnatichildrens.org/health/d/down

[9] Delabar JM, Theophile D, Rahmani Z, Chettouh Z, Blouin JL, Preiur M,Noel B, Sinet PM. Molecular mapping of 24 features of Down syndrome on chromosome 21.Eur J Hum Genet 1993; 1: 114-24.

[10] Du ZD, Roguin N, Barak M, Bihari SG, Ben-Elisha M. High prevalence of muscular ventricular septal defect in preterm neonates. Am J Cardiol. 1996; 78: 1183-85.

[11] Ferencz C, Loffredo CA, Correa-Villasenor A, Wilson PD, , editors. Perspective in pediatric cardiology. Vol 5. Armonk NY: The Baltimore-Washington infant study, 1997.

[12] Francis F, Lehrach H, Reinhardt R, Yaspo MI. The DNA sequence of human chromosome 21. Nature 2000; 405: 311-19.

[13] Hubert RS, Mitchell S, Chen X-N, Ekmekji K, Gadomski C, Sun Z, Noya D, Kim U-J, Chen C, Shizuya H, Simon M, de jong PJ, Korenberg JR. BAC and PAC contigs covering 3.5 Mb of the down syndrome congenital heart disease region between D21S55 and MX1 on chromosome 21. Genomics 1997; 41: 218-26.

[14] Hattori M, Fujiyama A, Taylor TD, Watanabe H, Yada T, Park HS, Toyoda A, Ishii K, Totoki Y, Choi DK, Soeda E, Ohki M, Takagi T, Sakaki T, Taudien S, Blechschmidt K,

Polley A, Menzel U, Delabar J, Kumpf K, Lehmann R, Patterson D, Reichwald K, Rump A, Schillhabel M, Schudy A, Zimmermann W, Rosenthal A, Kudoh J, Shibuya K, Kawasaki K, Asakawa S, Shintani A, Sasaki T, Nagamine K, Mitsuyama S, Antonarakis SE, Minoshima S, Shimizu N, Nordsick G, Hornischer K, Bendt P, Scharfe M, Schn O, Desario A, Reichelt J, Kaur G, Blocker H, Ramser J, Beck A, Klages S, Hennig S, Rielssenmann I, Dagand F, Haaf T, wehrmeyer S, Borzym K, Gardiner k, Nizetic D, Francis F, Lehrach H, Reirhardt R, Yas Po MI. The DNA sequence of human chromosome 21. Nature 2000;405:311-19.

[15] Hassold TA, and Sherman S. Down syndrome; Genetic recombination and origin of the extra chromosome 21. Clin Genet, 2000; 57: 95-100.

[16] Hoffman JI. Congenital heart disease: incidence and inheritance. Pediatr Clin North Am. 1990; 37: 25-43.

[17] Hoffman JI, Kaplan S, Liberthson RR. Prevalence of congenital heart disease. Am Heart J. 2004; 147: 425-39.

[18] Korenberg JR, Kawashima H, Pulst SM, Ikeuchi T, Ogasawara SA, Yamatoto K, Schonberg SA. Molecular definition of a region of chromosome 21 that causes features of the Down syndrome phenotype. Am J Hum Genet 1990; 47: 236-46.

[19] Korenberg JR, Bradley C, Disteche C. Down syndrome: molecular mapping of the congenital heart disease and duodenal stenosis. Am J Hum Genet 1992; 50: 294-302.

[20] Korenberg JR, Chen X-N, Schipper R, Sun Z, Gonsky RGerwehr S, Carpenter N, Daumer C, Dignan P, Disteche C, Graham JM, Hudgins L, McGiillivray B, Miyazaki K, Ogasawara N, Park JP, Pagon R, Pueschel S, Sack G, Say B, Schuffenhaur S, Soukup S, Yamanaka T. Down symdrome phenotypes: the consequences of chromosomal imbalance. Proc Natl Acad Sci U S A 1994;91:4997-5001.

[21] Moller JH, Allen HD, Clerk EB, Dajani AS, Golden A, Hayman LL, Lauer RM, Marmer EL, McAnulty JH, Oparil S. Report of the task force on children and youth: American heart association. Circulation. 1993; 88: 2479-86.

[22] McCormick MK, Schinzel A, Petersen MB, Stetten G, Driscoll DJ, Cantu ES,Tranebjaerg L, Mikkelsen M, Watkins PC, Antonarakis SE. Molecular genetic approach to the characterization of the" Down syndrome region" of chromosome 21. Genomics 1989; 5: 325-31.

[23] Payne M, Johnson MC, Grant JW, and Strauss AW. 1995. Towards a molecular understanding of congenital heart disease . Circulation. 91: 494-504.

[24] Piperpont ME, Craig T, Basson D, Benson W, Jr. Bruce DG, Giglia TM, Goldmuntz E, McGee G, Craig A Sable, Srivastava D, and Catherine L. Webb. Genetic Basis for Congenital Heart Defects: Current Knowledge: Circulation 2007; 115: 3015-3038.

[25] Rahmani Z, Blouin JI, Creau-Goldberg N Watkins PC, Mattei JF, Poissonnier M,Prieur M, Chettouh Z, Nicole A, Aurias A, Sinet P, Delabar J.Critical role of the

D21S55 region on chromosome 21 in the pathogenesis of Down syndrome. Proc Natl Acad Sci U S A 1989; 86: 5958-62.

[26] Ramakrishnan V. Research Article: Genetic aspects of congenital heart disease in Down syndrome. Inter J Cur Res 2011; 3(6): 165-70.

[27] Roguin N, Du ZD, Barak M, Nasser N, hershkowitz S, Milgram E. High prevalence of muscular ventricular septal defect in neonates. J Am Coll Cardiol. 1995; 26: 1545-48.

[28] Rodriguez LH, and Reyes JN. Cardiopatias en el syndrome de Down. Bol Med Hosp Infant Mex. 1984; 41: 622-25.

[29] Shashi V, Berry MN, Covitz W. A combination of physical examination and ECG detects the majority of hemodynamically significant heart defects in neonates with Down syndrome. Am J Med Genet 2002 Mar 15;108(3):205-8.

[30] Stoll C, Alembik Y, Dott B, Roth MP. 1998. Study of Down syndrome in 238,942 consecutive births. Ann Genet. 41: 44-51.

[31] T R J Tubman, M D Shields, B G Craig, H C Mulholland, N c Nevin. Congenital Heart Disease in Down syndrome; two year prospective early screening study. B M J, Volume 302, 15 June, 1991, 1425-27.

[32] Van Praagh R, Papagiannis J, Bar-EI YI, Schwint OA. The heart in Down syndrome: Pathologic anatomy. In: Marino B, Pueschel SM, editors. Heart disease in persons with Down syndrome. Baltimore, MD: Paul H Brookers Publishing Co. 1996: 69-110.

[33] Yamakawa K, Huo YK, Haendelt MA, Hubert R, Chen X-N, Lyones GE, Korenberg JR. DSCAM: a novel member of the immunoglobulin super family maps in a Down syndrome region and is involved in the development of the nervous system. Hum Mol Genet 1998; 7: 227-37.

Chapter 7

Myeloid Leukemia Associated with Down Syndrome

Kazuko Kudo

Additional information is available at the end of the chapter

http://dx.doi.org/10.5772/52784

1. Introduction

Children with Down syndrome (DS) have a 10- to 20-fold increased risk of developing acute leukemia. [1-4] The relative risk of developing acute megakaryoblastic leukemia (AMKL) is estimated to be 500 times higher in children with DS than in those without DS. Interestingly, five to 10 % of neonates with DS develop transient abnormal myelopoiesis (TAM). In most cases, it resolves spontaneously within 3 months. However, approximately 15% of the severe cases are fatal and 20% of patients develop AMKL until 3 year-old (Fig.1). AMKL in DS has a number of distinct features and it is now considered a specific subtype of acute myeloid leukemia (AML) in the 4th edition of the World Health Organization (WHO) classification called Myeloid Leukemia of Down syndrome (ML-DS).

2. Acute Myeloid Leukemia (AML)

The majority of cases of AML with DS (70-100%) are megakaryoblastic [5] and occur within the first 4 years of life. [6] The characteristic antecedent preleukaemic TAM is observed in 20–30% of cases. Overt leukemia in DS children is preceded in 20- 60% of cases by an indolent myelodysplasia, characterised by thrombocytopenia and bone marrow fibrosis, which may last several months before overt AML. [1, 7] The median age at presentation of AML is 1.8 years. [7] The bone marrow aspirate shows dysplasia, increased blasts, abnormal megakaryocytes and variable myelofibrosis.[5, 7-8] Immunophenotypically, ML-DS blasts typically express megakaryocytic (CD42b and CD41) and erythroid markers (CD36 and Glycophorin A) as well as the T cell marker, CD7. [9]Neither the favorable cytogenetic changes, such as t(8;21), t(15;17), t(9;11) and inv(16), nor the AMKL-associated translocations, t(1;22) and t(1;3), occur in ML-DS.[1] Additional copies of chromosome 8 and/or 21 (in addition to the +21c, 10-15%), monosomy 7 and –5/5q- (together in 10–20%) are observed. [10]

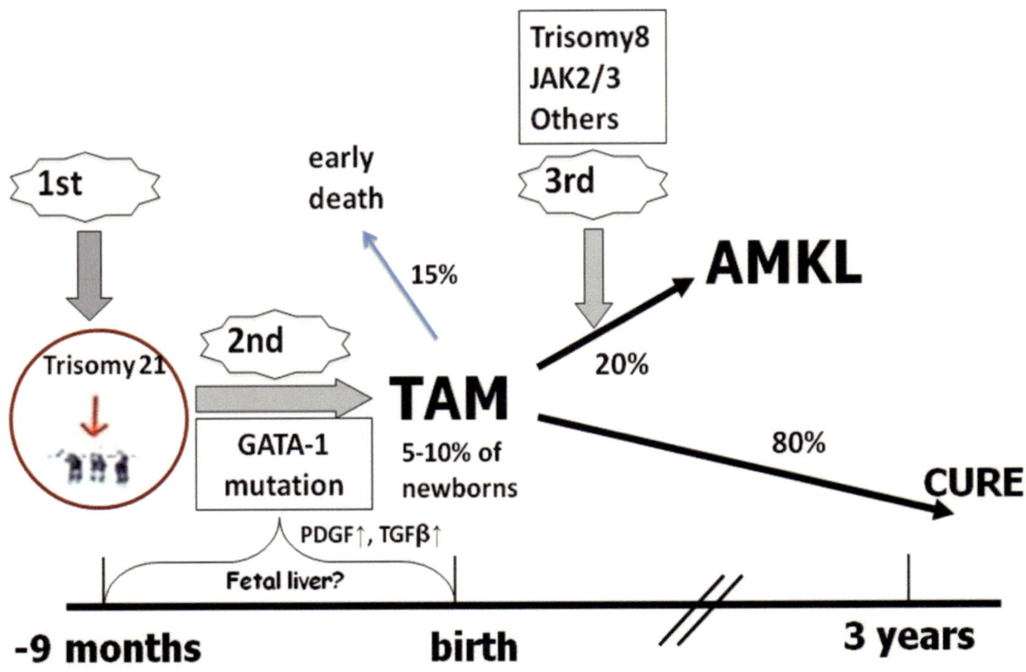

Figure 1. Multi-step model of myeloid leukemogenesis in DS. Trisomy 21 enhances the proliferation of fetal liver megakaryo-erythroid progenitors via PDGF and/or TGF beta. The acquisition of GATA1 mutation further enhances the clonal proliferation of immature magakaryoblasts diagnosed at birth as TAM. GATA1 mutations are necessary but insufficient for the development of AMKL. Additional genetic events such as trisomy 8, or JAK2/3 mutations have been proposed in progression from TAM to AMKL.

2.1. Treatment for AML-DS

Conventional treatment of AML-DS has been associated with excessive treatment-related mortality (TRM), cardiac toxicity due to anthracyclines and serious infections. Zwaan et al demonstrated a 12-fold increase in sensitivity to cytarabine in DS-AML cells compared with non-DS AML cells, as well as increased sensitivity to anthracyclines (two- to seven-fold) and etoposide (20-fold).[11] Several collaborative study groups have adapted their standard AML protocol for AML-DS by reducing the dose of drugs (Table 1).[5, 8, 12-17] In the Children's Oncology Group (COG) trial A2971 (n=132), [13] etoposide, dexamethasone, and the maintenance course were eliminated from the previous CCG2891 protocol. COG A2971 achieved a 5-year EFS rate of 79% plus or minus 7% (versus 77% plus or minus 7% in the CCG2891 trial) while maintaining a low induction failure rate of 6.4%, attaining a 0% CNS relapse rate, and sustaining an acceptably low 5-year postremission. In the AML-BFM98 study (n=66), [7] AML-DS patients were treated with reduced doses of anthracyclines and cytarabine compared with the previous AMLBFM93 protocol (n = 44). The cumulative doses of anthracyclines and cytarabine were 220 to 240mg/m2 and 23 to 29g/m2 in the BFM98 study, and 440mg/m2 and

23.3 g/m2 in the AMLBFM93 study, respectively. Outcome improved significantly for patients treated in the AMLBFM98 study, with a 3-year EFS of 91% plus or minus 4% versus 70% plus or minus 7% in the AMLBFM93 study.

					Drugs administered			
Protocol	No of patients	EFS (%)	Relapse (%)	death in CCR (%)	Cytarabine (g/m2)	Daunorubicin (mg/m2)	Mitoxantrone (mg/m2)	Etoposide (mg/m2)
POG9421[12]	57	77 (5y)	7	14	20.7	135	80	1,000
CCG2891[5]	161	77 (6y)	14	4	15.8	320	0	1,600
COG-A2971[13]	132	79 (5y)	11	3	24.8	80	0	0
NOPHO-AML93[14]	41	85 (8y)	7	5	49.6	150	30	1,600
AML-BFM98[7]	67	89 (3y)	6	5	23-29	Ida; 26-36	0-14	950
MRC-AML10/12[8]	46	74 (5y)	3	15	7.8	300	50	1,500
AT-DS(Japan)[15]	33	80 (8y)	6	9	4.2	100-400	0	2,700
AML99 DS[16]	72	83 (4y)	12.5	1.4	3.5	THP; 250	0	2,250
JCCLSG 9805DS[17]	24	83 (5y)	0	13	12.6	THP; 135	10	200

POG, Pediatric Oncology Group; CCG, Children's Cancer Group; COG, Children's Oncology Group; NOPHO, Nordic Society for Paediatric Haematology and Oncology; BFM, Berlin-Frankfurt-Munster; MRC, Medical Research Council; JCCLSG; Japan Children's Cancer and Leukemia Study Group DS, Down syndrome; Ida, Idarubicin; THP, pirarubicin

Table 1. Comparison of the results in DS-AML patients

A treatment regimen specifically designed for AML-DS has been used in Japan since the mid- 1980s.[15, 16] AML 99 DS protocol consisted of pirarubicin (25 mg/m2/d, on days 1 and 2), which was estimated to be equivalent as 25mg/m2/d of daunomycin (DNR), cytarabine (100 mg/m2/d on day 1 through 7), and etoposide (150 mg/m2/d on day 3 through 5). Pirarubicin is much less cardiotoxic and more myelosuppressive than daunorubicin.A total of 70 of the 72 patients (97.2%) achieved a CR. The 4-year EFS was 83.3% plus or minus 9.1% and the 4-year OS was 83.7% plus or minus 9.5%. The regimen-related toxicities were relatively tolerable. Only one patient died as a result of pneumonia in the second course of intensification. The 3-year EFS in the five patients with monosomy 7 was significantly worse than in the 65 patients without monosomy 7 (40,0% plus or minus 26.3% v 86.2% plus or minus 8.8%). Future treatment protocols could include adherence to a very low-intensity chemotherapy for the majority of ML-DS patients, identification of the subgroup with a poor prognosis using minimal residual disease (MRD), and stratification of these patients to receive a more intensive chemotherapy containing high-dose and/or continuous infusion of intermediate-dose cytarabine.

3. Transient Abnormal Myelopoiesis (TAM)

Transient abnormal myelopoiesis (TAM), also known as transient leukemia (TL) or transient myeloproliferative disorder (TMD) occurs in approximately 10% of infants with DS.[1, 4] TAM was considered to be ''self-limiting''; the prognosis of TAM was favorable, except for the risk of the subsequent development of acute leukemia. Most of newborns are asymptomatic and only present with circulating blast cells, with or without leucocytosis. Other clinical features include hepatomegaly, splenomegaly, serous effusions and, in up to 10% of patients, liver fibrosis due to blast cell infiltration that can rarely cause fulminant liver failure. Leucocytosis and thrombocytopenia are common. About a quarter of patients have abnormal liver transaminases and abnormal laboratory coagulation tests. The blast cells in TAM usually have the 'blebby' appearance characteristic of megakaryoblasts and typically express CD41, CD42b. Most neonates with TAM do not need chemotherapy as the clinical and laboratory abnormalities spontaneously resolve within 3–6 months after birth. However, symptomatic babies with TAM, especially those with high blast counts or liver dysfunction, may benefit from low-dose cytarabine.

In 2006, Children's Oncology Group (COG) reported a prospective study of the natural history of 48 children with DS and TAM. [18] Early death occurred in 17% of infants and was significantly correlated with higher WBC count at diagnosis, increased bilirubin and liver enzymes, and failure to normalize the blood count. Recurrence of leukemia occurred in 19% of infants at a mean of 20 months. In the AML-BFM study, 22 children among total 146 children (15%) died within the first 6 months. The 5-year OS and EFS were 85% plus or minus 3% and 63% plus or minus 4%, respectively. [19]A total of 28 children received a short course of cytarabine treatment. Interestingly, EFS and OS did not differ significantly in the treated versus the untreated group. Among the 124 children who survived the first 6 months of life, 29 (23.4%) subsequently developed ML-DS. The 5-year EFS after diagnosis of ML-DS for all 29 patients was 91% plus or minus 5%, which is significantly higher than the 5-year EFS of those of ML-DS patients without documented TAM (70% plus or minus 4%). According to the retrospective study from Japan, estimated gestational age (EGA), higher WBC counts and higher direct bilirubin levels were significant predictive factors for poor prognosis. [20, 21] Muramatsu et al devised a simple risk stratification system based on the EGA and the peak WBC count. The high-risk group (HR) was defined as preterm infants with WBC >100 x 10^9/l, the intermediate-risk group (IR) was defined as preterm infants with WBC <100 x 10^9/l and term infants with WBC >100 x 10^9/l, and the low-risk group (LR) was defined as term infants with WBC< 100 x 10^9/l. In the LR group, only three of 39 patients (7.7 %) died early. Based on their data, patients in the LR group should receive no interventions. However, since the probability of early death in patients in the HR group exceeded 50%, active intervention including low dose cytarabine should be tried in the context of a clinical trial for these patients.

3.1. Treatment for TAM

In patients with a severe form of TAM, the main causes of death in early life are progressive hepatic fibrosis, cardiopulmonary failure, and disseminated intravascular coagulation. These complications may be caused by blast cell infiltration into visceral organs. In the Pediatric Oncology Group (POG) study 9481, 10 mg/m2 per dose or 1.2–1.5 mg/kg per dose was given subcutaneously or intravenously by slow injection twice a day for 7 days (Table 2). [18] In the AML-BFM study, 0.5–1.5 mg/kg was administered for 3–12 days. [19] As TAM blasts are highly sensitive to cytarabine, there is generally a rapid response, characterized by the disappearance of peripheral blasts by day 7 of treatment.

Study group	No of patients	Early death (%)	Leukemia (%)	OS (%)	No of treated patients	Cytarabine
POG9481[18]	48	17	19	78 (3y)	2	10mg/m2 x 2 x 1-2 days
AML-BFM[19]	146	15	23.4*	85 (5y)	28	0.5-1.5 mg/kg x 3-12 days
COGA2971[20]	135	21	16	77 (3y)	29	3.33mg/kg/24 hrs x 5 days
Tokai (Japan)[21]	70	23	22*	74.3(1y)	3	0.7 mg/kg x 5days, 10mg/m^2 x 2/day
Kikuchi (Japan)[22]	73	22	23	71.2(3y)	9	

POG, Pediatric Oncology Group; BFM, Berlin-Frankfurt-Munster;

COG, Children's Oncology Group; *. Alive > 6 mo

Table 2. The outcomes of transient abnormal myelopoiesis with Down syndrome.

Although TAM resolves in the majority of DS infants, 20– 30% subsequently develop ML-DS, usually within in the first 4 years of life. [18-22] In the COG study 2971, twenty-one patients among total 135 TAM patients (16%) developed ML-DS, including 3 received cytarabine.[20] The development of AMKL after remission of TAM has been interested as a model of myeloid leukaemogenesis, presumably from a subclone of persisting TMD cells that acquire a selective advantage. This hypothesis can be verified by monitoring minimal residual disease, either by immunophenotype or quantitative GATA1[23] polymerase chain reaction.

Author details

Kazuko Kudo

Address all correspondence to: kazukok@sch.pref.shizuoka.jp

Division of Hematology and OncologyShizuoka Children's Hospital, Urushiyama, Aoi-ku, Shizuoka, Japan

References

[1] Lange B: The management of neoplastic disorders of haematopoiesis in children with Down's syndrome. Br J Haematol 110(3): 512-24, 2000

[2] Zwaan CM, Reinhardt D, Hitzler J, et al: Acute leukemias in children with Down syndrome. Hematol Oncol Clin North Am 24(1): 19-34, 2010

[3] Izraeli S, Rainis L, Hertzberg L, et al. Trisomy of chromosome 21 in leukemogenesis. Blood Cells Mol Dis 39(2): 156-9, 2007

[4] Roy A, Roberts I, Norton A, et al. Acute megakaryoblastic leukaemia (AMKL) and transient myeloproliferative disorder (TMD) in Down syndrome: a multi-step model of myeloid leukaemogenesis. Br J Haematol. 2009 Oct;147(1):3-12. Epub 2009 Jul 6. Review.

[5] Gamis AS, Woods WG, Alonzo TA, et al. Increased age at diagnosis has a significantly negative effect on outcome in children with Down syndrome and acute myeloid leukemia: a report from the Children's Cancer Group Study 2891. J Clin Oncol. 2003 Sep 15; 21(18): 3415-22.

[6] Hasle H, Abrahamsson J, Arola M,et al. Myeloid leukemia in children 4 years or older with Down syndrome often lacks GATA1 mutation and cytogenetics and risk of relapse are more akin to sporadic AML. Leukemia. 2008 Jul; 22(7): 1428-30.

[7] Creutzig U, Reinhardt D, Diekamp S, et al: AML patients with Down syndrome have a high cure rate with AML-BFM therapy with reduced dose intensity. Leukemia 19(8): 1355-60, 2005

[8] Rao A, Hills RK, Stiller C, et al. Treatment for myeloid leukaemia of Down syndrome: population-based experience in the UK and results from the Medical Research Council AML 10 and AML 12 trials. Br J Haematol. 2006 Mar; 132(5): 576-83.

[9] Yumura-Yagi K, Hara J, Kurahashi H, et al. Mixed phenotype of blasts in acute megakaryocytic leukaemia and transient abnormal myelopoiesis in Down's syndrome. Br J Haematol. 1992 Aug;81(4):520-5.

[10] Forestier E, Izraeli S, Beverloo B, et al. Cytogenetic features of acute lymphoblastic and myeloid leukemias in pediatric patients with Down syndrome: an iBFM-SG study. Blood. 2008 Feb 1;111(3):1575-83. Epub 2007 Oct 30.

[11] Zwaan CM, Kaspers GJ, Pieters R, et al. Different drug sensitivity profiles of acute myeloid and lymphoblastic leukemia and normal peripheral blood mononuclear cells in children with and without Down syndrome. Blood. 2002 Jan 1; 99(1):245-51.

[12] O'Brien MM, Taub JW, Chang MN, et al. Cardiomyopathy in children with Down syndrome treated for acute myeloid leukemia: a report from the Children's Oncology Group Study POG 9421. J Clin Oncol. 2008 Jan 20; 26(3):414-20.

http://dx.doi.org/10.5772/52784

[13] Sorrell AD, Alonzo TA, Hilden JM, et al. Favorable survival maintained in children who have myeloid leukemia associated with Down syndrome using reduced-dose chemotherapy on Children's Oncology Group trial A2971: A report from the Children's Oncology Group.Cancer 2012 .Mar 5 [Epub ahead of print]

[14] Abildgaard L, Ellebaek E, Gustafsson G, et al: Optimal treatment intensity in children with Down syndrome and myeloid leukaemia: data from 56 children treated on NOPHO-AML protocols and a review of the literature. Ann Hematol 85(5): 275-80, 2006

[15] Kojima S, Sako M, Kato K, et al: An effective chemotherapy regimen for acute myeloid leukemia and myelodysplastic syndrome with Down's syndrome. Leukemia 14: 786-91, 2000

[16] Kudo K, Kojima S, Tabuchi K, et al: Prospective study of a pirarubicin, intermediate-dose cytarabine, and etoposide regimen in children with Down syndrome and acute myeloid leukemia: the Japanese Childhood AML Cooperative Study Group. J Clin Oncol 25(34): 5442-7, 2007

[17] Taga T, Shimomura Y, Horikoshi Y, et al: Continuous and high-dose cytarabine combined chemotherapy in children with Down syndrome and acute myeloid leukemia: Report from the Japanese Children's Cancer and Leukemia Study Group (JCCLSG) AML 9805 Down Study. Pediatr Blood Cancer 2011; 57(1): 36-40.

[18] Massey GV, Zipursky A, Chang MN,et al: A prospective study of the natural history of transient leukemia (TL) in neonates with Down syndrome (DS): Children's Oncology Group (COG) study POG-9481. Blood 107(12): 4606-13, 2006

[19] Klusmann JH, Creutzig U, Zimmermann M, et al: Treatment and prognostic impact of transient leukemia in neonates with Down syndrome Blood 111(6): 2991-8, 2008

[20] Gamis AS, Alonzo TA, Gerbing RB, et al. Natural history of transient myeloproliferative disorder clinically diagnosed in Down syndrome neonates: a report from the Children's Oncology Group Study A2971. Blood. 2011 Dec 22; 118(26):6752-9; quiz 6996. Epub 2011 Aug 17.

[21] Muramatsu H, Kato K, Watanabe N, et al: Risk factors for early death in neonates with Down syndrome and transient leukaemia. Br J Haematol 142(4): 610-5, 2008

[22] Kikuchi A: Transient abnormal myelopoiesis in Down's syndrome. JPH23: 58-61, 2009

[23] Wechsler J, Greene M, McDevitt MA et al: Acquired mutations in GATA 1 in the megakaryoblastic leukemia of Down syndrome. Nat Genet 32: 148-52, 2002

Section 3

Genetics of Down Syndrome

Chapter 8

Molecular Pathways of Down Syndrome Critical Region Genes

Ferdinando Di Cunto and Gaia Berto

Additional information is available at the end of the chapter

http://dx.doi.org/10.5772/53000

1. Introduction

1.1. Identification and annotation of the DSCR

Down syndrome (DS) is a very complex disorder that requires, even more than other human genetics diseases, a "system level" understanding [1,2], both under the clinical and under the molecular genetics perspectives. Under the clinical point of view, all individuals affected by Down syndrome are characterized by learning disabilities, distinctive facial features, and low muscle tone (hypotonia) in early infancy. However, in most cases the clinical picture is complicated by additional problems, such as heart defects, leukemia, and early-onset Alzheimer's disease [3,4]. The degree to which an individual is affected by these characteristics varies from mild to severe. After the pioneering description by J.L. Down in 1866, almost one century was needed to decipher the etiology of the syndrome. The work of Lejeune proved that DS was caused by an extra copy of chromosome 21 (HSA21) [5], thus providing the first evidence for a genetic basis of intellectual disability. The main implication of this seminal discovery is that the complex phenotype seen in DS patients [6] must be caused by overdosage of HSA21 genes. However, it also raised the outstanding questions of whether one or few HSA21 genes may play a dominant role in the syndrome and whether specific HSA21 genes could contribute to specific phenotypic tracts. Answering these questions is still of paramount importance, because the identification of one or few 'dominant' molecular players could pave the road for the development of targeted therapeutic approaches. The development of molecular karyotyping has provided strong support to the view that a restricted region of HSA21, commonly referred to as Down Syndrome Crtitical Region (DSCR) might be responsible for the different phenotypes that characterize DS. In 1976 Poissonnier and coworkers, by using chromosome staining methods, found that one DS patient not possessing an extra HSA21 had only a partial trisomy, involving 21q22.1 and 21q22.2 bands [7]. Afterwards, it turned out that partial trisomies are responsible for approximately 1% of DS cases [8,9]. These patients show variable phenotypes, depending on the extension of the triplicated region. Therefore, partial trisomies of genes carried by chromosome 21 have been extremely valuable in investigating the involvement in DS. The analysis of 10 partial trisomy patients, [10] suggested that two regions of chromosome 21 were linked to most of the Jackson signs [3], including cognitive disorders. These regions, referred to has DCR-1 and DCR-2, respectively, encompassed the 21q22.2 band and were located around the D21S55 Site Targeted Sequence (STS) and between D21S55 and the MX1 gene, respectively. Korenberg and coworkers studied a different population and observed that the proximal and distal regions of the 21q arm were also associated with the full DS phenotype [11]. Although these studies confirmed the strong association of DS phenotypes with the DCR-1 region, they also suggested that DS is a contiguous gene syndrome, arguing against a single DS chromosomal region responsible for most of the DS phenotypic features [11]. More recently, an additional causal link of the region located between D21S17 and ETS2 to clinical features of DS was confirmed through lattice analysis [12]. Although the notion of a DSCR has gained wide acceptance in DS research, it must be underscored that some of the data that support it remain controversial and that its existence has recently come under considerable question. Indeed, a detailed study of segmental trisomy 21 in DS subjects, performed by using array comparative genome hybridization (GCH), excludes the implication of a single but rather suggest that multiple regions of HSA21 contribute to many of the phenotypes of DS, including intellectual disability DSCR [13]. Despite these apparent inconsistencies, we think that, in practical terms, the crucial point is not to prove whether one or more "critical region" exist, but rather to understand which dosage-sensitive genes contribute to specific DS phenotypes. Indeed, it is quite clear that the classical "reductionist" approach of identifying one or few master genes, which has been very successful in the case of Mendelian disorders, is not appropriate to unravel the extremely more complicated case of DS. In this case, the overall phenotype is certainly produced by the combined action of several genes, causing complex rearrangements of different molecular networks [14]. The relevance of the mentioned studies has been to restrict the list of HSA21 genes that may contribute more significantly to the clinical manifestations.

For these motivations, in Tables 1 and 2 we adopt an inclusive definition of the DSCR, which extends from the RCAN1 gene to the MX1 gene. This definition takes into account not only the putative borders that have been identified in the mentioned studies, but also the fact that the RCAN1 gene as been commonly considered as part of the DSCR, even though a precise mapping on the current release of the human genome sequence (HG19) would locate it outside the centromeric border defined by [12]. Obviously, the usefulness of this information will strongly depend on the degree of functional characterization of the genes comprised in the interval. Under this respect, as it is generally true for the human genome, it must be recognized that our knowledge is still quite limited.

HSA21 was one of the first human chromosomes to be fully sequenced [15]. Nevertheless, the list of the possible functional sequences located in the DSCR has progressively changed, not only for the uncertainty of defining precise borders, but especially for the changes in the current view of what a human gene is. Obviously, the initial emphasis has been to identify the protein-

http://dx.doi.org/10.5772/53000

coding sequences, whose number is approximately of 40, on the basis of a comprehensive definition of the DSCR and of the present annotation of the human genome (Table 1). However, systematic studies performed in the last few years revealed that many genomic sequences that have been initially considered as "junk DNA", are endowed with extremely relevant functional potential [16]. Indeed, genome-wide interrogations have revealed that a large majority of the human genome is transcribed and that a significant proportion of transcripts appears to be non-protein coding (ncRNA). Although it is well recognized that some ncRNAs play essential enzymatic activities in translation, splicing and ribosome biogenesis, the functions of most ncRNAs are still unknown. It is now believed that they could participate in complex regulatory circuits responsible for the fine-tuning of gene expression at both the transcriptional and post-transcriptional levels [16]. The best known ncRNAs are miRNAs, ~22 nucleotide-long molecules that mediate post-transcriptional gene silencing by binding complementary sequences located in the 3′ UTR of the mRNAs. Long intergenic ncRNAs (lincRNA) represent a less characterized but more abundant and heterogeneous class, and comprise transcripts longer than 200 nt involved in many biological processes, including transcriptional control, epigenetic modification and post-transcriptional control on mRNAs [16]. A recent discovery demonstrated that both mRNAs and ncRNAs can deploy their functions by contributing to an extensive RNA-RNA interaction network, based on the competition of these molecules for the binding of shared miRNAs (the ceRNA hypothesis) [17-20]. Importantly, transcribed pseudogenes could also be involved in these complex regulatory interactions [21]. In light of this growing complexity, we think that the presence of many 'non conventional' sequences within the DSCR should be taken into consideration when exploring the molecular consequences of an increased dosage of this region. We provide an updated list of them in Table 2.

DCR	Gene Name	Entrez Gene ID	Main molecular function	Essential references	Expression in adult brain
1	RCAN1	1827	CaN inhibitor	See main text	Yes
1	CLIC6	54102	Channel	See main text	Yes
1	RUNX1	861	Transcription factor	See main text	Yes
1	SETD4	54093	Unknown	No information	Yes
1	CBR1	873	Enzyme	[165]	Yes
1	CBR3	874	Enzyme	[165]	
1	DOPEY2	9980	Unknown	[166]	Yes
1	MORC3	23515	RNA-binding	[167]	
1	CHAF1B	8208	Chromatin assembly	[168]	Yes
1	CLDN14	23562	Tight junctions component	[169]	
1	SIM2	6493	Transcription factor	See main text	Yes
1	HLCS	3141	Enzyme	[170]	Yes

DCR	Gene Name	Entrez Gene ID	Main molecular function	Essential references	Expression in adult brain
1	DSCR6	53820	Unknown	[171]	Yes
1	PIGP	51227	Enzyme	[172]	Yes
1	TTC3	7267	E3 ligase	See main text	Yes
1	DSCR3	10311	Unknown	[173]	Yes
1	DYRK1A	1859	Protein kinase	See main text	Yes
1-2	KCNJ6	3763	Channel	See main text	
1-2	DSCR4	10281	Unknown	[174]	
1-2	DSCR8	84677	Unknown	[175]	
1-2	KCNJ15	3772	Channel	[176]	
1-2	ERG	2078	Transcription factor	See main text	Yes
1-2	ETS2	2114	Transcription factor	See main text	Yes
2	PSMG1	8624	Chaperone	[177]	Yes
2	BRWD1	54014	Transcription factor	See main text	Yes
2	HMGN1	3150	Transcription factor	See main text	Yes
2	WRB	7485	Protein trafficking	[178]	Yes
2	LCA5L	150082	Ciliary protein	[179]	
2	SH3BGR	6450	Unknown	No information	Yes
2	B3GALT5	10317	Enzyme	[180]	
2	C21orf88	114041	Unknown	No information	Yes
2	IGSF5	150084	Adhesion molecule	[181]	
2	PCP4	5121	Unknown	[182]	Yes
2	DSCAM	1826	Adhesion molecule	[183]	
2	BACE2	25825	Protease	See main text	Yes
2	FAM3B	54097	Cytokine	[184]	
2	MX2	4600	Unknown	[185]	
2	MX1	4599	Unknown	[185]	Yes

Table 1. Summary of the protein-coding genes contained by the DSCR. The first column indicates whether the genes belong to the DCR-1, to the DCR-2 or to the overlap region. The evidence for expression in adult brain is derived from the EVOC data [186] contained in the Ensembl genome browser. Genes are given in their physical order, starting from the more centromeric sequence.

http://dx.doi.org/10.5772/53000

DCR	Gene Name	Ensembl ID	Entrez Gene ID	HSA21 coordinates	Gene Biotype	Evidence of expression (EST)
1	LINC00160	ENSG00000230978	54064	36096105 - 36109478	lincRNA	
1	AP000330.8	ENSG00000234380	100506385	36118054 - 36157183	Antisense	
1	AF015262.2	ENSG00000234703		36508935 - 36511519	lincRNA	+
1	RPL34P3	ENSG00000223671	54026	36844395 - 36844730	Pseudogene	+
1	EZH2P1	ENSG00000231300	266693	36972030 - 36972320	Pseudogene	
1	AF015720.3	ENSG00000230794		37085437 - 37105240	processed transcript	+
1	MIR802	ENSG00000211590	768219	37093013 - 37093106	miRNA	
1	RPS20P1	ENSG00000229761	54025	37097045 - 37097398	Pseudogene	
1	PPP1R2P2	ENSG00000234008	54036	37259493 - 37260105	Pseudogene	
1	AP000688.8	ENSG00000231106		37377636 - 37379899	lincRNA	+
1	RPL23AP3	ENSG00000214914	8489	37388377 - 37388844	Pseudogene	++
1	RIMKLBP1	ENSG00000189089	54031	37422512 - 37423675	Pseudogene	
1	AP000688.11	ENSG00000236677		37432730 - 37436706	Antisense	+
1	U6	ENSG00000200213	1497008	37438843 - 37438950	snRNA	
1	AP000688.14	ENSG00000230212	100133286	37441940 - 37498938	sense intronic	
1	AP000688.15	ENSG00000236119		37455157 - 37462712	lincRNA	+
1	AP000688.29	ENSG00000233393		37477179 - 37481988	lincRNA	+
1	MEMO1P1	ENSG00000226054	728556	37502669 - 37504208	Pseudogene	
1	CBR3-AS1	ENSG00000236830	100506428	37504065 - 37528605	lincRNA	
1	RPS9P1	ENSG00000214889	8410	37504748 - 37505330	Pseudogene	
1	RPL3P1	ENSG00000228149	8488	37541268 - 37542478	Pseudogene	
1	Metazoa_SRP	ENSG00000265882		37585858 - 37586136	miscellaneous RNA	
1	snoU13	ENSG00000238851		37630724 - 37630829	snoRNA	
1	SRSF9P1	ENSG00000214867	54021	37667471 - 37668000	Pseudogene	
1	AP000692.9	ENSG00000228107		37732928 - 37734338	processed transcript	+
1	ATP5J2LP	ENSG00000224421	54100	37761176 - 37761410	Pseudogene	
1	AP000695.6	ENSG00000230479		37802658 - 37853368	Antisense	+
1	AP000695.4	ENSG00000233818		37818029 - 37904706	Antisense	
1	PSMD4P1	ENSG00000223741	54035	37858281 - 37859709	Pseudogene	+
1	AP000696.2	ENSG00000231324		38004979 - 38009331	lincRNA	++
1	AP000697.6	ENSG00000224269		38071073 - 38073864	Antisense	+
1	HLCS-IT1	ENSG00000237646	100874294	38176285 - 38178585	sense intronic	++
1	RN5S491	ENSG00000199806	100873733	38224211 - 38224328	rRNA	
1	AP000704.5	ENSG00000224790		38338812 - 38344128	lincRNA	++
1	Y_RNA	ENSG00000207416		38359039 - 38359151	miscellaneous RNA	
1	MRPL20P1	ENSG00000215734	359737	38366943 - 38367375	Pseudogene	
1	U6	ENSG00000212136	1497008	38417830 - 38417936	snRNA	
1	TTC3-AS1	ENSG00000228677	100874006	38559967 - 38566227	Antisense	++
1	DSCR9	ENSG00000230366	257203	38580804 - 38594037	lincRNA	

DCR	Gene Name	Ensembl ID	Entrez Gene ID	HSA21 coordinates	Gene Biotype	Evidence of expression (EST)
1	Metazoa_SRP	ENSG00000263969		38587906 - 38588202	miscellaneous RNA	
1	AP001432.14	ENSG00000242553		38593720 - 38610045	lincRNA	+
1-2	KCNJ6-IT1	ENSG00000233213	100874329	39089405 - 39091872	sense intronic	+
1-2	AP001427.1	ENSG00000264691		39334968 - 39335068	miRNA	+
1-2	DSCR4-IT1	ENSG00000223608	100874327	39378846 - 39382920	sense intronic	+
1-2	snoU13	ENSG00000238581		39559551 - 39559656	snoRNA	
1-2	DSCR10	ENSG00000233316	259234	39578250 - 39580738	lincRNA	
1-2	AP001434.2	ENSG00000226012		39609139 - 39610123	lincRNA	+
1-2	SPATA20P1	ENSG00000231123	100874060	39610149 - 39610586	Pseudogene	
1-2	AP001422.3	ENSG00000231231		39695557 - 39705343	lincRNA	++
1-2	SNRPGP13	ENSG00000231480	100874428	39874369 - 39874545	Pseudogene	
1-2	LINC00114	ENSG00000223806	400866	40110825 - 40140898	lincRNA	
2	AP001042.1	ENSG00000229986		40218171 - 40220568	lincRNA	
2	AF064858.6	ENSG00000205622	400867	40249215 - 40328392	lincRNA	
2	AP001043.1	ENSG00000229925		40260696 - 40275829	processed transcript	+
2	SNORA62	ENSG00000252384		40266709 - 40266791	snoRNA	
2	RPSAP64	ENSG00000227721		40266841 - 40267176	Pseudogene	
2	AP001044.2	ENSG00000234035		40285093 - 40287072	lincRNA	+
2	AF064858.7	ENSG00000232837		40346355 - 40349700	lincRNA	+
2	AF064858.8	ENSG00000235888		40360633 - 40378079	lincRNA	+
2	AF064858.11	ENSG00000237721		40378574 - 40383255	lincRNA	+
2	AF064858.10	ENSG00000237609		40400461 - 40401053	lincRNA	+
2	RPL23AP12	ENSG00000228861	391282	40499494 - 40499966	Pseudogene	+
2	PCBP2P1	ENSG00000235701	54040	40543056 - 40544032	Pseudogene	
2	TIMM9P2	ENSG00000232608	100862727	40588550 - 40589432	Pseudogene	
2	BRWD1-IT1	ENSG00000237373		40589019 - 40591731	processed transcript	+
2	METTL21AP1	ENSG00000229623	100421629	40607312 - 40607946	Pseudogene	
2	BRWD1-AS1	ENSG00000238141	100874093	40687633 - 40695144	Antisense	+
2	Y_RNA	ENSG00000252915		40716463 - 40716554	miscellaneous RNA	
2	snoU13	ENSG00000238556		40717300 - 40717383	snoRNA	
2	RNF6P1	ENSG00000227406	100420924	40745689 - 40748992	Pseudogene	
2	MYL6P2	ENSG00000235808	100431168	40860253 - 40860686	Pseudogene	++
2	RPS26P4	ENSG00000228349	692146	40863470 - 40863824	Pseudogene	+
2	AF121897.4	ENSG00000235012		40897510 - 40901782	Pseudogene	
2	AF064860.5	ENSG00000225330		41002198 - 41098012	processed transcript	+
2	AF064860.7	ENSG00000231713		41099682 - 41102607	lincRNA	+
2	MIR4760	ENSG00000263973	100616148	41584279 - 41584358	miRNA	
2	DSCAM-AS1	ENSG00000235123	100506492	41755010 - 41757285	Antisense	
2	SNORA51	ENSG00000207147		41885071 - 41885206	snoRNA	

DCR	Gene Name	Ensembl ID	Entrez Gene ID	HSA21 coordinates	Gene Biotype	Evidence of expression (EST)
2	AF064863.1	ENSG00000221396		41949429 - 41949538	miRNA	+
2	DSCAM-IT1	ENSG00000233756	100874326	41987304 - 42002693	sense intronic	++
2	YRDCP3	ENSG00000230859	100861429	42235920 - 42236399	Pseudogene	
2	LINC00323	ENSG00000226496	284835	42513427 - 42520060	Antisense	
2	MIR3197	ENSG00000263681	100423023	42539484 - 42539556	miRNA	
2	AL773572.7	ENSG00000225745		42548249 - 42558715	processed transcript	++
2	BACE2-IT1	ENSG00000224388	282569	42552024 - 42552553	Antisense	+
2	AP001610.5	ENSG00000228318		42813321 - 42814669	Antisense	+

Table 2. Summary of the non-protein-coding elements contained by the DSCR. The first column indicates whether the genes belong to the DCR-1, to the DCR-2 or to the overlap region. Elements are given in their physical order, starting from the more centromeric sequence. Genomic coordinates refer to the HG19 version of the human genome sequence. The evidence for expression is derived from the ESTs linked to the Ensembl genome browser. + = at least one EST sequence supporting the Ensemble prediction. ++ prediction supported by several EST sequences.

2. Functional analysis of the DSCR through mouse models

Animal models are essential to understand the molecular pathogenesis of DS. Moreover, although none of them can faithfully mimic the human situation, they are crucial for the preclinical development of new therapeutic strategies. The availability of sophisticated tools for mouse genetics and the conserved synteny between mouse chromosome 16 (MMU16) and HSA21 have provided the basis for the development of many mouse models of DS, allowing to test the critical region concept and to perform a genetic dissection of the complex DS phenotype.

The first mouse models have been obtained by studying the effects of partial trisomies of MMU16 derived from Robertsonian translocations. These mice live until adulthood and show many clinical phenotypes similar to DS patients, in particular the neuropathological and neurobiological alterations, including learning and behavioral abnormalities [22-25]. The most studied mouse model for DS is theTs65Dn mouse, which possesses an extra copy of the distal 13 Mbp part of MMU16, including ~ 104 mouse genes orthologous to those on HSA21 [23]. These mice show a number of developmental and functional parallels with DS, including craniofacial abnormalities and behavioural changes [26-32]. Moreover, they show alterations in the structure of dendritic spines in cortex and hippocampus [33] and reduced long-term potentiation (LTP) in the hippocampus and fascia dentata (FD) [34-36].

Ts1Cje mice, which are trisomic for a shorter but fully overlapping segment of MMU16 (~81 genes), show similar changes, usually to a lesser degree [24,25,37,38]. Comparison of the behavioral performances of the Ts1Cje and Ts65Dn showed that the learning deficits of Ts1Cje mice are similar to those of Ts65Dn. The data obtained from these models strongly supported the concept of DSCR, because they indicated that conserved genes are capable to influence cognition through their dosage lie in a region spanning from Sod1 to Mx1, which contains the mouse counterpart of the human DCR-1.

Probably, the most elegant studies that have addressed the role of the mouse genome region syntenic to the human DSCR are those undertaken by Roger H. Reeves and coworkers. Using chromosome engineering, this group has generated a mouse line referred to as Ts1Rhr, trisomic for a segment closely corresponding to the DCR-1 region, as defined by [10] and [11] and including 33 genes [39]. Moreover, they obtained the corresponding deletion, resulting in the monosomic line Ms1Rhr. Interestingly, the first results produced by the analysis of these models did not confirm strongly the DSCR hypothesis. Indeed, the craniofacial dysmorphologies of Ts1Rhr are less marked and distinct from those detected in Ts65Dn and Ts1Cje mice [39]. Furthermore, no differences were initially detected between Ts1Rhr and normal controls in the Morris water maze, in the induction of LTP in the hippocampal CA1 Region and in the hippocampal and in cerebellum volume [39-41]. These results seemed to suggest that triplication of the Ts1Rhr segment is not sufficient to produce these correlates of DS phenotypes. However, the intercross of the monosomic line Ms1Rhr with the Ds65Dn line, which restored in a disomic condition for DCR-1 genes, generated mice showing normal performances in the Morris water maze, indicating that trisomy of DCR-1 is necessary for these cognitive phenotypes [41]. Importantly, a more recent report established that, if the Ts1Rhr mutation is analyzed on the same genetic background of the Ts65Dn and Ts1Cje mice and with more stringent tests, important cognitive and synaptic neurobiological phenotypes can be detected [42]. In particular, 20 of 48 phenotypes, many of which are shared with Ts65Dn mice, distinguished Ts1Rhr animals from their 2N controls. In addition to the genetic background difference, it must be noticed that the task used in this work was less stressful and more sensitive than the water maze, which may further account for the initial discrepancy [42]. These phenotypes were correlated with changes in synaptic density and in dendritic spine morphology, further indicating that DCR-1 genes strongly contribute to these abnormalities [42]. In conclusion, taken together, these results provide strong support to the view that increased dosage of DCR1 genes is necessary and sufficient to confer to mice some of the neurobiological phenotypes characteristic of DS.

The use of mouse genetic tools has allowed the production of even more restricted models, addressing the role of specific subregions of the human or mouse DSCR, or even the role of single DSCR genes. For instance, the isolation from the DSCR of huge genomic clones maintained as Yeast Artificial Chromosomes (YAC) or as Bacterial Artificial Chromosomes (BAC) and their microinjection in mouse oocytes has allowed the generation of transgenic lines covering the entire length of the human DSCR [43-45]. The characterization of these mice has shown that the approach can be very useful to study the function of specific genes. However, it became also clear that this strategy is of limited usefulness to establish genes contribution to the phenotype. For instance, BAC transgenesis allowed the production of a mouse line carrying a single extra copy of the DYRK1A gene [46]. Interestingly, these mice showed impaired cognitive behaviours, but they were characterized by increased hippocampal LTP, while all the models discussed above show depressed hippocampal LTP [46]. The same conclusion applies even better to the models obtained through classical transgenesis approaches, in which a single human or mouse gene is inserted in the mouse genome in the form of a cDNA driven by a non-physiological promoter [47].

On the other hand, the combination of gene targeting technologies with the "classical" DS model discussed above allows a subtractive strategy, providing the most stringent test to address the relevance of single genes for the overall phenotype. Indeed, once a null allele for a DSCR gene is available, a compound mutant can be generated, carrying the specific mutation in a trisomic background. The subtractive approach allowed to detect a significant rescue of the phenotype in the case of some DS-related genes, belonging to the DSCR as in the case of DSCR1[48], Olig1 and Olig2 [49], or even external to it, as in the case of APP [50,51].

3. Functional role of DSCR genes in DS intellectual disability: Towards the identification of drugable pathways

In the following section we will summarize the most relevant functional information available on DSCR genes, trying to especially underscore their implication in molecular networks relevant to intellectual disability. As it is obvious from the previous sections, this discussion will involve not only genes that strictly belong to the DSCR, but also their interactions with other HSC21 genes, whose functional involvement is supported by abundant literature. In particular, we will try to discuss as much as possible the single DSCR genes on the basis of their common features. The essential information about genes not included in this section is reported in Tables 1 and 2. While deploying this summary, we will also provide a perspective of how this information can be useful for progressing towards the development of new therapeutic strategies that may take into account the complex nature of DS.

3.1. Pathogenesis of intellectual disability in DS

In order to evaluate the possible degree of functional involvement for specific genes, it is very important to briefly analyze the principal biological processes that have been to cognitive impairment in the DS. To this regard, studies performed both in humans and in animal models have shown that trisomy 21 leads to an unbalance of key cellular events, such as neuronal cell proliferation and differentiation, which can be detected during development and post-natal life using morphological methods [52,53]. Importantly, these defects may coexist with or may be causally related to functional deficits, that can be revealed using sophisticated physiological methods [52,53]. Reduced neurons number is found in cortex, hippocampus and cerebellum of DS brain and are accompanied by impaired neuronal function. Brain hypocellularity is acquired during early developmental stages and is paralleled by impaired cognitive development leading to intellectual disabilities. Further deterioration of cognitive abilities occurs in adolescence and adulthood, possibly due to degenerative mechanisms [28]. Although the syndrome invariably results in AD-like neuropathology, the actual onset of dementia is quite variable. The availability of genetic models of trisomy 21 has been instrumental in gaining insights into the pathogenic mechanisms leading to DS cognitive disability. Morphological abnormalities of neuronal dendritic compartment are paralleled by functional electrophysiological deficits and impairment of learning and memory, pointing to the existence of defective neural network connectivity and faulty neuronal communication as primary determinants of DS cognitive disabilities [34-38,42,54]. Such pathological scenario arises from a combination of neurodevelopmental abnormalities and neurodegenerative processes. Addressing which processes are irreversible and which ones can be prevented or reverted by manipulating genes and pathways is of paramount importance for the development of new therapeutic strategies. Although the crossover between neurogenesis dysfunction and neurodegeneration is still poorly understood, it is likely that common pathways differentially affect various cellular functions during development and aging. Thus, the developmental aspects are fundamental in defining the most important functional consequences of the genetic imbalance in DS at the cognitive level. However, the IQ of DS patients decreases in the first decade of life, indicating that the maturation of central nervous system is compromised [8]. Indeed, on one side, different observations suggest that neurogenesis impairment starting from the earliest stages of development may underlie the widespread brain atrophy of DS, the delayed and disorganized lamination in the DS fetal cortex [55] and hippocampal hypoplasia [56]. On the other, postmortem studies show that DS patients start their lives with an apparently normal neuronal architecture that progressively degenerates. During the peak period of dendritic growth and differentiation (2.5 months old infants), no significant differences were detected in dendritic differentiation between euploid and DS cases in pyramidal neurons of prefrontal cortex [57]. Similarly, DS infants younger than 6 months showed greater dendritic branching and length than normal infants [58] [59] in contrast to the reduced number of dendrites and degenerative changes in DS children older than two years [60].

3.2. Transcription factors and co-factors encoded by the DSCR

The DSCR contains 6 genes encoding for transcription factors (Table 1), which are likely to play crucial roles in determining DS phenotypes, considering their potential to affect many cellular networks. Two of them, ERG and ETS2 belong to the erythroblast transformation-specific (ETS) family. Members of this family are key regulators of embryonic development, cell proliferation, differentiation, angiogenesis, inflammation, and apoptosis [61]. ERG is required for vascular cell remodeling and hematopoesis [62,63], while ETS2 has been linked to thymocytes development and apoptosis [64]. Together with RUNX1 [65], these proteins are very likely to contribute to the hematological abnormalities that characterize DS, but not to contribute significantly to ID. In contrast, BRWD1 and HGMN1 are two proteins highly expressed in brain that is involved in chromatin-remodeling [66,67]. Importantly, HGMN1 has been found to regulate the expression of the ID gene MeCP2 [67]. Under the same perspective, another interesting candidate is the bHLH factor SIM2 that together with its paralog SIM1 is the homolog of *Drosophila* single-minded (sim) gene. The *Drosophila* sim gene encodes a transcription factor that is a master regulator of fruit fly neurogenesis [68], raising the possibility that SIM2 could perform a similar function in mammals. However, a role of SIM2 in mammalian neurogenesis has not been so far confirmed, while this gene has been shown to repress myogenesis in mouse [69]. Besides to directly regulating transcription, DSCR genes could strongly modulate the activity of transcription factors encoded by other loci. The best characterized example is RCAN1, which was initially named DSCR1 [70]. The gene name was then changed after realizing that the encoded protein inhibits calcineurin-dependent transcriptional responses by binding to the catalytic domain of calcineurin A and interfering with the phosphorylation of the NFAT transcription factor [71,72]. RCAN1 is overexpressed in DS brain [14,73] and seems to play a key role in the regulation of mitochondrial function and oxidative stress. Indeed, the *Drosophila* homolog of RCAN1 especially affects the activity of the mitochondrial ADP/ATP translocator [74]. Moreover, it has been shown that, when RCAN1 is overexpressed in PC12 cells, it induces the expression of superoxide dismutase type 1 (SOD1) [75], which is encoded by another HSA21 gene [15] and is upregulated in DS brain [76]. Importantly, RCAN1 acts as a stress response element: its acute overexpression protects cells from oxidative stress [77]. Indeed, RCAN1 overexpression may have beneficial effects by counteracting the oxidative damage associated with DS. Elevated levels of DNA damage, lipid peroxidation [78] and pro-oxidant state develop early in life in DS subjects [79]. Nevertheless, it is very likely that the benefits arising from these actions on oxidative stress may be overcome by the long-term detrimental effects on synaptic functions and neuronal survival due to the chronic RCAN1 overexpression, which will be discussed in sections 3.4 and 3.5.

3.3. Signaling proteins encoded by the DSCR

Modifications of the cellular cytoskeleton in response to extracellular stimuli, such as growth factor engagement and cell-cell contacts are essential for neuronal proliferation, for the formation of axons and Dendrites, for the differentiation and for the establishment, maintenance and remodeling of neuronal connections. Many of the well-characterized DSCR genes, such as DSCAM, CLDN14, PIGP, LCA5L, IGSF5 and FAM3B are implicated in these processes. However, the best characterized proteins belonging to this category are DYRK1A and TTC3.

3.3.1. DYRK1A

DYRK1A, dual-specificity tyrosine-phosphorilation-regulated kinase1A, encodes a protein kinase capable to phosphorylate serine, threonine and tyrosine residues, highly conserved at the aminoacidic level across vertebrates and invertebrates [80]. The orthologus *Drosophila* gene is involved in neuroblast proliferation and it is named *minibrain* (MNB), because null mutations affect post-embrionic neurogenesis, resulting in reduced brain size [81]. The highly conserved structure of this kinase and its mapping to the DSCR prompted extensive studies on its vertebrate homologues [82]. These studies have revealed that the dosage of DYRK1A is extremely important to normal brain development. Indeed, mice homozygous for a null mutation of DYRK1A die early in development and even heterozygous mice display reduced viability and a smaller brain, characterized by reduction of neuronal counts in specific regions [83]. Accordingly, truncation of the human MNB/DYRK1A gene has been reported to cause microcephaly [84,27]. Furthermore transgenic mice overexpressing DYRK1A show severe impairment in spatial learning and memory in the Morris water maze tests, indicating hippocampal and prefrontal cortical function alteration [45,85]. Moreover, these transgenic mice show abnormal LTP and LTD, indicating synaptic plasticity alterations [46]. These defects are similar to those found in murine models of DS with trisomy of chromosome 16, suggesting a causative role of DYRK1A in cognitive disorders present in DS patients. DYRK1A is expressed in the cortex, in the hippocampus and in the cerebellum [86,18] and is overexpressed in the mouse trisomic model Ts65Dn [87], in DS fetal brain and other trisomic tissues [88]. These data obtained from different experimental systems have revealed various possible functions of DYRK1A in central nervous system (CNS) development, including its influence on proliferation, neurogenesis, neuronal differentiation, cell death and synaptic plasticity [46, 89-92]. These multiple biological functions of DYRK1A are due to its interactions with numerous cytoskeletal, synaptic and nuclear proteins, including transcription and splicing factors [93]. Together with other studies [85,94-96], these data strongly support the involvement of Dyrk1A in several neuropathological phenotypes and in the cognitive deficits that characterize Down syndrome. More recently, the observation that DYRK1A is overexpressed in the adult DS brain [97] implicated this protein also in the DS neurodegenerative phenotype. In particular, DYRK1A overexpression appears to be the cause of gene dosage-dependent modifications of several mechanisms that may contribute to the early onset of neurofibrillary degeneration. In fact, it has been demonstrated that Dyrk1A phosphorylates tau at several sites *in vitro* [98] and such sites are phosphorylated in DS brain [99]. Dyrk1A-induced tau phosphorylation inhibits the biological activity of tau, primes it for further phosphorylation by glycogen synthetase-3β (GSK- 3β) and promotes its self-aggregation into neurofibrillary tangles (NFTs) [99]. Interestingly, besides to phosphorylating protein, DYRK1A also colocalizes with NFTs [100]. In addition, neuropathological and molecular studies indicate that overexpressed nuclear DYRK1A contributes to the modification of the alternative splicing of Tau leading to neurofibrillary degeneration [101,102]. Neurofibrillary degeneration is the leading cause of neuronal death and dementia in Alzheimer's disease (AD) and in DS/AD. The multi-pathway involvement of DYRK1A in neurofibrillary degeneration indicates that therapeutic inhibition of the activity of overexpressed DYRK1A may delay the age of onset and inhibit the progression of neurodegeneration in DS. To this regard, the studies recently performed by the group of Delabar [103] represent, arguably, the best example of how the functional knowledge about DSCR genes can be translated into new potential therapeutic strategy. Indeed, this research group has found that Epigallocatechin gallate (EGCG) - a member of a natural polyphenols family, found in great amount in green tea leaves - is a specific and safe DYRK1A inhibitor and that its administration can revert the brain defects induced by overexpression of DYRK1A [103]. Together with a previous report showing that EGCG administration may beneficially affect the LTP abnormalities detected in Ts65Dn mice [104], this study paved the way for the promotion of clinical trials, which are already in Phase 2 (see for instance http://clinicaltrials.gov/ct2/show/NCT01394796).

3.3.2. *TTC3*

Since its discovery in 1996, the TTC3 gene has been considered an important candidate for the CNS-related phenotypes that characterize DS, because of its mapping within the DSCR [105,106]. This hypothesis was further supported by the analysis of TTC3 expression during normal development. Indeed, during mouse and human brain embryogenesis, TTC3 expression shows regional and cellular specificities well correlated with the anatomical defects observed in DS patients [55,107]. In particular, TTC3 is expressed at highest levels in the post-mitotic areas of central nervous system (CNS), suggesting a role in neuronal cell differentiation [108,109]. Moreover, it has been reported that the expression of TTC3 is increased in tissues and in cells derived from DS experimental models [110] and from DS individuals [111,112]. In 2007, on the basis of both overexpression and knockdown experiments performed in PC12 neuroblastoma cells, we demonstrated that the TTC3 protein may play a pivotal role in regulating the differentiation program of neuronal cells, starting from the earliest stages [113]. More specifically, increased TTC3 function strongly prevents the neurite sprouting normally elicited by NGF-treatment, while TTC3 knockdown increases neurite length [113]. Importantly, TTC3 may affect not only the generation of neuronal processes, but also their maintenance (Berto et al., unpublished)., and its effects on neuronal differentiation are mediated by the activation of a specific pathway comprising the master cytoskeletal regulator RhoA and its effettor proteins, namely Citron-isoforms [113] Rho kinases (ROCKs) and LIM-kinase (Berto et al., in preparation), which have been implicated in all the different aspects of the neuronal differentiation program [114] and in different aspect of cognitive disorders [115]. Importantly, specific inhibitors of ROCKs, such as Fasudil, have been already approved by FDA, and therefore represent ideal candidates for testing in the experimental models [116]. In addition, a recent report by the group of Dr. M. Noguchi has shown that TTC3 can down-modulate the activity of the Akt kinases (AKTs), by promoting their ubiquitination and degradation [111]. This observation is particularly important, not only because AKTs have been shown to regulate neuronal survival [117], axonogenesis [118], dendritogenesis and synaptogenesis [119], but especially because these proteins are effectors of the PI3K pathway, which is the subject of extensive pharmacological investigation, in light of its centrality in cancer and inflammation research [120,121].

3.4. Gene networks affecting the excitatory-inhibitory balance in DS

The majority of forebrain is comprised of excitatory glutamatergic projection neurons and approximately 10% inhibitory γ-amminobutyric acid (GABA) interneurons. The normal functioning of the neural networks underlying cognitive functions depend on a finely-tuned balance of excitatory and inhibitory activities [122]. Accordingly, different reports have supported the possibility that cognitive impairment in DS models can be related to specific alterations of the excitatory/inhibitory balance, which may result from the direct action of DSCR genes or from more indirect mechanisms. For instance, it has been hypothesized that the increased dosage of HSA21 gene could favor the excitatory inputs in the hippocampus by increasing the activity of N-methyl-D-aspartate (NMDA) receptor (NMDAR), with potential effects on synaptic plasticity and neuron survival [123]. This theory was based on the observation that that several HSA21 genes, such as APP, SOD1, RCAN1 and DYRK1A, directly interact or indirectly affect the activity of the NMDARs. The best characterized pathway is that involving RCAN1, which regulates NMDARs by directly binding and inhibiting the calcineurin protein phosphatase (CaN) [71,77,124]. NMDARs are CaN targets [125] [126] and CaN inhibition leads to increased NMDARs [127] activity, by decreasing channel open probability and mean time [127]. On this basis Costa and co-workers hypothesized that the noncompetitive NMDA antagonist memantine, which acts as open channel blocker and is currently approved for AD therapy, could mimic the actions of CaN and restore normal NMDARs function, possibly improving learning and memory [123]. Indeed, memantine ameliorates contextual fear conditioning learning in 4–6- and 10–14-month old Ts65Dn mice when administered at 5 mg/kg by acute intraperitoneal injection before context exposure. Despite these studies, a recently published clinical trial reported that memantine is not an effective pharmacological treatment for cognitive decline or dementia in DS patients who are above 40 years old [128]. This suggests that therapies that are effective in DS models and in AD patients may not necessarily confer benefits in DS.

More consistent reports have shown that the LTP phenotypes and the reduced performance in cognitive tests observed in mouse models could be the result of excessive GABA-ergic responses, producing a net decrease of synaptic output [36,37,129]. This phenomenon could be a direct effect of the overexpression of at least three proteins encoded by the DSCR, namely the chloride channel CLIC6 and the rectifying potassium channels KCNJ6 and KCNJ15. Accordingly, primary hippocampal neurons derived from Ts65Dn mice display a significant increase in GABA-mediated GIRK currents, consistent with the increased expression of KCNJ6/GIRK2 [130]. However, some of the data are also consistent with an increased presynaptic availability of GABA [129], produced by undefined and probably indirect mechanisms. On this basis, several pharmacological interventions have been proposed to restore the excitatory-inhibitory imbalance by decreasing the excessive inhibition of GABAergic neurotransmission prevalent in DS mouse models [131]. In particular, Ts65Dn mice have been treated with non-competitive $GABA_A$ antagonists, pentylenetetrazol (PTZ) and picrotoxin (PTX), which inhibit $GABA_A$ receptors. Chronic treatment with PTZ reversed the deficits seen in the novel object recognition task (NORT) and spontaneous alternation tasks in Ts65Dn mice [129,132]. Surprisingly, the improvement in cognition and LTP was sustained for up to 2 months after initial treatment, suggesting a long-lasting effect on neuronal circuit modification. Chronic treatment with PTZ for 8 weeks in Ts65Dn mice did not modify sensorimotor abilities and locomotor activity in home cages. However it did rescue learning and memory performance in the Morris water maze (MWM) task [133]. Recently, chronic treatment in Ts65Dn mice with an inverse agonist selective for the $\alpha5$ subunit of the $GABA_A$ benzodiazepine receptor (α5IA) improved cognitive deficits in the MWM and normalized Sod1 overexpression with an enhancement in learning-evoked immediate early genes expression levels [134]. Encouraged by this body of evidence, Roche, a healthcare company, recently announced the commencement of a trial to examine the cognitive impact of reducing GABA-ergic neurotransmission in the hippocampus using a drug selective for the $\alpha5$ subunit of $GABA_A$ receptors (http://www.roche-trials.com).

Finally, the imbalance in excitatory/inhibitory ratio could be the result of abnormal neurogenesis. Indeed, reduced cell numbers in the DS hippocampus could be caused by impaired adult neurogenesis, which has been observed in Ts65Dn [135] [136] and Ts1Cje mice [137]. Therefore, approaches targeting neurogenesis seem very promising for DS therapy. Interestingly, a fascinating connection has been documented between the DSCR gene KCNJ6 and adult neurogenesis, mediated by serotonin signaling. DS has long been associated with defects in the serotonergic system [138]. In particular, the serotonin 5-HT1A receptor expression peaks earlier in developing DS brains and decreases to below normal levels by birth [139]. Moreover reduced 5-HT levels are present in adults with DS [140]. Since 5-HT depletion causes a permanent reduction in neuron number in the adult brain [138], it is conceivable that alterations in the serotonergic systems during early life stages may contribute to the reduced neurogenesis of the DS brain. Activity of the serotonin receptor 1A (5HTR1A) is required for adult neurogenesis in the hippocampus [141] and is mediated by the potassium channel KCNJ6. Overexpression of KCNJ6, as in the Ts65Dn, may over-inhibit presynaptic 5HTR1A, causing reduced levels of serotonin. Fluoxetine, an antidepressant that inhibits serotonin (5-HT) reuptake, inhibits KCNJ6 and increases presynaptic levels of serotonin. Consistent with this, it has been already demonstrated that fluoxetine is able to rescue neurogenesis in the adult Ts65Dn [135]. Recently, treatment during the early postnatal period restored neurogenesis and the total number of neurons in the dentate gyrus. This effect was accompanied by the full recovery of a cognitive task [142]. The releance of these data is even greater if considering that fluoxetin is an antidepressant widely used by adults and prescribed in children and adolescents [143] and that it does not seem to have negative effects on post-natal development [144].

3.5. The DSCR and Alzheimer-related molecular networks

Most DS patients experience a decline in cognition during adulthood, followed by the development of classical Alzheimer's disease (AD) neuropathology, characterized by the accumulation of amyloid plaques containing high levels of the A-beta fragments of the APP protein, by neurofibrillary tangles containing high levels of hyperphosphorylated Tau protein and by massive neurodegeneration [145]. Increased dosage of the APP gene, which is located outside the DSCR, is very likely the most important factor that underlies this phenomenon [146]. Indeed, increased dosage of APP is sufficient to strongly increase the risk of AD, since APP gene duplication has been detected as the mutation responsible for some early-onset familial cases of AD [147]. The link between AD and the APP gene has been further strengthened by the finding that an extra copy of APP seems to be necessary for the development of AD in DS. Indeed, it has been reported the case of an old patient affected by DS but not showing any signs of dementia [148]. At autopsy, plaques and tangles were absent in the brain of this individual. The patient had a segmental trisomy HSA21, not including the APP gene [148]. These data strongly support that the early onset of AD pathology in DS is in part due to overexpression of the APP gene. The data obtained from experimental models further support the crucial role of APP in DS [51]. Indeed, it has been shown that APP overexpression in Ts65Dn impairs the retrograde transport of nerve growth factor (NGF) from the hippocampus to the basal forebrain, causing the degeneration of BFCN [51], which significantly degenerates in Ts65Dn. Importantly, APP is one of the few genes for which a successful subtractive genetic approach has been reported, since restoring APP gene dosage to two copies in the Ts65Dn model corrected the water maze phenotype and prevented BFCN degeneration [50,51]. Finally, APP-mediated pathological mechanism may also contribute to the developmental abnormalities detected in mouse models, since it has been suggested that APP overexpression can result in increased Notch signaling pathway, which is crucial for neuronal and glial differentiation [149]. However, it is conceivable that also some of the DSCR genes may cooperate with APP in accelerating the AD-related neuropathological phenotypes observed in DS patients. In particular BACE2 could promote the beta-cleavage of APP, further increasing the amount of generated A-beta peptides [150-152]. DYRK1A can also play an important role, because it can stimulate the phosphorylation of APP and Tau, resulting in increased cleavage and aggregation, respectively [98,153]. Finally, Tau hyperphosphorylation can be stimulated by increased expression of RCAN1, since phosphorylated Tau is one of the substrates of calcineurin [154]. Moreover, it has been shown that this activity of RCAN1 can be modulated by DYRK1A [155] Therefore it is very likely that the development of new approaches aimed at targeting these proteins could turn out to be beneficial both for AD and for DS management.

3.6. DSCR-dependent RNA-networks

As it is generally the case for the human genome, besides to protein coding genes, the DSCR contains many sequences that have been so far almost completely neglected, because they are not predicted to encode for proteins [16]. However, as we show in Table 2, on the basis of the current knowledge, many of these loci display features indicating that they could be functionally relevant and could contribute to the pathogenesis of DS phenotypes. Indeed, besides to the two copies of snRNAs and five copies of snoRNAs associated to splicing factors, the DSCR contains many regions that are transcribed to produce processed transcripts, devoid of coding potential. Some of these sequences, such as antisense transcripts, processed pseudogenes and sequences located in proximity of promoters, are closely associated to functioning genes, and could be involved in their regulation, as it has been shown in many other cases [156-158]. In many other cases, the genes appear to produce llincRNAs, that could act in cis to modify chromatin structure, or in trans to modify gene expression at the transcriptional and post transcriptional level, as it has been shown in the cases of HOTAIR [159] and of LincRNA-p21 [160,161]. Although the function of these molecules is at the moment completely unknown, their study could be extremely interesting. Indeed many of these sequences have been implicated in the epigenetic and in the post-transcriptional control of gene expression. Moreover, since these sequences diverge much more rapidly than the sequences of protein-coding genes, it is very likely that they could be strongly implicated in the control of human-specific features and phenotypes. Therefore, it seems reasonable to anticipate that the functional study of lincRNA-encoding genes in DS models and the study of their variation in humans will be a fertile ground for future research. Finally, the DSCR contains at least three genes encoding miRNA precursors (probably five, if considering also those that have only been predicted). Interestingly, mir-802, which is encoded by the DSCR, and mir-155, which is located on HSA21 in a more centromeric position, have been shown to repress the expression of MeCP2 [162], whose inactivation is the cause of Rett syndrome. Since MeCP2 is also repressed by HMGN1, this study further underscore the potential relevance of MeCP2 repression in DS and provides a very interesting example of how the intertwining of transcription and post-transcriptional regulatory networks dependent on DSCR genes can produce intellectual disability. Considering the reported reversibility of MeCP2 downregulation phenotypes [163] and the great efforts that are being dedicated to identify drugable pathways downstream of MeCP2 [164], it is conceivable that the functional exploration of these networks in DS could be also relevant for the development of future therapies.

http://dx.doi.org/10.5772/53000

4. Concluding remarks

Functional information on HSA21 genes is still quite partial and mostly limited to a subset of protein-coding genes. However, the recent success in DS models of therapeutic strategies targeted either on specific DSCR genes, or even on much broader mechanisms, justifies to our opinion an optimistic view of the future. In particular, we think that it will be reasonable to expect that a high level of understanding of the complex networks implicating DSCR genes through systems biology approaches will provide very useful insight, which could be translated into new therapies that could turn out to be useful not only for DS, but also for other disorders such as Alzheimer's disease and Rett syndrome.

Acknowledgements

We are grateful to Dr. Christian Damasco for his help in the production of Tables 1 and 2. The financial contribution of the Jerome Lejeune Foundation FDC and GB is gratefully acknowledged.

Author details

Ferdinando Di Cunto* and Gaia Berto

*Address all correspondence to: ferdinando.dicunto@unito.it; gaia.berto@unito.it

University of Torino, Molecular Biotechnology Centre, Torino, Italy

References

[1] Piro RM (2012) Network medicine: linking disorders. Hum Genet.

[2] Chan SY, Loscalzo J (2012) The emerging paradigm of network medicine in the study of human disease. Circ Res 111: 359-374.

[3] Jackson JF, North ER, 3rd, Thomas JG (1976) Clinical diagnosis of Down's syndrome. Clin Genet 9: 483-487.

[4] Antonarakis SE, Epstein CJ (2006) The challenge of Down syndrome. Trends Mol Med 12: 473-479.

[5] Lejeune J, Gautier M, Turpin R (1959) Study of somatic chromosomes from 9 mongoloid children. C R Hebd Seances Acad Sci 248: 1721-1722.

[6] Antonarakis SE (1998) 10 years of Genomics, chromosome 21, and Down syndrome. Genomics 51: 1-16.

[7] Poissonnier M, Saint-Paul B, Dutrillaux B, Chassaigne M, Gruyer P, et al. (1976) Partial trisomy 21 (21q21 - 21q22.2). Ann Genet 19: 69-73.

[8] Dierssen M, Herault Y, Estivill X (2009) Aneuploidy: from a physiological mechanism of variance to Down syndrome. Physiol Rev 89: 887-920.

[9] Rachidi M, Lopes C, Vayssettes C, Smith DJ, Rubin EM, et al. (2007) New cerebellar phenotypes in YAC transgenic mouse in vivo library of human Down syndrome critical region-1. Biochem Biophys Res Commun 364: 488-494.

[10] Delabar JM, Theophile D, Rahmani Z, Chettouh Z, Blouin JL, et al. (1993) Molecular mapping of twenty-four features of Down syndrome on chromosome 21. Eur J Hum Genet 1: 114-124.

[11] Korenberg JR, Chen XN, Schipper R, Sun Z, Gonsky R, et al. (1994) Down syndrome phenotypes: the consequences of chromosomal imbalance. Proc Natl Acad Sci U S A 91: 4997-5001.

[12] Chabert C, Cherfouh A, Delabar JM, Duquenne V (2001) Assessing implications between genotypic and phenotypic variables through lattice analysis. Behav Genet 31: 125-139.

[13] Lyle R, Bena F, Gagos S, Gehrig C, Lopez G, et al. (2009) Genotype-phenotype correlations in Down syndrome identified by array CGH in 30 cases of partial trisomy and partial monosomy chromosome 21. Eur J Hum Genet 17: 454-466.

[14] Kahlem P, Sultan M, Herwig R, Steinfath M, Balzereit D, et al. (2004) Transcript level alterations reflect gene dosage effects across multiple tissues in a mouse model of down syndrome. Genome Res 14: 1258-1267.

[15] Hattori M, Fujiyama A, Taylor TD, Watanabe H, Yada T, et al. (2000) The DNA sequence of human chromosome 21. Nature 405: 311-319.

[16] Esteller M (2011) Non-coding RNAs in human disease. Nat Rev Genet 12: 861-874.

[17] Tay Y, Kats L, Salmena L, Weiss D, Tan SM, et al. (2011) Coding-independent regulation of the tumor suppressor PTEN by competing endogenous mRNAs. Cell 147: 344-357.

[18] Sumazin P, Yang X, Chiu HS, Chung WJ, Iyer A, et al. (2011) An extensive microRNA-mediated network of RNA-RNA interactions regulates established oncogenic pathways in glioblastoma. Cell 147: 370-381.

[19] Salmena L, Poliseno L, Tay Y, Kats L, Pandolfi PP (2011) A ceRNA hypothesis: the Rosetta Stone of a hidden RNA language? Cell 146: 353-358.

[20] Cesana M, Cacchiarelli D, Legnini I, Santini T, Sthandier O, et al. (2011) A long noncoding RNA controls muscle differentiation by functioning as a competing endogenous RNA. Cell 147: 358-369.

[21] Poliseno L, Salmena L, Zhang J, Carver B, Haveman WJ, et al. (2011) A coding-independent function of gene and pseudogene mRNAs regulates tumour biology. Nature 465: 1033-1038.

[22] Davisson MT, Gardiner K, Costa AC (2001) Report and abstracts of the ninth international workshop on the molecular biology of human chromosome 21 and Down syndrome. Bar Harbor, Maine, USA. 23-26 September 2000. Cytogenet Cell Genet 92: 1-22.

[23] Davisson MT, Schmidt C, Akeson EC (1990) Segmental trisomy of murine chromosome 16: a new model system for studying Down syndrome. Prog Clin Biol Res 360: 263-280.

[24] Sago H, Carlson EJ, Smith DJ, Kilbridge J, Rubin EM, et al. (1998) Ts1Cje, a partial trisomy 16 mouse model for Down syndrome, exhibits learning and behavioral abnormalities. Proc Natl Acad Sci U S A 95: 6256-6261.

[25] Sago H, Carlson EJ, Smith DJ, Rubin EM, Crnic LS, et al. (2000) Genetic dissection of region associated with behavioral abnormalities in mouse models for Down syndrome. Pediatr Res 48: 606-613.

[26] Demas GE, Nelson RJ, Krueger BK, Yarowsky PJ (1998) Impaired spatial working and reference memory in segmental trisomy (Ts65Dn) mice. Behav Brain Res 90: 199-201.

[27] Demas GE, Nelson RJ, Krueger BK, Yarowsky PJ (1996) Spatial memory deficits in segmental trisomic Ts65Dn mice. Behav Brain Res 82: 85-92.

[28] Holtzman DM, Santucci D, Kilbridge J, Chua-Couzens J, Fontana DJ, et al. (1996) Developmental abnormalities and age-related neurodegeneration in a mouse model of Down syndrome. Proc Natl Acad Sci U S A 93: 13333-13338.

[29] Hyde LA, Crnic LS (2001) Age-related deficits in context discrimination learning in Ts65Dn mice that model Down syndrome and Alzheimer's disease. Behav Neurosci 115: 1239-1246.

[30] Escorihuela RM, Fernandez-Teruel A, Vallina IF, Baamonde C, Lumbreras MA, et al. (1995) A behavioral assessment of Ts65Dn mice: a putative Down syndrome model. Neurosci Lett 199: 143-146.

[31] Escorihuela RM, Vallina IF, Martinez-Cue C, Baamonde C, Dierssen M, et al. (1998) Impaired short- and long-term memory in Ts65Dn mice, a model for Down syndrome. Neurosci Lett 247: 171-174.

[32] Reeves RH, Irving NG, Moran TH, Wohn A, Kitt C, et al. (1995) A mouse model for Down syndrome exhibits learning and behaviour deficits. Nat Genet 11: 177-184.

[33] Belichenko PV, Masliah E, Kleschevnikov AM, Villar AJ, Epstein CJ, et al. (2004) Synaptic structural abnormalities in the Ts65Dn mouse model of Down Syndrome. J Comp Neurol 480: 281-298.

[34] Siarey RJ, Stoll J, Rapoport SI, Galdzicki Z (1997) Altered long-term potentiation in the young and old Ts65Dn mouse, a model for Down Syndrome. Neuropharmacology 36: 1549-1554.

[35] Siarey RJ, Carlson EJ, Epstein CJ, Balbo A, Rapoport SI, et al. (1999) Increased synaptic depression in the Ts65Dn mouse, a model for mental retardation in Down syndrome. Neuropharmacology 38: 1917-1920.

[36] Kleschevnikov AM, Belichenko PV, Villar AJ, Epstein CJ, Malenka RC, et al. (2004) Hippocampal long-term potentiation suppressed by increased inhibition in the Ts65Dn mouse, a genetic model of Down syndrome. J Neurosci 24: 8153-8160.

[37] Siarey RJ, Villar AJ, Epstein CJ, Galdzicki Z (2005) Abnormal synaptic plasticity in the Ts1Cje segmental trisomy 16 mouse model of Down syndrome. Neuropharmacology 49: 122-128.

[38] Belichenko PV, Kleschevnikov AM, Salehi A, Epstein CJ, Mobley WC (2007) Synaptic and cognitive abnormalities in mouse models of Down syndrome: exploring genotype-phenotype relationships. J Comp Neurol 504: 329-345.

[39] Olson LE, Richtsmeier JT, Leszl J, Reeves RH (2004) A chromosome 21 critical region does not cause specific Down syndrome phenotypes. Science 306: 687-690.

[40] Aldridge K, Reeves RH, Olson LE, Richtsmeier JT (2007) Differential effects of trisomy on brain shape and volume in related aneuploid mouse models. Am J Med Genet A 143A: 1060-1070.

[41] Olson LE, Roper RJ, Sengstaken CL, Peterson EA, Aquino V, et al. (2007) Trisomy for the Down syndrome 'critical region' is necessary but not sufficient for brain phenotypes of trisomic mice. Hum Mol Genet 16: 774-782.

[42] Belichenko NP, Belichenko PV, Kleschevnikov AM, Salehi A, Reeves RH, et al. (2009) The "Down syndrome critical region" is sufficient in the mouse model to confer behavioral, neurophysiological, and synaptic phenotypes characteristic of Down syndrome. J Neurosci 29: 5938-5948.

[43] Smith DJ, Stevens ME, Sudanagunta SP, Bronson RT, Makhinson M, et al. (1997) Functional screening of 2 Mb of human chromosome 21q22.2 in transgenic mice implicates minibrain in learning defects associated with Down syndrome. Nat Genet 16: 28-36.

[44] Smith DJ, Rubin EM (1997) Functional screening and complex traits: human 21q22.2 sequences affecting learning in mice. Hum Mol Genet 6: 1729-1733.

[45] Smith DJ, Zhu Y, Zhang J, Cheng JF, Rubin EM (1995) Construction of a panel of transgenic mice containing a contiguous 2-Mb set of YAC/P1 clones from human chromosome 21q22.2. Genomics 27: 425-434.

[46] Ahn KJ, Jeong HK, Choi HS, Ryoo SR, Kim YJ, et al. (2006) DYRK1A BAC transgenic mice show altered synaptic plasticity with learning and memory defects. Neurobiol Dis 22: 463-472.

[47] Liu C, Belichenko PV, Zhang L, Fu D, Kleschevnikov AM, et al. (2011) Mouse models for Down syndrome-associated developmental cognitive disabilities. Dev Neurosci 33: 404-413.

[48] Baek KH, Zaslavsky A, Lynch RC, Britt C, Okada Y, et al. (2009) Down's syndrome suppression of tumour growth and the role of the calcineurin inhibitor DSCR1. Nature 459: 1126-1130.

[49] Chakrabarti L, Best TK, Cramer NP, Carney RS, Isaac JT, et al. (2010) Olig1 and Olig2 triplication causes developmental brain defects in Down syndrome. Nat Neurosci 13: 927-934.

[50] Cataldo AM, Petanceska S, Peterhoff CM, Terio NB, Epstein CJ, et al. (2003) App gene dosage modulates endosomal abnormalities of Alzheimer's disease in a segmental trisomy 16 mouse model of down syndrome. J Neurosci 23: 6788-6792.

[51] Salehi A, Delcroix JD, Belichenko PV, Zhan K, Wu C, et al. (2006) Increased App expression in a mouse model of Down's syndrome disrupts NGF transport and causes cholinergic neuron degeneration. Neuron 51: 29-42.

[52] Haydar TF, Reeves RH (2012) Trisomy 21 and early brain development. Trends Neurosci 35: 81-91.

[53] Antonarakis SE, Lyle R, Dermitzakis ET, Reymond A, Deutsch S (2004) Chromosome 21 and down syndrome: from genomics to pathophysiology. Nat Rev Genet 5: 725-738.

[54] Kleschevnikov AM, Belichenko PV, Faizi M, Jacobs LF, Htun K, et al. (2012) Deficits in Cognition and Synaptic Plasticity in a Mouse Model of Down Syndrome Ameliorated by GABAB Receptor Antagonists. J Neurosci 32: 9217-9227.

[55] Golden JA, Hyman BT (1994) Development of the superior temporal neocortex is anomalous in trisomy 21. J Neuropathol Exp Neurol 53: 513-520.

[56] Guidi S, Bonasoni P, Ceccarelli C, Santini D, Gualtieri F, et al. (2008) Neurogenesis impairment and increased cell death reduce total neuron number in the hippocampal region of fetuses with Down syndrome. Brain Pathol 18: 180-197.

[57] Vuksic M, Petanjek Z, Rasin MR, Kostovic I (2002) Perinatal growth of prefrontal layer III pyramids in Down syndrome. Pediatr Neurol 27: 36-38.

[58] Becker L, Mito T, Takashima S, Onodera K (1991) Growth and development of the brain in Down syndrome. Prog Clin Biol Res 373: 133-152.

[59] Takashima S, Becker LE, Armstrong DL, Chan F (1981) Abnormal neuronal development in the visual cortex of the human fetus and infant with down's syndrome. A quantitative and qualitative Golgi study. Brain Res 225: 1-21.

[60] Becker LE, Armstrong DL, Chan F (1986) Dendritic atrophy in children with Down's syndrome. Ann Neurol 20: 520-526.

[61] Hollenhorst PC, McIntosh LP, Graves BJ (2011) Genomic and biochemical insights into the specificity of ETS transcription factors. Annu Rev Biochem 80: 437-471.

[62] Dryden NH, Sperone A, Martin-Almedina S, Hannah RL, Birdsey GM, et al. (2012) The transcription factor Erg controls endothelial cell quiescence by repressing activity of nuclear factor (NF)-kappaB p65. J Biol Chem 287: 12331-12342.

[63] Martens JH (2011) Acute myeloid leukemia: a central role for the ETS factor ERG. Int J Biochem Cell Biol 43: 1413-1416.

[64] Fisher IB, Ostrowski M, Muthusamy N (2012) Role for Ets-2(Thr-72) transcription factor in stage-specific thymocyte development and survival. J Biol Chem 287: 5199-5210.

[65] Lam K, Zhang DE (2012) RUNX1 and RUNX1-ETO: roles in hematopoiesis and leukemogenesis. Front Biosci 17: 1120-1139.

[66] Huang H, Rambaldi I, Daniels E, Featherstone M (2003) Expression of the Wdr9 gene and protein products during mouse development. Dev Dyn 227: 608-614.

[67] Abuhatzira L, Shamir A, Schones DE, Schaffer AA, Bustin M (2011) The chromatin-binding protein HMGN1 regulates the expression of methyl CpG-binding protein 2 (MECP2) and affects the behavior of mice. J Biol Chem 286: 42051-42062.

[68] Martin-Bermudo MD, Carmena A, Jimenez F (1995) Neurogenic genes control gene expression at the transcriptional level in early neurogenesis and in mesectoderm specification. Development 121: 219-224.

[69] Havis E, Coumailleau P, Bonnet A, Bismuth K, Bonnin MA, et al. (2012) Sim2 prevents entry into the myogenic program by repressing MyoD transcription during limb embryonic myogenesis. Development 139: 1910-1920.

[70] Fuentes JJ, Pritchard MA, Planas AM, Bosch A, Ferrer I, et al. (1995) A new human gene from the Down syndrome critical region encodes a proline-rich protein highly expressed in fetal brain and heart. Hum Mol Genet 4: 1935-1944.

[71] Fuentes JJ, Genesca L, Kingsbury TJ, Cunningham KW, Perez-Riba M, et al. (2000) DSCR1, overexpressed in Down syndrome, is an inhibitor of calcineurin-mediated signaling pathways. Hum Mol Genet 9: 1681-1690.

[72] Rothermel B, Vega RB, Yang J, Wu H, Bassel-Duby R, et al. (2000) A protein encoded within the Down syndrome critical region is enriched in striated muscles and inhibits calcineurin signaling. J Biol Chem 275: 8719-8725.

[73] Ermak G, Morgan TE, Davies KJ (2001) Chronic overexpression of the calcineurin inhibitory gene DSCR1 (Adapt78) is associated with Alzheimer's disease. J Biol Chem 276: 38787-38794.

[74] Chang KT, Min KT (2005) Drosophila melanogaster homolog of Down syndrome critical region 1 is critical for mitochondrial function. Nat Neurosci 8: 1577-1585.

[75] Ermak G, Cheadle C, Becker KG, Harris CD, Davies KJ (2004) DSCR1(Adapt78) modulates expression of SOD1. Faseb J 18: 62-69.

[76] Gulesserian T, Seidl R, Hardmeier R, Cairns N, Lubec G (2001) Superoxide dismutase SOD1, encoded on chromosome 21, but not SOD2 is overexpressed in brains of patients with Down syndrome. J Investig Med 49: 41-46.

[77] Ermak G, Harris CD, Davies KJ (2002) The DSCR1 (Adapt78) isoform 1 protein calcipressin 1 inhibits calcineurin and protects against acute calcium-mediated stress damage, including transient oxidative stress. Faseb J 16: 814-824.

[78] Jovanovic SV, Clements D, MacLeod K (1998) Biomarkers of oxidative stress are significantly elevated in Down syndrome. Free Radic Biol Med 25: 1044-1048.

[79] Pallardo FV, Degan P, d'Ischia M, Kelly FJ, Zatterale A, et al. (2006) Multiple evidence for an early age pro-oxidant state in Down Syndrome patients. Biogerontology 7: 211-220.

[80] Okui M, Ide T, Morita K, Funakoshi E, Ito F, et al. (1999) High-level expression of the Mnb/Dyrk1A gene in brain and heart during rat early development. Genomics 62: 165-171.

[81] Tejedor F, Zhu XR, Kaltenbach E, Ackermann A, Baumann A, et al. (1995) minibrain: a new protein kinase family involved in postembryonic neurogenesis in Drosophila. Neuron 14: 287-301.

[82] Chen H, Antonarakis SE (1997) Localisation of a human homologue of the Drosophila mnb and rat Dyrk genes to chromosome 21q22.2. Hum Genet 99: 262-265.

[83] Fotaki V, Dierssen M, Alcantara S, Martinez S, Marti E, et al. (2002) Dyrk1A haploinsufficiency affects viability and causes developmental delay and abnormal brain morphology in mice. Mol Cell Biol 22: 6636-6647.

[84] Moller RS, Kubart S, Hoeltzenbein M, Heye B, Vogel I, et al. (2008) Truncation of the Down syndrome candidate gene DYRK1A in two unrelated patients with microcephaly. Am J Hum Genet 82: 1165-1170.

[85] Altafaj X, Dierssen M, Baamonde C, Marti E, Visa J, et al. (2001) Neurodevelopmental delay, motor abnormalities and cognitive deficits in transgenic mice overexpressing Dyrk1A (minibrain), a murine model of Down's syndrome. Hum Mol Genet 10: 1915-1923.

[86] Rahmani Z, Lopes C, Rachidi M, Delabar JM (1998) Expression of the mnb (dyrk) protein in adult and embryonic mouse tissues. Biochem Biophys Res Commun 253: 514-518.

[87] Guimera J, Casas C, Estivill X, Pritchard M (1999) Human minibrain homologue (MNBH/DYRK1): characterization, alternative splicing, differential tissue expression, and overexpression in Down syndrome. Genomics 57: 407-418.

[88] Lyle R, Gehrig C, Neergaard-Henrichsen C, Deutsch S, Antonarakis SE (2004) Gene expression from the aneuploid chromosome in a trisomy mouse model of down syndrome. Genome Res 14: 1268-1274.

[89] Park J, Oh Y, Yoo L, Jung MS, Song WJ, et al. (2010) Dyrk1A phosphorylates p53 and inhibits proliferation of embryonic neuronal cells. J Biol Chem 285: 31895-31906.

[90] Hammerle B, Elizalde C, Tejedor FJ (2008) The spatio-temporal and subcellular expression of the candidate Down syndrome gene Mnb/Dyrk1A in the developing mouse brain suggests distinct sequential roles in neuronal development. Eur J Neurosci 27: 1061-1074.

[91] Hammerle B, Ulin E, Guimera J, Becker W, Guillemot F, et al. (2011) Transient expression of Mnb/Dyrk1a couples cell cycle exit and differentiation of neuronal precursors by inducing p27KIP1 expression and suppressing NOTCH signaling. Development 138: 2543-2554.

[92] Yabut O, Domogauer J, D'Arcangelo G (2010) Dyrk1A overexpression inhibits proliferation and induces premature neuronal differentiation of neural progenitor cells. J Neurosci 30: 4004-4014.

[93] Galceran J, de Graaf K, Tejedor FJ, Becker W (2003) The MNB/DYRK1A protein kinase: genetic and biochemical properties. J Neural Transm Suppl: 139-148.

[94] Hammerle B, Elizalde C, Galceran J, Becker W, Tejedor FJ (2003) The MNB/DYRK1A protein kinase: neurobiological functions and Down syndrome implications. J Neural Transm Suppl: 129-137.

[95] Hammerle B, Carnicero A, Elizalde C, Ceron J, Martinez S, et al. (2003) Expression patterns and subcellular localization of the Down syndrome candidate protein MNB/DYRK1A suggest a role in late neuronal differentiation. Eur J Neurosci 17: 2277-2286.

[96] Martinez de Lagran M, Altafaj X, Gallego X, Marti E, Estivill X, et al. (2004) Motor phenotypic alterations in TgDyrk1a transgenic mice implicate DYRK1A in Down syndrome motor dysfunction. Neurobiol Dis 15: 132-142.

[97] Dowjat WK, Adayev T, Kuchna I, Nowicki K, Palminiello S, et al. (2007) Trisomy-driven overexpression of DYRK1A kinase in the brain of subjects with Down syndrome. Neurosci Lett 413: 77-81.

[98] Ryoo SR, Jeong HK, Radnaabazar C, Yoo JJ, Cho HJ, et al. (2007) DYRK1A-mediated hyperphosphorylation of Tau. A functional link between Down syndrome and Alzheimer disease. J Biol Chem 282: 34850-34857.

[99] Liu F, Liang Z, Wegiel J, Hwang YW, Iqbal K, et al. (2008) Overexpression of Dyrk1A contributes to neurofibrillary degeneration in Down syndrome. Faseb J 22: 3224-3233.

[100] Wegiel J, Dowjat K, Kaczmarski W, Kuchna I, Nowicki K, et al. (2008) The role of overexpressed DYRK1A protein in the early onset of neurofibrillary degeneration in Down syndrome. Acta Neuropathol 116: 391-407.

[101] Shi J, Zhang T, Zhou C, Chohan MO, Gu X, et al. (2008) Increased dosage of Dyrk1A alters alternative splicing factor (ASF)-regulated alternative splicing of tau in Down syndrome. J Biol Chem 283: 28660-28669.

[102] Yin X, Jin N, Gu J, Shi J, Gong CX, et al. (2012) Dual-specificity-tyrosine-phosphorylated and regulated kinase 1A (Dyrk1A) modulates serine-arginine rich protein 55 (SRp55)-promoted tau exon 10 inclusion. J Biol Chem.

[103] Guedj F, Sebrie C, Rivals I, Ledru A, Paly E, et al. (2009) Green tea polyphenols rescue of brain defects induced by overexpression of DYRK1A. PLoS One 4: e4606.

[104] Xie W, Ramakrishna N, Wieraszko A, Hwang YW (2008) Promotion of neuronal plasticity by (-)-epigallocatechin-3-gallate. Neurochem Res 33: 776-783.

[105] Ohira M, Ootsuyama A, Suzuki E, Ichikawa H, Seki N, et al. (1996) Identification of a novel human gene containing the tetratricopeptide repeat domain from the Down syndrome region of chromosome 21. DNA Res 3: 9-16.

[106] Tsukahara F, Urakawa I, Hattori M, Hirai M, Ohba K, et al. (1998) Molecular characterization of the mouse mtprd gene, a homologue of human TPRD: unique gene expression suggesting its critical role in the pathophysiology of Down syndrome. J Biochem 123: 1055-1063.

[107] Raz N, Torres IJ, Briggs SD, Spencer WD, Thornton AE, et al. (1995) Selective neuroanatomic abnormalities in Down's syndrome and their cognitive correlates: evidence from MRI morphometry. Neurology 45: 356-366.

[108] Lopes C, Rachidi M, Gassanova S, Sinet PM, Delabar JM (1999) Developmentally regulated expression of mtprd, the murine ortholog of tprd, a gene from the Down syndrome chromosomal region 1. Mech Dev 84: 189-193.

[109] Rachidi M, Lopes C, Gassanova S, Sinet PM, Vekemans M, et al. (2000) Regional and cellular specificity of the expression of TPRD, the tetratricopeptide Down syndrome gene, during human embryonic development. Mech Dev 93: 189-193.

[110] Saran NG, Pletcher MT, Natale JE, Cheng Y, Reeves RH (2003) Global disruption of the cerebellar transcriptome in a Down syndrome mouse model. Hum Mol Genet 12: 2013-2019.

[111] Suizu F, Hiramuki Y, Okumura F, Matsuda M, Okumura AJ, et al. (2009) The E3 ligase TTC3 facilitates ubiquitination and degradation of phosphorylated Akt. Dev Cell 17: 800-810.

[112] Toker A (2009) TTC3 ubiquitination terminates Akt-ivation. Dev Cell 17: 752-754.

[113] Berto G, Camera P, Fusco C, Imarisio S, Ambrogio C, et al. (2007) The Down syndrome critical region protein TTC3 inhibits neuronal differentiation via RhoA and Citron kinase. J Cell Sci 120: 1859-1867.

[114] Govek EE, Newey SE, Van Aelst L (2005) The role of the Rho GTPases in neuronal development. Genes Dev 19: 1-49.

[115] Newey SE, Velamoor V, Govek EE, Van Aelst L (2005) Rho GTPases, dendritic structure, and mental retardation. J Neurobiol 64: 58-74.

[116] Gupta V, Ahsan F (2010) Inhalational therapy for pulmonary arterial hypertension: current status and future prospects. Crit Rev Ther Drug Carrier Syst 27: 313-370.

[117] Dudek H, Datta SR, Franke TF, Birnbaum MJ, Yao R, et al. (1997) Regulation of neuronal survival by the serine-threonine protein kinase Akt. Science 275: 661-665.

[118] Grider MH, Park D, Spencer DM, Shine HD (2009) Lipid raft-targeted Akt promotes axonal branching and growth cone expansion via mTOR and Rac1, respectively. J Neurosci Res 87: 3033-3042.

[119] Majumdar D, Nebhan CA, Hu L, Anderson B, Webb DJ (2011) An APPL1/Akt signaling complex regulates dendritic spine and synapse formation in hippocampal neurons. Mol Cell Neurosci 46: 633-644.

[120] Harris SJ, Foster JG, Ward SG (2009) PI3K isoforms as drug targets in inflammatory diseases: lessons from pharmacological and genetic strategies. Curr Opin Investig Drugs 10: 1151-1162.

[121] Courtney KD, Corcoran RB, Engelman JA (2010) The PI3K pathway as drug target in human cancer. J Clin Oncol 28: 1075-1083.

[122] Castillo PE, Chiu CQ, Carroll RC (2011) Long-term plasticity at inhibitory synapses. Curr Opin Neurobiol 21: 328-338.

[123] Costa AC, Scott-McKean JJ, Stasko MR (2008) Acute injections of the NMDA receptor antagonist memantine rescue performance deficits of the Ts65Dn mouse model of

Down syndrome on a fear conditioning test. Neuropsychopharmacology 33: 1624-1632.

[124] Chang KT, Min KT (2009) Upregulation of three Drosophila homologs of human chromosome 21 genes alters synaptic function: implications for Down syndrome. Proc Natl Acad Sci U S A 106: 17117-17122.

[125] Krupp JJ, Vissel B, Thomas CG, Heinemann SF, Westbrook GL (2002) Calcineurin acts via the C-terminus of NR2A to modulate desensitization of NMDA receptors. Neuropharmacology 42: 593-602.

[126] Rycroft BK, Gibb AJ (2004) Inhibitory interactions of calcineurin (phosphatase 2B) and calmodulin on rat hippocampal NMDA receptors. Neuropharmacology 47: 505-514.

[127] Lieberman DN, Mody I (1994) Regulation of NMDA channel function by endogenous Ca(2+)-dependent phosphatase. Nature 369: 235-239.

[128] Hanney M, Prasher V, Williams N, Jones EL, Aarsland D, et al. (2012) Memantine for dementia in adults older than 40 years with Down's syndrome (MEADOWS): a randomised, double-blind, placebo-controlled trial. Lancet 379: 528-536.

[129] Kleschevnikov AM, Belichenko PV, Gall J, George L, Nosheny R, et al. (2012) Increased efficiency of the GABAA and GABAB receptor-mediated neurotransmission in the Ts65Dn mouse model of Down syndrome. Neurobiol Dis 45: 683-691.

[130] Best TK, Siarey RJ, Galdzicki Z (2007) Ts65Dn, a mouse model of Down syndrome, exhibits increased GABAB-induced potassium current. J Neurophysiol 97: 892-900.

[131] Rissman RA, Mobley WC (2011) Implications for treatment: GABAA receptors in aging, Down syndrome and Alzheimer's disease. J Neurochem 117: 613-622.

[132] Fernandez F, Morishita W, Zuniga E, Nguyen J, Blank M, et al. (2007) Pharmacotherapy for cognitive impairment in a mouse model of Down syndrome. Nat Neurosci 10: 411-413.

[133] Rueda N, Florez J, Martinez-Cue C (2008) Chronic pentylenetetrazole but not donepezil treatment rescues spatial cognition in Ts65Dn mice, a model for Down syndrome. Neurosci Lett 433: 22-27.

[134] Braudeau J, Dauphinot L, Duchon A, Loistron A, Dodd RH, et al. (2011) Chronic Treatment with a Promnesiant GABA-A alpha5-Selective Inverse Agonist Increases Immediate Early Genes Expression during Memory Processing in Mice and Rectifies Their Expression Levels in a Down Syndrome Mouse Model. Adv Pharmacol Sci 2011: 153218.

[135] Clark S, Schwalbe J, Stasko MR, Yarowsky PJ, Costa AC (2006) Fluoxetine rescues deficient neurogenesis in hippocampus of the Ts65Dn mouse model for Down syndrome. Exp Neurol 200: 256-261.

[136] Rueda N, Mostany R, Pazos A, Florez J, Martinez-Cue C (2005) Cell proliferation is reduced in the dentate gyrus of aged but not young Ts65Dn mice, a model of Down syndrome. Neurosci Lett 380: 197-201.

[137] Ishihara K, Amano K, Takaki E, Shimohata A, Sago H, et al. (2010) Enlarged brain ventricles and impaired neurogenesis in the Ts1Cje and Ts2Cje mouse models of Down syndrome. Cereb Cortex 20: 1131-1143.

[138] Whitaker-Azmitia PM (2001) Serotonin and brain development: role in human developmental diseases. Brain Res Bull 56: 479-485.

[139] Bar-Peled O, Gross-Isseroff R, Ben-Hur H, Hoskins I, Groner Y, et al. (1991) Fetal human brain exhibits a prenatal peak in the density of serotonin 5-HT1A receptors. Neurosci Lett 127: 173-176.

[140] Risser D, Lubec G, Cairns N, Herrera-Marschitz M (1997) Excitatory amino acids and monoamines in parahippocampal gyrus and frontal cortical pole of adults with Down syndrome. Life Sci 60: 1231-1237.

[141] Banasr M, Hery M, Printemps R, Daszuta A (2004) Serotonin-induced increases in adult cell proliferation and neurogenesis are mediated through different and common 5-HT receptor subtypes in the dentate gyrus and the subventricular zone. Neuropsychopharmacology 29: 450-460.

[142] Bianchi P, Ciani E, Guidi S, Trazzi S, Felice D, et al. (2010) Early pharmacotherapy restores neurogenesis and cognitive performance in the Ts65Dn mouse model for Down syndrome. J Neurosci 30: 8769-8779.

[143] Boylan K, Romero S, Birmaher B (2007) Psychopharmacologic treatment of pediatric major depressive disorder. Psychopharmacology (Berl) 191: 27-38.

[144] Bairy KL, Madhyastha S, Ashok KP, Bairy I, Malini S (2007) Developmental and behavioral consequences of prenatal fluoxetine. Pharmacology 79: 1-11.

[145] Tyrrell J, Cosgrave M, McCarron M, McPherson J, Calvert J, et al. (2001) Dementia in people with Down's syndrome. Int J Geriatr Psychiatry 16: 1168-1174.

[146] Millan Sanchez M, Heyn SN, Das D, Moghadam S, Martin KJ, et al. (2011) Neurobiological elements of cognitive dysfunction in down syndrome: exploring the role of APP. Biol Psychiatry 71: 403-409.

[147] Rovelet-Lecrux A, Hannequin D, Raux G, Le Meur N, Laquerriere A, et al. (2006) APP locus duplication causes autosomal dominant early-onset Alzheimer disease with cerebral amyloid angiopathy. Nat Genet 38: 24-26.

[148] Prasher VP, Farrer MJ, Kessling AM, Fisher EM, West RJ, et al. (1998) Molecular mapping of Alzheimer-type dementia in Down's syndrome. Ann Neurol 43: 380-383.

[149] Fischer DF, van Dijk R, Sluijs JA, Nair SM, Racchi M, et al. (2005) Activation of the Notch pathway in Down syndrome: cross-talk of Notch and APP. Faseb J 19: 1451-1458.

[150] Stockley JH, O'Neill C (2007) The proteins BACE1 and BACE2 and beta-secretase activity in normal and Alzheimer's disease brain. Biochem Soc Trans 35: 574-576.

[151] Ahmed RR, Holler CJ, Webb RL, Li F, Beckett TL, et al. (2010) BACE1 and BACE2 enzymatic activities in Alzheimer's disease. J Neurochem 112: 1045-1053.

[152] Holler CJ, Webb RL, Laux AL, Beckett TL, Niedowicz DM, et al. (2012) BACE2 expression increases in human neurodegenerative disease. Am J Pathol 180: 337-350.

[153] Ryoo SR, Cho HJ, Lee HW, Jeong HK, Radnaabazar C, et al. (2008) Dual-specificity tyrosine(Y)-phosphorylation regulated kinase 1A-mediated phosphorylation of amyloid precursor protein: evidence for a functional link between Down syndrome and Alzheimer's disease. J Neurochem 104: 1333-1344.

[154] Lloret A, Badia MC, Giraldo E, Ermak G, Alonso MD, et al. (2011) Amyloid-beta toxicity and tau hyperphosphorylation are linked via RCAN1 in Alzheimer's disease. J Alzheimers Dis 27: 701-709.

[155] Jung MS, Park JH, Ryu YS, Choi SH, Yoon SH, et al. (2011) Regulation of RCAN1 protein activity by Dyrk1A protein-mediated phosphorylation. J Biol Chem 286: 40401-40412.

[156] Hirotsune S, Yoshida N, Chen A, Garrett L, Sugiyama F, et al. (2003) An expressed pseudogene regulates the messenger-RNA stability of its homologous coding gene. Nature 423: 91-96.

[157] Magistri M, Faghihi MA, St Laurent G, 3rd, Wahlestedt C (2012) Regulation of chromatin structure by long noncoding RNAs: focus on natural antisense transcripts. Trends Genet 28: 389-396.

[158] Kurokawa R (2011) Promoter-associated long noncoding RNAs repress transcription through a RNA binding protein TLS. Adv Exp Med Biol 722: 196-208.

[159] Kogo R, Shimamura T, Mimori K, Kawahara K, Imoto S, et al. (2011) Long noncoding RNA HOTAIR regulates polycomb-dependent chromatin modification and is associated with poor prognosis in colorectal cancers. Cancer Res 71: 6320-6326.

[160] Yoon JH, Abdelmohsen K, Srikantan S, Yang X, Martindale JL, et al. (2012) LincRNA-p21 Suppresses Target mRNA Translation. Mol Cell.

[161] Huarte M, Guttman M, Feldser D, Garber M, Koziol MJ, et al. (2010) A large intergenic noncoding RNA induced by p53 mediates global gene repression in the p53 response. Cell 142: 409-419.

[162] Kuhn DE, Nuovo GJ, Terry AV, Jr., Martin MM, Malana GE, et al. (2010) Chromosome 21-derived microRNAs provide an etiological basis for aberrant protein expression in human Down syndrome brains. J Biol Chem 285: 1529-1543.

[163] Robinson L, Guy J, McKay L, Brockett E, Spike RC, et al. (2012) Morphological and functional reversal of phenotypes in a mouse model of Rett syndrome. Brain.

[164] Weng SM, Bailey ME, Cobb SR (2011) Rett syndrome: from bed to bench. Pediatr Neonatol 52: 309-316.

[165] Malatkova P, Maser E, Wsol V (2010) Human carbonyl reductases. Curr Drug Metab 11: 639-658.

[166] Rachidi M, Delezoide AL, Delabar JM, Lopes C (2009) A quantitative assessment of gene expression (QAGE) reveals differential overexpression of DOPEY2, a candidate gene for mental retardation, in Down syndrome brain regions. Int J Dev Neurosci 27: 393-398.

[167] Mimura Y, Takahashi K, Kawata K, Akazawa T, Inoue N (2010) Two-step colocalization of MORC3 with PML nuclear bodies. J Cell Sci 123: 2014-2024.

[168] Mello JA, Sillje HH, Roche DM, Kirschner DB, Nigg EA, et al. (2002) Human Asf1 and CAF-1 interact and synergize in a repair-coupled nucleosome assembly pathway. EMBO Rep 3: 329-334.

[169] Wilcox ER, Burton QL, Naz S, Riazuddin S, Smith TN, et al. (2001) Mutations in the gene encoding tight junction claudin-14 cause autosomal recessive deafness DFNB29. Cell 104: 165-172.

[170] Bao B, Pestinger V, Hassan YI, Borgstahl GE, Kolar C, et al. (2011) Holocarboxylase synthetase is a chromatin protein and interacts directly with histone H3 to mediate biotinylation of K9 and K18. J Nutr Biochem 22: 470-475.

[171] Shibuya K, Kudoh J, Minoshima S, Kawasaki K, Asakawa S, et al. (2000) Isolation of two novel genes, DSCR5 and DSCR6, from Down syndrome critical region on human chromosome 21q22.2. Biochem Biophys Res Commun 271: 693-698.

[172] Watanabe R, Murakami Y, Marmor MD, Inoue N, Maeda Y, et al. (2000) Initial enzyme for glycosylphosphatidylinositol biosynthesis requires PIG-P and is regulated by DPM2. Embo J 19: 4402-4411.

[173] Nakamura A, Hattori M, Sakaki Y (1997) Isolation of a novel human gene from the Down syndrome critical region of chromosome 21q22.2. J Biochem 122: 872-877.

[174] Du Y, Zhang J, Wang H, Yan X, Yang Y, et al. (2011) Hypomethylated DSCR4 is a placenta-derived epigenetic marker for trisomy 21. Prenat Diagn 31: 207-214.

[175] de Wit NJ, Cornelissen IM, Diepstra JH, Weidle UH, Ruiter DJ, et al. (2005) The MMA1 gene family of cancer-testis antigens has multiple alternative splice variants:

characterization of their expression profile, the genomic organization, and transcript properties. Genes Chromosomes Cancer 42: 10-21.

[176] Okamoto K, Iwasaki N, Doi K, Noiri E, Iwamoto Y, et al. (2012) Inhibition of Glucose-Stimulated Insulin Secretion by KCNJ15, a Newly Identified Susceptibility Gene for Type 2 Diabetes. Diabetes 61: 1734-1741.

[177] Hirano Y, Hendil KB, Yashiroda H, Iemura S, Nagane R, et al. (2005) A heterodimeric complex that promotes the assembly of mammalian 20S proteasomes. Nature 437: 1381-1385.

[178] Vilardi F, Lorenz H, Dobberstein B (2011) WRB is the receptor for TRC40/Asna1-mediated insertion of tail-anchored proteins into the ER membrane. J Cell Sci 124: 1301-1307.

[179] den Hollander AI, Koenekoop RK, Mohamed MD, Arts HH, Boldt K, et al. (2007) Mutations in LCA5, encoding the ciliary protein lebercilin, cause Leber congenital amaurosis. Nat Genet 39: 889-895.

[180] Seko A, Kataoka F, Aoki D, Sakamoto M, Nakamura T, et al. (2009) Beta1,3-galactosyltransferases-4/5 are novel tumor markers for gynecological cancers. Tumour Biol 30: 43-50.

[181] Hirabayashi S, Tajima M, Yao I, Nishimura W, Mori H, et al. (2003) JAM4, a junctional cell adhesion molecule interacting with a tight junction protein, MAGI-1. Mol Cell Biol 23: 4267-4282.

[182] Harashima S, Wang Y, Horiuchi T, Seino Y, Inagaki N (2011) Purkinje cell protein 4 positively regulates neurite outgrowth and neurotransmitter release. J Neurosci Res 89: 1519-1530.

[183] Xu Y, Ye H, Shen Y, Xu Q, Zhu L, et al. (2011) Dscam mutation leads to hydrocephalus and decreased motor function. Protein Cell 2: 647-655.

[184] Robert-Cooperman CE, Carnegie JR, Wilson CG, Yang J, Cook JR, et al. (2010) Targeted disruption of pancreatic-derived factor (PANDER, FAM3B) impairs pancreatic beta-cell function. Diabetes 59: 2209-2218.

[185] Muller M, Winnacker EL, Brem G (1992) Molecular cloning of porcine Mx cDNAs: new members of a family of interferon-inducible proteins with homology to GTP-binding proteins. J Interferon Res 12: 119-129.

[186] Kelso J, Visagie J, Theiler G, Christoffels A, Bardien S, et al. (2003) eVOC: a controlled vocabulary for unifying gene expression data. Genome Res 13: 1222-1230.

Chapter 9

Risk Factors for Down Syndrome Birth: Understanding the Causes from Genetics and Epidemiology

Sujay Ghosh and Subrata Kumar Dey

Additional information is available at the end of the chapter

http://dx.doi.org/10.5772/52903

1. Introduction

Aneuploidy can be defined as presence of erroneous number of chromosome in organisms and in human aneuploidy is the major cause of birth wastage. Among all known recognizable human aneuploidies, trisomy 21 shows the highest frequency of occurrence, estimating approximately 1 in 700 live-births (Kanamori *et al.*, 2000). The trisomy 21 condition originates due to non-separation or nondisjunction (NDJ) of chromosome 21(Ch21) during gametogenesis and as a result disomic gametes with two copies of a particular chromosome are formed and upon fertilization by haploid gamete from opposite sex lead to the formation and implantation of trisomic fetus. The trisomy 21 condition is popularly known as Down syndrome (DS) after the name of John Langdon Down who described the syndrome for the first time in 1866 (Down, 1866). Beside chromosomal NDJ, a small proportion of DS occurs due to post zygotic mitotic error or translocation of chromosome 21 to other autosomes.

Within the category of free trisomy 21 due to NDJ, overwhelming majority of errors occurs in maternal oogenesis particularly at meiosis I (MI) stage (Table 1). A little fraction of NDJ errors arise at paternal spermatogenesis. This preferential occurrence of maternal meiotic error is probably due to the mechanism of oocyte maturation in the ovary. Meiosis is initiated in the human foetal ovary at 11–12 weeks of gestation (Gondos *et al.*, 1986), but becomes arrested after completion of homologous chromosome pairing and recombination. This meiotic-halt lasts for several years until the elevated level of LH and FSH resume the process at the onset of puberty. Then the oocyte completes meiosis I (MI) and enters meiosis II (MII) and again undergoes a phase of pause. It completes the meiosis II after the sperm enter its cytoplasm following fertilization. Thus, the oocyte, whose ovulation marks the menarche, remains in pause for shortest period and that ovulates just preceding menopause experiences longest period of arrest. This long tenure of oocyte development makes it vulnerable to acquire environmental hazards within its microenvironment which inevitably increases the risk of chromosomal NDJ.

Parental Origin	Meiotic Origin of Nondisjunction	Frequency	Maternal Age at Conception (Years±SD)	Paternal Age at Conception (Years±SD
Maternal	Meiosis I	79.03%	29.07±6.11	34.98±3.88
	Meiosis II	29.97%	32.54±2.45	35.02±4.66
Paternal	Meiosis I	39.23%	24.07±6.22	33.02±5.9
	Meiosis II	59.26%	28.03±4.6	34.09±3.9
Post Zygotic Mitotic Error		2.2%	29.66±7.3	32.08±5.32

Table 1. Distribution of mean parental age for Down syndrome birth and nondisjunctional errors of chromosome 21 stratified by parent and meiotic stage of origin

In search of etiology of Ch21 NDJ, researchers have unambiguously identified two risk factors namely advancing maternal age and altered pattern of meiotic recombination. Beside these two risk factors, other environmental and behavioural factors have also been identified as risk of Ch21 NDJ and they exhibit several degrees of interactions with advancing maternal age and recombination pattern of Ch21. These make the etiology of DS birth a puzzle in the field of medical genetics.

2. Genetic risk factors

2.1. Advanced maternal age and related hypotheses

The age of the mother at the time of the conception of a fetus with DS is, by far, the most significant risk factor for meiotic NDJ of Ch21. As a woman ages, her risk for having a fetus with trisomy 21 significantly increases. This association was noted initially by Penrose in 1933 (Penrose, 1933). For all the populations studied so far, estimated mean maternal age of conception of DS baby is higher than that of controls i.e., having euploid baby and women with MII NDJ is older than women affected with MI NDJ.

Several hypotheses have been put forward to explain the link between advancing maternal age and higher incidence of aneuploid oocyte formation but no one has proved to be completely satisfactory. The most popular hypothesis (Gondos *et al.*, 1986) holds that the protracted tenure of oogenesis interrupted with meiotic halts (Figure 1), probably makes the eggs more vulnerable to the aging effect than sperms. This long period of oocyte maturation results in the aging associated deteriorative changes to accumulate over time either in the oocyte or its milieu. Examples of such factors would be a diminishing amount of a meiotic proteins, like those maintaining sister chromatid adhesion (Hodges *et al*., 2005; Hunt & Hassold, 2008) or meiotic checkpoints components (Garcia-Cruz *et al*., 2010) or weakening of centromere cohesion due to age-related reduction in centromere associated proteins MCAK (Eichenlaub-Ritter *et al*. 2010). This list of age related risks may also include the accumulation of environmentally induced damage to the meiotic machinery over time or genetic changes such as mitochondrial deletions (Van Blerkom, 2011). Among all these variables, the spindle assembly check point (SAC) components and sister chromatid cohesion (SCC) were investigated thoroughly (Chiang *et al*.; 2010), as they are prospective genetic candidates that may explain the aging effect on aneuploid oocyte formation. The SAC is a molecular machine that ensures proper chromosome separation in both mitosis and meiosis. In meiosis SAC prevents anaphase until all chromosomes properly attach to the spindle. The SAC includes *MAD2L1, BUB1B*, and *TTK* (Hached *et al*., 2011; Niault *et al*., 2007) which show decline in concentration with age in mouse leading to misaligned chromosomes (Pan *et al*., 2008) and errors in SAC function contribute in age-related aneuploidy. Disrupted spindles, misaligned chromosomes and decreased expression of SAC components *Mad2L1* and *Bub1* have evident in aged human oocytes (Mc Guinness *et al*., 2009; Steuerwald *et al*., 2001) and these findings are consistent with aging hypothesis. On the other hand, the SSC mediates physical pairing of duplicated chromosomes which is essential for appropriate distribution of chromosomes. The cohesion along chromosome arms keeps the bivalents intact in MI and centromere cohesion holds sister chromatids together in MII. A defect in cohesion distal to crossover sites may result in a shift in chiasmata placement (alternatively known as 'chiasma slippage') or even premature bivalent separation in MI, whereas reduced centromere cohesion may result in premature separation of sister chromatids in MII (Steuerwald *et al*., 2001). The loss of cohesion with maternal age for distally placed chiasma (Subramanian and Bickel, 2008) is consistent with the idea that cohesion defects may contribute to age related aneuploidy (Chiang *et al*., 2012). Another component that supposed to decline with age and contributes significantly to aging effect on DS birth is the meiosis surveillance system of ovary that ensures achiasmate chromosome segregation (Oliver *et al*., 2008). Chiasma formation and subsequent recombination are prerequisite of faithful separation of homologues at meiotic anaphase. Absences of chiasma, faulty configurations of chiasma and reduction in chiasma frequency have been attributed to NDJ of Ch21 and subsequent DS birth (Lamb *et al*., 2005; Ghosh *et al*., 2010). A high proportion of achiasmate Ch21 tetrad was reported among the mothers of DS having age >35 year (Oliver *et al*., 2008). As the decision regarding chiasma formation is taken in foetal ovary, high frequency of achisamate nondisjoined Ch21 in older oocyte can only be explained by down regulation of surveillance system. Human proteins involved in segregation of nonexchange chromosome show down regulation with increasing ovarian age (Steuerwald *et al*., 2001; Baker *et al*., 2004).

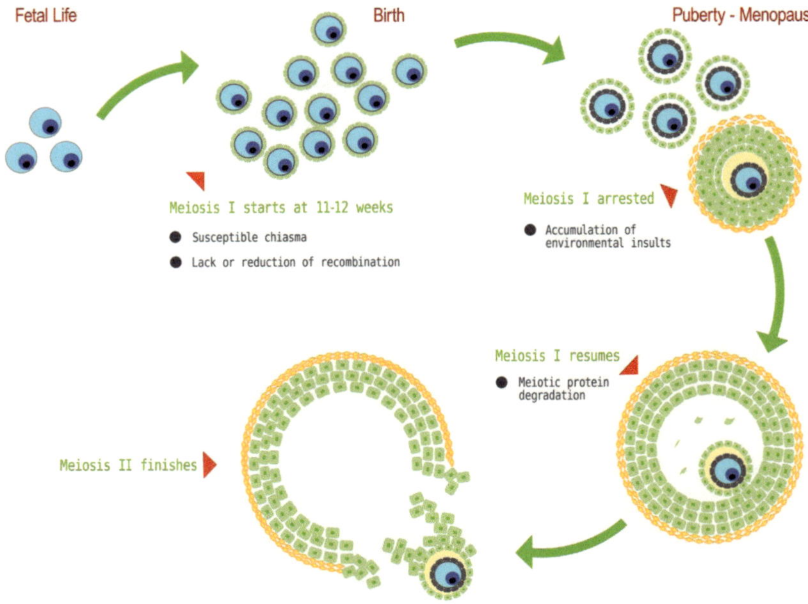

Figure 1. Time line for oocyte development in human and probable time of occurrence of risk factors for chromosome 21 nondisjunction.

A second hypothesis relates the "biological aging" or "ovarian aging" with the increasing rate of meiotic errors (Warburton, 1989; 2005). The central theme of this hypothesis is the prediction that biological aging is different among women of the same chronological age and that the frequency of trisomic conceptions depends upon the biological age of the woman rather than the chronological age (Warburton, 2005). The biological age of women can usually be assessed by counting the falling number of antral follicles with chronological age together with decrease in total oocyte pool size (Scheffer *et al.* 1999; Kline *et al.* 2004). These altogether alter the optimum hormonal balance in ovary, which is marked by falling concentration of serum inhibin A and B, decline in estrogens surge and elevated level of FSH (Warburton, 2005). This change in hormone balance is related to increased rate of aneuploidy at advanced maternal age. Support to this prediction is available from the experiment on mouse model (Robert *et al.* 2005). Alternative to this prediction was provided in the 'limited oocyte pool hypothesis' (Warburton, 2005), which stated that with biological age there is a decrease in the number of antral follicles, leaving only the premature or post mature oocyte to ovulate. The "biological aging" hypothesis predicts that women with a trisomic conception should on the average have an older "ovarian age" than other women of the same chronological age with a normal conception (Warburton, 2005) and women having trisomic pregnancy have average earlier (~1 year) age of menopause (Kline *et al.*, 2000). If these were the facts, one would expect that after a trisomic conception, the risk of a subsequent trisomy for any chromosome should be higher than the maternal age-related risk. Support to this prediction comes from the recent data from prenatal diagnosis after a previous trisomic conception which shows that the risk of a subsequent trisomy birth is about 1.7 times the maternal age-related risk (Warburton *et al.*, 2005). Mathematical model proposed by Kline and Levin (1992) estimated that women with trisomy pregnancy experience 0.9 years early menopause which suggests that such women suffer from advanced ovarian aging than the women with chromosomally normal pregnancies. Population sample survey for calculating the median age of menopause among the women with trisomic pregnancy loss also suggested an early cessation of menstrual cycle among them than the mothers with chromosomally normal foetus (Kline *et al.*, 2000). Elevated level of FSH is reported among the women with DS pregnancy (Nasseri *et al.*, 1991; van Montfrans *et al.*, 2002) which suggests precocious aging among them. Very recently, Kline *et al.* (2011) conducted the survey on the hormonal level of women with trisomic pregnancy and supported the *'reduced oocyte pool hypothesis'*, suggesting that some women have smaller follicle content than the others of same chronological age. The former group are susceptible for rapid ovarian aging and associated trisomic conceptions. All these findings suggest intuitive existence of some predisposing factors among some women for their earlier aging that relates their trisomic conception too.

The third hypothesis is concerned with 'genetic age' of women and stated that it is the genetic aging that underlies the all kind of degenerative changes in ovary and oocyte. The hypothesis was proposed by Ghosh *et al.*, (2010). The authors estimated the telomere length of peripheral lymphocyte of women with DS child and compared with age matched controls. They found that beyond of age 29 years the DS bearing mothers exhibit rapid telomere shortening and hence rapid genetic aging than the controls. The authors inferred that DS bearing younger mothers do not experience any accelerated genetic aging; it is only the chronological older age when DS bearing mothers suffer from rapid genetic and molecular aging than the age matched mothers of euploid child. The authors proposed 'Genetic aging hypothesis' which stated that some women are predisposed to rapid genetic and molecular aging and its effect is exacerbated at advance age when age-related deteriorative changes also affect the chromosome separation system leading to NDJ. The notion has suggested some intuitive link between telomere maintenance system (i.e., system of molecular aging) and chromosome segregating apparatus at molecular level.

2.2. Altered pattern of recombination and its interaction with maternal age

Aside from maternal age, there is only one other factor that has been shown to associate increased susceptibility of maternal NDJ, namely altered recombination patterns. Warren *et al.* (1987) provided the first evidence to suggest that a proportion of maternal NDJ errors were associated with reduced recombination along Ch 21. Further examination has shown that, in addition to the absence of an exchange along the nondisjoined Ch 21, the placement of an exchange is an important susceptibility factor for NDJ. Examination of recombination along the maternal nondisjoined Ch 21 has suggested three susceptible exchange patterns: 1) no exchange leads to an increased risk of MI errors, 2) a single telomeric exchange leads to an increased risk of MI errors, and 3) a pericentromeric exchange leads to an increased risk of so-called MII errors. These patterns are similar to those observed in model organisms where absence or reduced recombination, along with sub-optimally placed recombinant events, increases the likelihood of NDJ (Rasooly *et al.*, 1991; Moore *et al.*, 1994; Sears *et al.*1995; Zetka and Rose, 1995; Koehler *et al.*, 1996; Ross *et al.*, 1996; Krawchuk and Wahls, 1999). Exchanges too close to the centromere or single exchange too close to the telomere seem to confer chromosomal instability.

Subsequently, researchers have identified a potential interaction between maternal age and pattern of recombination. The study on US population (Sherman *et al.*, 1994) provided the first evidence in this regard and proved an age related reduction in recombination frequency among the MI cases, with older women (35 yrs. and more) having less recombination along 21q than younger women (< 35 yrs.), as suggested by estimated length (cM) of age-specific linkage map of Ch21. In exploring the interaction between maternal age and recombination and to gain further insight into the potential mechanisms of abnormal chromosome segregation, comparison had been made for frequency and location of meiotic exchanges along 21q (Lamb et al. 2005) among women of various ages who had an infant with DS due to a maternal MI error. While there was no significant association between maternal age and overall frequency of exchange, the placement of meiotic exchange differed significantly by age of conception. In particular, single telomeric recombination event was present in highest proportion among the youngest age group (80%), while the proportion in the oldest group of women and in control group were almost equal (14% and 10% respectively). Moreover, studies (Lamb *et al.*, 1996, 2005) suggested that in maternal MI error cases, majority of single exchanges were located in the telomeric end of Ch21, whereas the single exchange within the peri-centromeric region was associated with maternal MII errors. In the independent age-stratified analysis on the US population by Oliver *et al.*, (2008) and on the Indian population by Ghosh et al., (2009) a universal pattern of interactions among maternal age groups, chiasma placement and amount of meiotic recombination has been discovered. In these studies a major fraction of MI errors was recorded due to absence of any detectable exchange between non-sister chromatids of nondisjoined homologues. A trend of decreasing frequency of achiasmate meiosis (meiosis without recombination) with increasing maternal age is also observed in both the studies (Oliver *et al.*, 2008; Ghosh *et al.*, 2009), which suggests achiasmate meiosis without any recombination is maternal age-independent risk. According to the model of maternal risk factors for DS birth proposed by Oliver *et al.*, (2008) and supported by (Ghosh *et al.* 2009, Ghosh *et al.*,. 2010) that any risk factor which is maternal age independent should present in highest frequency in the younger mother, the age group in which other risk factors are usually absent. In contrast, any risk factors whose frequency increases with increasing maternal age is regarded as maternal age dependent risk factor as its effect gets exacerbated in interaction with increasing maternal age. The chiasma stabilizes the tetrad and counter balances the pull from opposite poles which ensure the faithful segregation of homologues. In absence of chiasma, the chromosomes move randomly at MI, resulting in formation of disomic gametes. As the chiasma formation takes place in foetal ovary, the achisamate chromosome containing disomic oocyte may ovulate at any time in reproductive life and hence it is maternal age independent risk factor of Ch21 NDJ.

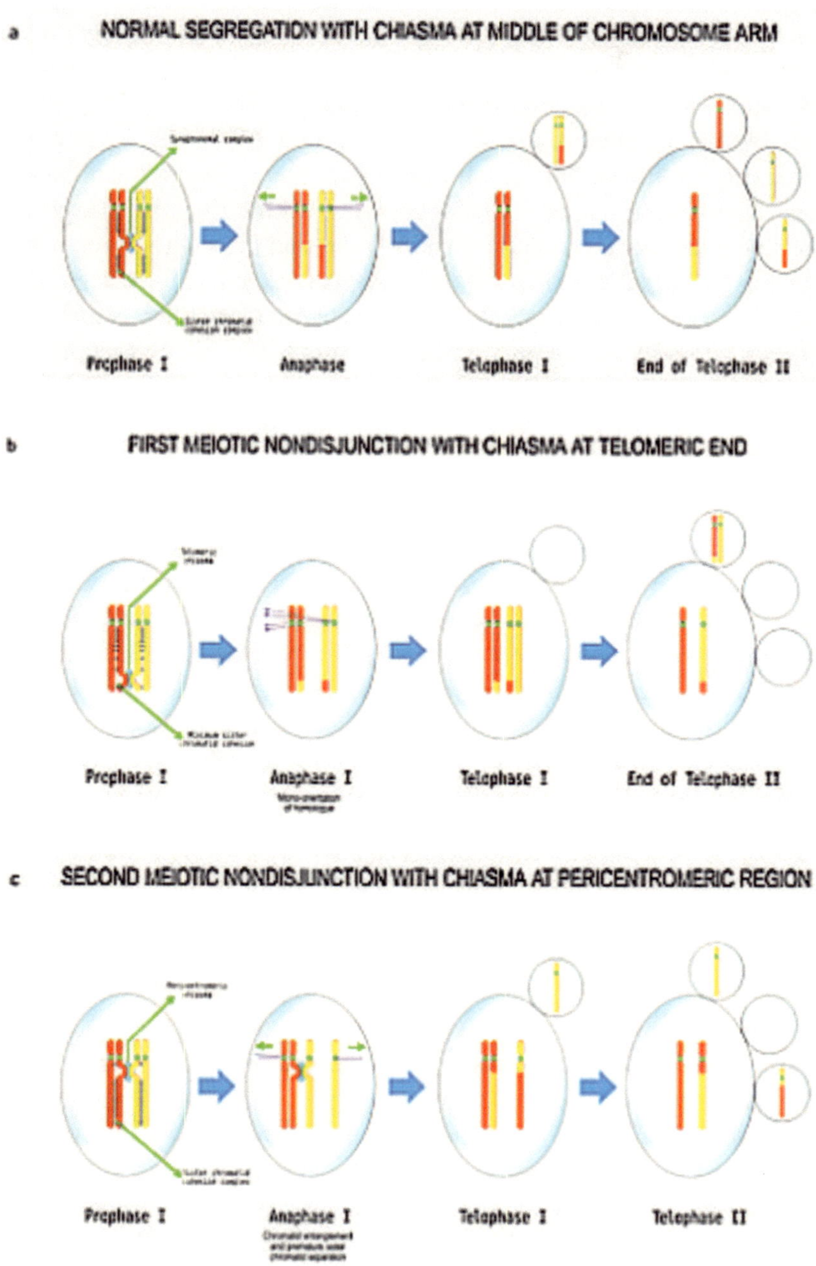

Figure 2. Model for mechanism of nondisjunction of chromosome 21: a) Normal segregation of chromosomes; b) First meiotic nondisjunction; c) Second meiotic nondisjunction. The first meiotic nondisjunction involves telomeric chiasma with premature sister chromatid separation followed by mono-orientation of homologous chromosome at MI. The second meiotic nondisjunction involves peri-centromeric chiasma formation with chromosome entanglement. Noted that the error actually arises at MI but its effect appeared at MII.

In both the studies on US and Indian populations (Oliver *et al.*, 2008; Ghosh *et al.*, 2009), the single telomeric chiasma and subsequent recombination were found in highest frequency among the women of younger age group i.e., age group below 29 years, who had a NDJ error at meiosis I stage of oogenesis and there was a gradual decrease in telomeric chiasma frequency with advancing maternal age. This observation suggests that the single telomeric chiasma formation is the risk of NDJ of Ch 21 even in younger women who otherwise do not suffer from deterioration related to the aging. Thus within the total risk probability of Ch21 NDJ, the single telomeric chiasma formation represent the highest proportion among the younger women of MI NDJ category. Two important inferences have been drawn from this finding. The first one is that the single telomeric chiasma formation is maternal age independent risk of Ch21 NDJ. The second is that the single telomeric chiasma probably induces some structural instability of Ch21 that segregates randomly at meiosis I which takes place in fetal ovary.

Understanding the exact mechanism how does single telomeric chiasma cause chromosomal mis-segregation has been obtained from the observations in model organisms like *Drosophila* (Koehler *et al.*, 1996), *Saccharomyces* (Ross *et al.* 1996) and *Caenorhabditis elegans* (Zetka and Rose, 1995). As the telomeric chiasma located far from the kinetochore, the point of spindle-attachment links the homologues less efficiently and orients each kinetochore to the same spindle pole and prevents bi-orientation of homologues (Nicklas, 1974; Hawley *et al.*, 1994; Koehler *et al.*, 1996). Most likely, this susceptibility is related to the minimal amount of sister chromatid cohesion complex (Figure 2b) remaining distal to the exchange event (Orr-Weaver, 1996). Alternatively, the integrity of chiasma may be compromised when a minimum amount of cohesin remains to hold homologue together. Thus bivalent may act as pair of functional univalent during MI, as has been evident in human oocyte (Angell, 1994; 1995).

Another chiasma configuration that poses susceptibility for NDJ of Ch21 is the pericentromeric exchange. In both the studies on US and Indian DS populations (Oliver *et al.*, 2008; Ghosh *et al.*, 2009), highest frequency of pericentromeric exchange was scored in older women having age >34 years. A trend of gradual increase in centromeric chiasma frequency with increasing age was recorded in both the studies with gradual shifting of chiasma from middle of the chromosome in younger age group to more proximal to centromere in older age group. In explaining the effect on chromosome segregation that single centromeric chiasma imparts two hypotheses have been put forward by the authors. The chiasma that is positioned very close to centromere may cause 'chromosomal entanglement' at MI, with the bivalent being unable to separate, passing intact to MII metaphase plate (Lamb *et al.*, 1996). Upon MII division, the bivalent divides reductionally, resulting in disomic gamete with identical centromeres (Figure 2c). In this manner, proximal pericentromeric exchange, which occurs at MI, is resolved and visualized as MII error. According to an alternate model, studied in *Drosophila* (Koehler *et al.*, 1996), proximal chiasma leads to a premature sister chromatid separation just prior to anaphase I. Resolution of chiasma requires the release of sister chromatid cohesion distal to the site of exchange (Hawley *et al.*, 1994). Attempt to resolve chiasma that is very close to centromere could result in premature separation of chromatids (Figure 2c). If the sister chromatids migrate to a common pole at MI, they have 50% probability to move randomly into the same product of meiosis at MII, resulting in an apparent MII NDJ. Similar observation is reported from the study in Yeast in which centromere-proximal crossover promotes local loss of sister-chromatid cohesion (Rockmill *et al.*, 2006). Studies of NDJ in both humans (Angell, 1995) and *Drosophila* (Miyazaki & Orr-Weaver, 1992) have provided preliminary supports for this model.

The effect of pericentromeric exchange on meiotic chromosome separation gets exacerbated with maternal age related insults in ovarian environment, as suggested by greater proportion of DS births among older women who have experienced the particular pattern of chiasma formation. This relationship can be interpreted in two different ways: 1) pericentromeric exchange set up a sub-optimal configuration that initiates or exacerbates the susceptibility to maternal age-related risk factors, perhaps leading to an increase in premature sister chromatid segregation or 2) a pericentromeric exchange protect the bivalent against age related risk factor, allowing proper segregation of homologues, but not the sister chromatids at MII (Oliver *et al.*, 2008). The former explanation is likely to the '*two hit model*' proposed previously by Lamb *et al.*, (1996). Alternatively, a pericentromeric exchange may protect the bivalent from maternal age related risk factors. The effect of degradation of centromere or sister chromatid cohesion complexes or of spindle proteins with age of oocyte may lead to premature sister chromatid separation. Perhaps the pericentromeric exchanges help to stabilize the compromised tetrad through MI. This would lead to an enrichment of MII errors among the older oocytes which is a maternal age dependent risk for NDJ of Ch21.

As far as effect of multiple chiasmata formation on the nondisjoined Ch 21 is concerned, two important reports have been published very recently. In their study Ghosh *et al.* (2010) found that two or more chiasmata formation is prevalent particularly in older age group (≥ 34 years). This infers that the older oocyte suffers from nondisjunctional errors even when Ch21 experiences formation of two or more chiasmata which are believed to be protective of NDJ; this is due to aging effects that imparts various degenerative changes in ovary. Analyzing the effect of multiple chiasmata of the 21q, Oliver *et al.* (2011) found a decrease in the interval between two simultaneous chisamata on the chromosome that disjoined at MI and this closeness is due to shifting of distal chiasma towards centromere. The author argued that as the proximal chiasma remains at its usual position, similar to that on the normally disjoined chromosome, it is the distal chiasma whose dislocation towards the proximal chiasma nullifies the 'good-effect' of the latter that is needed for faithful segregation of the chromosome. The Ch21 experiences such distal chiasma dislocation in association with correctly placed proximal chiasma disjoines erroneously at MI. Moreover, the authors found more intimate positioning of proximal chiasma with the centromere of the chromosomes with two exchanges and this tendency increases with advancing age. This pattern is very similar to the single chiasma shifting related to MII errors reported in earlier studies (Oliver et al., 2008; Ghosh et al., 2009). Moreover, the authors further extend their realization that the centromeric chiasma may not be protective of NDJ, the notion previously assumed both by Oliver *et al.* (2008) and Ghosh *et al.* (2009).

2.3. Genetic polymorphism and increasing susceptibility of Down syndrome birth

Maternal genetic factors such as polymorphism of certain gene probably make them susceptible for NDJ error. Experimental organisms have been used to identify genes that are important in the proper segregation of chromosomes. The potential candidates are those genes involved in the meiotic process such as homologue pairing, assembly of the synaptonemal complex, chiasmata formation and chiasma positioning, sister chromatid cohesion, spindle formation. Genetic variations of these genes are predisposing factors for chromosome NDJ.

The gene that has been identified first in this category is *MTHFR* (methylene tetrahydrofolate reductase), which is not directly related to the meiotic process. The case-control study by James *et al.*, (1999) provided primary evidence that the 677C→T polymorphism in the *MTHFR* gene increases the risk of having a child with DS (Odds Ratio = 2.6) in North American population. This polymorphism is associated with elevated plasma homocysteine and/or low folate status (Sherman *et al.*, 2005). Folate is essential for the production of S-adenosylmethionine, which is the primary methyl donor (Figure 3a) for epigenetic DNA methylation essential for gene expression regulation and maintenance of chromosomal integrity at centromere (James *et al.*, 1999; Dworkin *et al.*, 2009; Sciandrello *et al.*, 2004). Folate deficiency reduces S-adenosylmethionine synthesis, leading to DNA hypomethylation (Pogribny *et al.*, 1997; Beetstra *et al.*, 2005; Wang *et al.*, 2004). The pericentromeric hypomethylation could impair the heterochromatin formation and kinetochore establishment (Figure 3b)resulting in chromosomal NDJ (James *et al.*, 1999). This happens because the stable centromeric chromatin depends on the epigenetic inheritance of specific centromeric methylation patterns and it binds with specific methyl-sensitive proteins in order to maintain the higher-order DNA architecture necessary for kinetochore assembly (Migliore *et al.*, 2009).

This initial report had inspired several follow-up studies on the *MTHFR* 677C→T polymorphism, as well as several other allelic variants in the folate pathway genes to identify genetic risk factors for having a child with DS. But the results are inconsistent (James *et al.* 2004a, 2004b), especially those that have evaluated genotype alone without biomarkers of metabolic phenotype. Those who have examined blood homocysteine levels, a broad-spectrum indicator of nutritional and/or genetic impairment in folate/B12 metabolism have documented a significantly higher level among the mothers of children with DS compared with control mothers from the same country. One possible explanation for the inconsistent results among the numerous studies may reflect the complex interaction between effects of genetic variants and nutritional intake (James *et al.*, 2004b). Nevertheless, support to the notion regarding the association between MTHFR 677C-T polymorphism and risk of DS birth was provided by other studies in different populations. Wang *et al.*, (2004) reported significant increase in the risk of DS conception among Chinese women bearing two polymorphisms namely, polymorphisms of *MTHFR* 677C→T and the polymorphism *MTRR* (Methionine synthase reductase) 66A→G. The estimated risks were more than three folds and five folds for *MTHFR* (Odd Ratio=3.7; 95% CI, 1.78~8.47) and *MTRR* (Odd Ratio= 5.2; 95% CI, 1.90~14.22) respectively. The combined presence of both polymorphisms was associated with a greater risk of DS than the presence of either alone, with an odds ratio of 6.0 (95% CI, 2.058~17.496). The study on Italian population also agreed the link between DS birth and *MTHFR* and *MTRR* polymorphisms (Coppedè *et al.*, 2010). Cyril *et al.*, (2009) conducted such association study on Indian women and confirmed the association of *MTHFR* 677C→T polymorphism with DS birth risk.

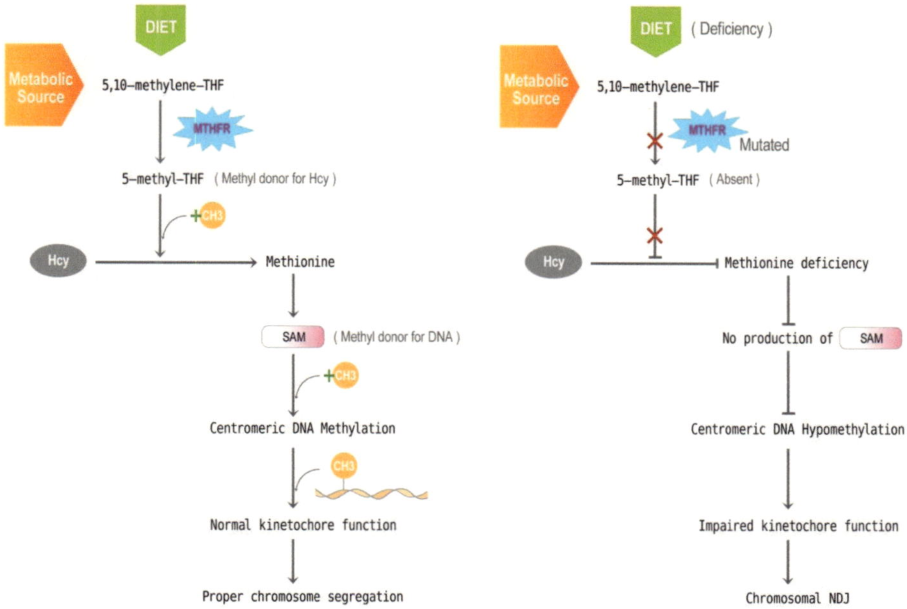

Figure 3. Role of *MTHFR* gene in folate metabolism pathway and effect of its polymorphism on chromosome 21 segregation. a) The left panel shows wild *MTHFR* genes and its involvement in chromosome segregation system; b) The mutation in MTHFR gene disrupts the folate metabolism pathway leading to missegregation of chromosome.

The other way to find out the genes involved in human NDJ is to analyze the association of consanguinity and trisomy 21(Sherman *et al.*, 2005). If such an association really does exist, it would provide evidence for a genetic effect for NDJ. The study of Alfi *et al.*, (1980) provided one of the earlier reports suggesting an association between increased consanguinity among parents of individuals with DS in a study population in Kuwait. Authors postulated the existence of a gene that increases the risk for mitotic NDJ. Alternatively, they suggested that increased rates of consanguinity among parents would be correlated with those in grandparents and therefore, an autosomal recessive gene may be postulated to be involved in meiotic NDJ in the homozygous parents. But the reports from subsequent studies in other populations are contradictory and did not find any evidence for an association between consanguinity and human NDJ (Devoto *et al.*, 1985; Hamamy *et al.*, 1990; Roberts *et al.*, 1991; Basaran *et al.*, 1992; Zlotogora, 1997; Sayee & Thomas, 1998; Rittler *et al.*, 2001).

Lastly, differences in the prevalence of DS among different racial groups may provide indirect evidence for genetic factors involved in human NDJ. However, such studies are difficult to conduct and to interpret. Differences (or similarities) may reflect the maternal age distribution of the population, accuracy of diagnosis, cultural preference and/or access to selective prenatal termination of pregnancies with trisomic fetuses, and as yet unidentified environmental factors (Sherman *et al.*, 2005). Only one such study by Allen *et al.*, (2009) reported demographic differences in mean maternal age of DS conception recorded in two different sample sets from USA. This study included DS samples from Atlanta Down syndrome project and National Down syndrome project and found that mothers enrolled in National Down syndrome project were on an average older than those of Atlanta. Moreover, the authors have also reported some ethnic differences in maternal age distribution. The Atlanta Down syndrome project had a higher proportion of cases and controls that were black and a significantly smaller proportion of Hispanics than did the National Down syndrome project. Comparison of mean maternal ages indicated variation by ethnic groups. In both the Atlanta Down syndrome project and National Down syndrome project, white mothers tended to be older than their black or Hispanic counterparts. Specifically, for both cases and controls, white mothers were found to be significantly older than black mothers ($P< 0.01$) and Hispanic mothers ($P< 0.01$); blacks and Hispanics were not significantly different from each other ($P>0.05$). To confirm such effect of demographic and ethnic differences on the etiology of DS birth, further large scale population based studies are needed to be conducted.

2.4. Paternal risk factor for chromosome 21 nondisjunction

The paternal error constitutes nearly 5 to 10% of total occurrence of live born DS cases, depending upon the populations studied. Unlike maternal cases the studies on the etiology of paternal NDJ are limited by insufficient sample size. The first significant report was provided by Savage *et al.*, (1998) who found reduction in recombination in MI nondisjoined cases, but not in MII errors. Moreover, the authors inferred that altered chiasma positioning may not associate with NDJ in spermatogenesis, as the authors recorded very concordant pattern of chiasma distribution among DS cases and control. In their extension study with more paternally derived samples, Oliver *et al.*, (2009) determined that majority of Ch21 NDJ errors in spermatogenesis occurs at MII (32%MI:68%MII), and the authors did not found significant reduction in recombination either in MI or in MII errors. Moreover, their sample did not exhibit any advanced age effect for either of meiotic outcome groups. The authors argued that the time scale of spermatogenesis is much shorter starting at puberty runs continuously without meiotic halt and this explains why advancing paternal age does not exacerbate and associate Ch21 NDJ in spermatogenesis. This study is significant in the realization that etiology of Ch21 NDJ differs in two sexes and case of paternal errors remains an enigma. In general the frequency of recombination for normally segregating chromosome is less in male than in female. But further reduction in recombination frequency may not cause NDJ in male. Moreover, epidemiological study on the risk factors for paternal NDJ of Ch21 is yet to be conducted.

3. Habitual risk factor for chromosome 21 nondisjunction

Beside maternal age and altered pattern of recombination, set of prospective environmental or habitual risk factors have been identified in several epidemiological studies. These factors

http://dx.doi.org/10.5772/52903

show various degrees of associations with DS birth. The list includes maternal cigarette smoking, use of oral contraceptive, peri-conceptional alcohol consumption by mother, exposure to radiation and low socio-economic status. Number of studies reported a negative association between maternal smoking around the time of conception and the risk for DS birth (Kline *et al.*, 1983, 1993; Hook & Cross, 1985, 1988; Shiono *et al.*, 1986; Chen *et al.*, 1999). One explanation for the negative association was that trisomic conceptuses were selectively lost prenatally among women who smoke (Hook and Cross, 1985; Kline *et al.*, 1993). But evidence against this speculation is also available (Cuckle *et al.*, 1990; Kallen, 1997; Torf & Christianson, 2000). Study conducted by Yang *et al.*, (1999) suggested that maternal-smoking was significantly associated with MII error and probably due to compromise in blood and oxygen supply surrounding the developing follicles. Besides smoking, the other maternal risk factor for which epidemiological studies have been conducted most is oral contraceptive. The use of oral contraceptive by women at the time of conception is subject of speculation as risk for DS births (Yang *et al.*, 1999). The study by Martinez-Frias *et al.*, (2001) showed that the risk for DS in infants born to mothers with less than 35 years of age (as a group) who became pregnant while taking oral-contraceptive is near the risk for mothers of DS with more than 35 years of age. In their epidemiological study, Yang *et al.*, (1999) found that women having simultaneous habits of smoking and using oral contraceptive have seven folds increased risk of having DS pregnancy and they argued that this is due to anoxic condition in ovarian microenvironment related to toxicant induced reduction in blood flow surrounding ovary. This speculation is similar to that proposed by Gaulden (1992) to explain the cause of maternal-age related NDJ. She suggested that the follicular microcirculation may be compromised in an aging ovary because of abnormal hormone signaling. Although sufficient evidence is lacking (Henderson *et al.*, 2007), alcohol consumption by women increases the chance of having DS pregnancy as suggested by Kaufman (1983).

Very recently, population based epidemiological study by Ghosh *et al.*, (2011) analyzed the effect of chewing tobacco and contraceptive pill use on the Ch21 NDJ in interaction with known risk variables like maternal age, meiotic stage of NDJ and pattern of recombination i.e., amount of exchange and positioning of chiasma on the recombining homologues. Various logistic regression models have been designed to examine every possible interaction among all above mentioned risk factors. Smokeless chewing tobacco was associated with significant risk for MII NDJ and achiasmate (nonexchange) MI error among the younger mothers. For both of these groups, the highest frequency of tobacco user was recorded in young age group (≤28 yrs) with successive gradual decrease in middle (29-34 years) and old (≥35 years) age group. According to risk prediction model (mentioned above) of DS birth, the chewing tobacco may impart some maternal age-independent risk of DS birth. In explaining the possible adverse influence of chewing tobacco on subcellular components of oocyte, the authors speculated that, regardless of oocyte age and the amount and location of recombination, tobacco probably affects some molecular system common both to meiosis I and meiosis II stages, for example the spindle apparatus. Conversely, the prevalence of oral contraceptive pill exhibited a trend of increasing frequency of occurrence with advancing maternal age, suggesting maternal age dependent risk of contraceptive pill in both the meiotic I and meiotic II error groups. Moreover, both risk factors, when present together, exhibited a strong age-dependent effect.

4. Epidemiology of environmental pollutants associated with Down syndrome birth

The epidemiological evidences in favour of the association between DS birth and environmental pollution are also surprisingly high, although controversial. Several pollution events are known to be followed by higher incidence of DS birth in an affected geographical locality. Early reports in the 1950s from USA suggested that fluoridation of water supplies might result in an increase in the frequency of DS birth (Dolk & Vrijheid, 2003). Subsequent comparison of overall DS birth rates in fluoridated and non-fluoridated areas in Massachusetts found no evidence for a difference (Needleman *et al.*, 1974). In this study prevalence rates of DS at birth were compared for Massachusetts residents ingesting fluoridated and non-fluoridated water. The observations included nearly all children born alive with DS in Massachusetts during the 17-year period 1950–1966. A rate of 1.5 cases per 1000 births was found both for fluoride-related births and appropriate comparison groups. Analysis of data from 51 American cities also found no difference in maternal age-specific DS rates between fluoridated and non-fluoridated areas (Erickson, 1980).

Similarly, water contamination with pesticide trichlorfon has been reported to cause an outbreak of DS birth incidence. It was reported in the village of Hungary in 1990s (Czeizel *et al.*, 1993) to increase in teratogenic births, including that of DS. In Woburn, Massachusetts, toxic chemicals (industrial solvents, mainly trichloroethylene) from a waste disposal site were detected in municipal drinking water wells (Dolk & Vrijheid, 2003) and people of this area reported increased incidence of several congenital anomalies. Lagakos *et al.*, (1986) followed up this finding by compiling an exposure score for residential zones in Woburn, using information on what fraction of the water supply in each zone had come from the contaminated wells annually since the start of the wells. The authors found a positive correlation between contaminated water use and higher birthrate of DS in this locality.

The increase in DS birth incidence due to accidental exposure to radioactive materials or radiation remains as a subject of research interest for long time. The disaster at nuclear power plant of Chernobyl, located in former Soviet Union, now at Ukraine, is the worst nuclear accident of the century. The immediate fallout of the incidence was the exposure of a large number of people to the various degree of ionizing radiation, which created a new situation for epidemiological investigation. The accidental event prompted numerous studies on the genetic effects of low dose ionizing radiation in man and almost all studies reported a significant increase in Down syndrome birth along with other birth defects in the parts of Germany, Scandinavia and the Lothian region of central Scotland, nine months after the disaster (Burkart *et al.*, 1997; Sperling *et al.*, 1994; Verger, 1997). This incidence was suggestive for the deleterious effect of ionizing radiation on the chromosome segregation system in oocyte of the women who are exposed to the radiation. After conducting month wise birth prevalence study on DS birth in West Germany from January 1980 to December 1989, Sperling *et al.*, (1994) suggested that low dose of ionizing radiation might cause birth of cluster of trisomy21 children in that area. Further they hypothesized that the effect of radiation got worse owing to error susceptible process of oogenesis and rapid accumulation of radioactive iodine (I^{131}) in body, as the people of that area suffered from iodine deficiency. Although the notion is intuitive, it is very compelling and needs further scientific investigation. Similarly, the effect of irradiation to which the women remained exposed for medical purpose has also been evaluated as DS birth risk in few studies (Uchida *et al.*, 1979; Strigini *et al.*, 1990; Padmanabhan *et al.*, 2004), which suggest radiation may affect the younger women more severely and may increase the chance of having DS conception.

5. Future research

Attempt to resolve the etiology of DS birth is a continuous process and we hope this will bring new insight in the understanding the hidden truth in near future. But the problem lies in its multi factorial nature (Table 2) which inevitably suggests necessity of multi-faceted research efforts from the several directions. For example, it is needed to analyze the polymorphisms of certain genes that regulate meiotic recombination or genes that control maternal molecular aging or those who are involved in faithful chromosome segregation system in meiosis. In searching the cause of recombination anomaly, *PRDM9* would be the good target of investigation, as it is a documented regulator of mammalian recombination (Borel *et al.*, 2012). Telomere maintenance system and their genetic components such as *TERT* and *TERC* may be the other targets of research and exploration of these genes would help us to realize the cause of molecular aging and related genetic susceptibility of NDJ. The component of sister chromatid cohesion complex and their role in chromosome segregation have been evident in mammals and non-mammalian model organisms. Their functional impairment is known to associate with increased rate of chromosomal missegregation and aneuploidy. But their role and allelic variations have not been explored in the context of Ch21 NDJ and subsequent DS birth. Apart from genetic components, several environmental influences are known to associate with DS birth as risk factors. But proper molecular study on how their adverse effect interacts and imperils faithful chromosome separation apparatus is tantalizingly low. At this level it is almost certain that environmental hazards or aneugen in various forms are associated with accidental increase in DS birth rate at different parts of world. But scientific evidence in favor of their interaction with genetic component is lacking and needs in depth study. If these could be resolved properly in future great advances will be made in the field of medical science and potential couple would enjoy their parenthood with physically and mentally healthy babies.

Risk Factors	**Relation with maternal age**	**Interaction with other risk factors**	**Meiotic stage of errors**	**Reference**
Reduced meiotic recombination	Maternal age independent	Not clear, possibly affected by genetic polymorphisms influence chiasma formation	MI	Lamb et al. (2005), Oliver et al. (2008), Ghosh et al. (2009), Ghosh et al. (2011).
Telomeric single chiasma	Maternal age independent	Not evident	MI	Oliver et al. (2008), Ghosh et al. (2009).
Pericentromeric single chiasma	Maternal age dependent	The risk exacerbates with increasing maternal age	MII	Oliver et al. (2008), Ghosh et al. (2009).
Shifting of distal chiasma towards proximal one when two simultaneous recombination occur	Maternal age independent	Not evident	MI	Oliver et al. (2011)
Shifting of proximal chiasma towards centromere when two simultaneous recombination occur	Maternal age dependent	The risk exacerbates with increasing maternal age	MII	Oliver et al. (2011)
Genetic polymorphisms: MTHFR 677C→T, MTRR 66A→G	Possibly maternal age independent	Not evident	Not analyzed	James et al. (2004), Wang et al. (2004).
Maternal cigarette smoking	Maternal age independent	Not evident	Not analyzed	Kline et al. (1983), Hook & Cross (1985); Yang et al. (1999).
Maternal chewing tobacco use	Maternal age independent	Possibly affects system that ensure non recombinant chromosome segregation and some components common to both MI and MII phases	Both MI and MII	Ghosh et al. (2011)
Maternal oral contraceptive use	Debatable	Supposed to affect ovarian hormone level	MII	Martı´nez-Frı´as et al (2001), Ghosh et al. (2011)
Combined exposure to tobacco and oral contraceptive	Maternal age dependent	The risk exacerbates with increasing maternal age	Both MI and MII	Yang et al. (1999). Ghosh et al. (2011)
Maternal low socioeconomic exposure	Maternal age independent	Not evident	MII	Christianson et al. (2004)

Table 2. Summary of maternal risk factors for Ch21 nondisjunction and their probable mode of action

Acknowledgements

We are extremely grateful to Prof. Eleanor Feingold, Pittsburgh University, USA and Prof. Stephanie Sherman, Emory University, Atlanta, USA for their cooperation in Down syndrome research.

Author details

Sujay Ghosh[1,2] and Subrata Kumar Dey[1]

*Address all correspondence to: g.sujoy.g@gmail.com

1 Centre for Genetic Studies, Department of Biotechnology, School of Biotechnology and Biological Sciences, West Bengal University of Technology, Salt Lake City, Kolkata, West Bengal, India

2 Genetics Research Unit, Department of Zoology, Sundarban Hazi Desarat College (Affiliated to University of Calcutta), Pathankhali, West Bengal, India

References

[1] Alfi, O. S., Chang, R., & Azen, S. P. (1980). Evidence for genetic control of nondisjunction in man. Am J Hum Genet , 32, 477-483.

[2] Allen, E. G., Freeman, S. B., Druschel, C., Hobbs, C. A., O'Leary, L. A., Romitti, P. A., Royle, M. H., Torfs, C. P., & Sherman, S. L. (2009). Maternal age and risk for trisomy 21 assessed by the origin of chromosome nondisjunction: a report from the Atlanta and National Down Syndrome Projects. Hum Genet , 125, 41-52.

[3] (Angell, R. (1994). Higher rates of aneuploidy in oocytes from older women. Hum Reprod 9:1199-2000). 9, 1199-2000.

[4] Angell, R. (1995). Mechanism of chromosome nondisjunction in human oocytes. Prog Clin Biol Res , 393, 13-26.

[5] Baker, D. J., Jeganathan, K. B., Cameron, J. D., Thompson, M., Juneja, S., Kopecka, A., Kumar, R., Jenkins, R. B., de Groen, P. C., Roche, P., & van Deursen, J. M. (2004). BubR1 insufficiency causes early onset of aging associated phenotypes and infertility in mice. Nat Genet , 36, 744-749.

[6] Basaran, N., Cenani, A., Sayli, B. S., Ozkinay, C., Artan, S., Seven, H., Basaran, A., & Dincer, S. (1992). Consanguineous marriages among parents of Down patients. Clin Genet , 42, 13-15.

[7] Beetstra, S., Thomas, P., Salisbury, C., Turner, J., & Fenech, M. (2005). Folic acid deficiency increases chromosomal instability, chromosome 21 aneuploidy and sensitivity to radiation-induced micronuclei. *Mutation Research*, 578, 317-326.

[8] Borel, C., Cheung, F., Stewart, H., Koolen, D. A., Phillips, C., Thomas, N. S., Jacobs, P. A., Eliez, S., & Sharp, A. J. (2012). Evaluation of PRDM9 variation as a risk factor for recurrent genomic disorders and chromosomal non-disjunction. Hum Genet , 131, 1519-24.

[9] Burkart, W., Grosche, B., & Schoetzau, A. (1997). Down syndrome clusters in Germany after the Chernobyl accident. Radiat Res , 147, 321-328.

[10] Burkart, W., Grosche, B., & Schoetzau, A. (1997). Down syndrome clusters in Germany after the Chernobyl accident. BMJ , 309, 158-162.

[11] Chen, C. L., Gilbert, T. J., & Daling, J. R. (1999). Maternal smoking and Down syndrome: the confounding effect of maternal age. Am J Epidemiol , 149, 442-446.

[12] Chiang, T., Duncan, F. E., & Schindler, K. (2010). Evidence that weakened centromere cohesion is a leading cause of age-related aneuploidy in oocytes. Curr Biol , 20, 1522-1528.

[13] Christianson, R. E., Sherman, S. L., & Torfs, C. P. (2004). Maternal meiosis II nondisjunction in trisomy 21 is associated with maternal low socioeconomic status. Genet Med , 6, 487-494.

[14] Cuckle, H. S., Alberman, E., Wald, N. J., Royston, P., & Knight, G. (1990). Maternal smoking habits and Down's syndrome. Prenat Diagn , 10, 561-567.

[15] Czeizel, A. E., Elek, C., Gundy, S., Métneki, J., Nemes, E., Reis, A., Sperling, K., Tímár, L., Tusnády, G., & Virágh, Z. (1993). Environmental trichlorfon and cluster of congenital abnormalities. *Lancet*, 341, 539-542.

[16] Devoto, M., Prosperi, L., Bricarelli, F. D., Coviello, D. A., Croci, G., Zelante, L., Ferranti, G., Tenconi, R., Stomeo, C., & Romeo, G. (1985). Frequency of consanguineous marriages among parents and grandparents of Down patients. Hum Genet , 70, 256-258.

[17] Dey, S. K., & Ghosh, S. (2011). Etiology of Down syndrome: Risk of Maternal age and altered meiotic recombination for chromosome 21 nondisjunction. In: S.K. Dey, ed. (2011). Genetics and Etiology of Down Syndrome. Croatia: InTech., 23-36.

[18] Dolk, H., Vrijheid, M., & (2003, . (2003). The impact of environmental pollution on congenital anomalies.Br Med Bull, , 68, 25-45.

[19] Dworkin, A. M., Huangb, T. H. M., & Toland, A. E. (2009). Epigenetic alterations in the breast: Implications for breast cancer detection, prognosis and treatment. *Seminars in Cancer Biology*, 19, 165-171.

[20] Eichenlaub-Ritter, U., Staubach, N., & Trapphoff, T. (2010). Chromosomal and cytoplasmic context determines predisposition to maternal age-related aneuploidy: brief

overview and update on MCAK in mammalian oocytes. Biochem Soc Trans , 38, 1681-1686.

[21] Erickson, J. D. (1980). Down syndrome, water fluoridation, and maternal age. Teratology , 198021, 177-180.

[22] Garcia-Cruz, R., Brieno, , Roig, I., et al. (2010). Dynamics of cohesin proteins REC8, STAG3, SMC1 beta and SMC3 are consistent with a role in sister chromatid cohesion during meiosis in human oocytes. H. um Reprod , 25, 2316-2327.

[23] Gaulden, M. E. (1992). Maternal age effect: the enigma of Down syndrome and other trisomic conditions.Mutat Res , 296, 69-88.

[24] Ghosh, S., Hong, C. S., Feingold, E., Ghosh, P., Ghosh, P., Bhaumik, P., & Dey, S. K. (2011). Epidemiology of Down syndrome: new insight into the multidimensional interactions among genetic and environmental risk factors in the oocyte. Am J Epidemiol , 174, 1009-1016.

[25] Ghosh, S., Bhaumik, P., Ghosh, P., & Dey, S. K. (2010). Chromosome 21 nondisjunction and Down syndrome birth in an Indian cohort: analysis of incidence and aetiology from family linkage data. Genet Res (Camb) , 92, 189-197.

[26] Ghosh, S., Feingold, E., & Dey, S. K. (2009). Etiology of Down Syndrome: Evidence for Consistent Association among Altered Meiotic Recombination, Nondisjunction and Maternal Age Across Populations. Am J Med Genet 149A, , 1415-1420.

[27] Ghosh, S., Feingold, E., Chakraborty, S., & Dey, S. K. (2010). Telomere length is associated with types of chromosome 21 nondisjunction: a new insight into the maternal age effect on Down syndrome birth. Hum Genet , 127, 403-409.

[28] Gondos, B., Westergaard, L., & Byskov, A. G. (1986). Initiation of oogenesis in the human fetal ovary: ultrastructural and squash preparation study. Am J Obstet Gynecol , 155, 189-195.

[29] (Hached, K., Xie, S.Z. & Buffin, E. (2011). Mps1 at kinetochores is essential for female mouse meiosis I. Development 138, 2261-2271). , 138, 2261-2271.

[30] Hamamy, H. A., al, Hakkak. Z. S., & al, Taha. S. (1990). Consanguinity and the genetic control of Down syndrome. Clin Genet , 37, 24-29.

[31] Hawley, R. S., Frazier, J. A., & Rasooly, R. (1994). Separation anxiety: the etiology of nondisjunction in flies and people. Hum Mol Genet , 3, 1521-1528.

[32] Henderson, J., Gray, R., & Brocklehurst, P. (2007). Systematic review of effects of low-moderate prenatal alcohol exposure on pregnancy outcome. BJOG , 114, 243-252.

[33] Hodges, C. A., Revenkova, E., Jessberger, R., Hassold, T. J., Hunt, P. A., (2005, , & , S. M. (2005). SMC1beta-deficient female mice provide evidence that cohesins are a missing link in age-related nondisjunction. Nat Genet , 3, 1351-1355.

[34] Hook, E. B., & Cross, P. K. (1985). Cigarette smoking and Down syndrome. Am J Hum Genet 37, 1:216-1224.

[35] Hook, E. B., & Cross, P. K. (1988). Maternal cigarette smoking, Down syndrome in live births, and infant race. Am J Hum Genet , 42, 482-489.

[36] Hunt, A., Hassold, T. J., & (2008, . (2008). Human female meiosis: What make a good egg go bad? Trend Genet , 24, 86-93.

[37] James, S. J., Pogribna, M., Pogribny, I. P., Melnyk, S., Hine, R. J., Gibson, J. B., Yi, P., Tafoya, D. L., Swenson, D. H., Wilson, V. L., & Gaylor, D. W. (1999). Abnormal folate metabolism and mutation in the methylenetetrahydrofolate reductase gene may be maternal risk factors for Down syndrome. American Journal Clinical Nutrition , 70, 495-501.

[38] James, S. J. (2004a). Maternal metabolic phenotype and risk of Down syndrome: beyond genetics. Am J Med Genet A , 127, 1-4.

[39] James, S. J. (2004b). Response to letter: Down syndrome and folic acid deficiency. Am J Med Genet A , 131, 328-329.

[40] James, S. J., Pogribna, M., Pofribny, I. P., Melnyk, S., Hine, R. J., Gibson, J. B., Yi, P., Swenson, D. H., Wilson, V. L., & Gaylor, D. W. (1999). Abnormal folate metaboloism and mutation in the methylenetetrahydrofolate reductase gene may be maternal risk factors for Down syndrome. Am J Cli Nut , 70, 495-501.

[41] Källén, K. (1997). Down's syndrome and maternal smoking in early pregnancy. Genet Epidemiol , 14, 77-84.

[42] Kanamori, G., Witter, M., Brown, J., & Williams-Smith, L. (2000). Otolaryngolog manifestations of Down Syndrome. Otolaryngol Clin North Am , 33, 1285-1292.

[43] Kaufman, M. (1983). Ethanol induced chromosomal abnormalities at conception. Nature, 302, 258-260.

[44] Kline, J., & Levin, B. (1992). Trisomy and age at menopause: predicted associations given a link with rate of oocyte atresia. Pediatr Perinat Epidemiol , 6, 225-239.

[45] Kline, J., Kinney, A., Levin, B., & Warburton, D. (2000). Trisomic pregnancy and earlier age at menopause. Am J Hum Genet , 67, 395-404.

[46] Kline, J., Kinney, A., Reuss, M. L., Kelly, A., Levin, B., Ferin, M., & Warburton, D. (2004). Trisomic pregnancy and the oocyte pool. Hum Reprod , 19, 1633-1643.

[47] Kline, J., Levin, B., Shrout, P., Stein, Z., Susser, M., & Warburton, D. (1983). Maternal smoking and trisomy among spontaneously aborted conceptions. Am J Hum Genet , 35, 421-431.

[48] Koehler, K. E., Hawley, R. S., Sherman, S., & Hassold, T. (1996). Recombination and nondisjunction in humans and flies. Hum Mol Genet , 5, 1495-1504.

[49] Krawchuk, M. D., & Wahls, W. P. (1999). Centromere mapping functions for aneuploid meiotic products: Analysis of rec8, rec10 and rec11 mutants of the fission yeast Schizosaccharomyces pombe. Genetic , 153, 49-55.

[50] Lagakos, S. W., Wessen, B. J., et al. (1986). An analysis of contaminated well water and health effects in Woburn, Massachusetts. J Am Stat Assoc, , 81, 583-596.

[51] Lamb, N. E., Freeman, S. B., Savage-Austin, A., Pettay, D., Taft, L., Hersey, J., Gu, Y., Shen, J., Saker, D., May, K. M., Avramopoulos, D., Petersen, M. B., Hallberg, A., Mikkelsen, M., Hassold, T. J., & Sherman, S. L. (1996). Susceptible chiasmate configurations of chromosome 21 predispose to non-disjunction in both maternal meiosis I and meiosis II. Nat Genet , 14, 400-405.

[52] Lamb, N. E., Sherman, S. L., & Hassold, T. J. (2005). Effect of meiotic recombination on the production of aneuploid gametes in humans. Cytogenet Genome Res , 111, 250-255.

[53] Lejeune, J., Gauthier, M., & Turpin, R. (1959). Les chromosomes humains en culture de tissues. C R Acad Sci Paris , 248, 602-603.

[54] Martínez-Frías, M. L., Bermejo, E., Rodríguez-Pinilla, E., & Prieto, L. (2001). Periconceptional exposure to contraceptive pills and risk for Down syndrome. J Perinatol , 21, 288-292.

[55] Mc Guinness, B. E., Anger, M., Kouznetsova, A., Gil-Bernabé, A. M., Helmhart, W., Kudo, N. R., Wuensche, A., Taylor, S., Hoog, C., Novak, B., & Nasmyth, K. (2009). Regulation of APC/C activity in oocytes by a Bub1-dependent spindle assembly checkpoint. Curr Biol , 19, 369-380.

[56] Migliore, L., Migheli, F., & Coppedè, F. (2009). Susceptibility to aneuploidy in young mothers of Down syndrome children. Scientific World Journal , 9, 1052-1060.

[57] Moore, D. P., Miyazaki, W. Y., Tomkiel, J. E., & Orr-Weaver, T. L. (1994). Double or nothing: a Drosophila mutation affecting meiotic chromosome segregation in both females and males. Genetics , 136, 953-964.

[58] Nasseri, A., Mukherjee, T., Grifo, J. A., Noyes, N., Krey, L., & Copperman, A. B. (1999). Elevated day 3 serum follicle stimulating hormone and/or estradiol may predict fetal aneuploidy. Fertil Steril , 71, 715-718.

[59] Needleman, H. L., Pueschel, S. M., & Rothman, K. J. (1974). Fluoridation and the occurrence of Down's syndrome. N Engl J Med , 291, 821-823.

[60] Niault, T., Hached, K., Sotillo, R., Sorger, P. K., Maro, B., Benezra, R., & Wassmann, K. (2007). Changing Mad2 levels affects chromosome segregation and spindle assembly checkpoint control in female mouse meiosis I. PLoS One 2, e1165.

[61] Nicklas, R. B. (1974). Chromosome segregation mechanisms. Genetics , 78, 205-213.

[62] Oliver, T. R., Bhise, A., Feingold, E., Tinker, S., Masse, N., & Sherman, S. L. (2009). Investigation of factors associated with paternal nondisjunction of chromosome 21. Am J Med Genet A 149A, , 1685-1690.

[63] Oliver, T. R., Feingold, E., Yu, K., Cheung, V., Tinker, S., Yadav-Shah, M., Masse, N., & Sherman, S. L. (2008). New insights into human nondisjunction of chromosome 21 in oocytes. PLoS Genet 4, e1000033.

[64] Orr-Weaver, T. (1996). Meiotic nondisjunction does the two-step. Nat Genet , 14, 374-376.

[65] Padmanabhan, V. T., Sugunan, A. P., Brahmaputhran, C. K., Nandini, K., & Pavithran, K. (2004). Heritable anomalies among the inhabitants of regions of normal and high background radiation in Kerala: results of a cohort study, 1988-1994. Int J Health Serv , 34, 483-515.

[66] Penrose, L. S. (1933). The relative effect of paternal and maternal age in Mongolism. J Genet , 27, 219-224.

[67] Pogribny, I. P., Muskhelishvili, L., Miller, B. J., & James, S. J. (1997). Presence and consequence of uracil in preneoplastic DNA from folate/methyl-deficient rats, Carcinogenesis , 18, 2071-2076.

[68] Rasooly, R. S., New, C. M., Zhang, P., Hawley, R. S., & Baker, B. S. (1991). The lethal (1) TW-6cs mutation of Drosophila melanogaster is a dominant antimorphic allele of nod and is associated with a single base change in the putative ATP-binding domain. Genetics , 129, 409-422.

[69] Reuss, M. L., Kline, J., Santos, R., Levin, B., & Timor-Tritsch, I. (1996). Age and the ovarian follicle pool assessed with transvaginal ultrasonography. Am J Obstet Gynecol , 174, 624-627.

[70] Rittler, M., Liascovich, R., Lopez-Camelo, J., & Castilla, E. E. (2001). Parental consanguinity in specific types of congenital anomalies. Am J Med Genet , 102, 36-43.

[71] Roberts, D. F., Roberts, M. J., & Johnston, A. W. (1991). Genetic epidemiology of Down's syndrome in Shetland. Hum Genet , 87, 57-60.

[72] Roberts, R., Iatropoulou, A., Ciantar, D., Stark, J., Becker, D. L., Franks, S., & Hardy, K. (2005). Follicle-stimulating hormone affects metaphase I chromosome alignment and aneuploidy in mouse oocytes matured in vitro. Biol Reprod , 72, 107-118.

[73] Ross, L. O., Maxfield, R., & Dawson, D. (1996). Exchanges are not equally able to enhance meiotic chromosome segregation in yeast. Proc Natl Acad Sci USA , 93, 4979-4983.

[74] Savage, A. R., Petersen, M. B., Pettay, D., Taft, L., Allran, K., Freeman, S. B., Karadima, G., Avramopoulos, D., Torfs, C., Mikkelsen, M., Hassold, T. J., & Sherman, S. L. (1998). Elucidating the mechanisms of paternal non-disjunction of chromosome 21 in humans. Hum Mol Genet , 7, 1221-1227.

[75] Sayee, R., & Thomas, I. M. (1998). Consanguinity, non-disjunction, parental age and Down's syndrome. J Indian Med Assoc , 96, 335-337.

[76] Scheffer, G. J., Broekmans, F. J., Dorland, M., Habbema, J. D., Looman, C. W., & te, Velde. E. R. (1999). Antral follicle counts by transvaginal ultrasonography are related to age in women with proven fertility. Fertil Steril , 72, 845-851.

[77] Sciandrello, G., Caradonna, F., Mauro, M., & Barbata, G. (2004). Arsenic-induced DNA hypomethylation affects chromosomal instability in mammalian cells. Carcinogenesis , 25, 413-417.

[78] Sears, D. D., Hegemann, J. H., Shero, J. H., & Hieter, P. (1995). Cis-acting determinants affecting centromere function, sister-chromatid cohesion and reciprocal recombination during meiosis in Saccharomyces cerevisiae. Genetics , 139, 1159-1173.

[79] Sherman, S. L., Freeman, S. B., Allen, E. G., & Lamb, N. E. (2005). Risk factors for nondisjunction of trisomy 21.Cytogenet Genome Res , 111, 273-280.

[80] Sherman, S. L., Petersen, M. B., Freeman, S. B., Hersey, J., Pettay, D., Taft, L., Frantzen, M., Mikkelsen, M., & Hassold, T. J. (1994). Non-disjunction of chromosome 21 in maternal meiosis I: evidence for a maternal age-dependent mechanism involving reduced recombination. Hum Mol Genet , 3, 1529-1535.

[81] Shiono, P. H., Klebanoff, M. A., & Berendes, H. W. (1986). Congenital malformations and maternal smoking during pregnancy. Teratology , 34, 65-71.

[82] Sperling, K., Pelz, J., Wegner, R. D., Dörries, A., Grüters, A., & Mikkelsen, M. (1994). Significant increase in trisomy 21 in Berlin nine months after the Chernobyl reactor accident: temporal correlation or causal relation? BMJ. , 309, 158-162.

[83] Steuerwald, N., Cohen, J., Herrera, R. J., Sandalinas, M., Brenner, C. A., & (2001, . (2001). Association between spindle assembly checkpoint expression and maternal age in human oocytes. Mol Hum Reprod , 7, 49-55.

[84] Strigini, P., Sansone, R., Carobbi, S., & Pierluigi, M. (1990). Radiation and Down's syndrome. Nature 347, 717.

[85] Subramanian, V. V., & Bickel, S. E. (2008). Aging predisposes oocytes to meiotic nondisjunction when the cohesin subunit SMC1 is reduced. PLoS Genet 4, e1000263.

[86] Torfs, C. P., & Christianson, R. E. (2000). Effect of maternal smoking and coffee consumption on the risk of having a recognized Down syndrome pregnancy. Am J Epidemiol , 152, 1185-1191.

[87] Uchida, I. A. (1979). Radiation-induced nondisjunction. Environ Health Perspect , 31, 13-17.

[88] Van Blerkom, J. (2011). Mitochondrial function in the human oocyte and embryo and their role in developmental competence. Mitochondrion , 11, 797-813.

[89] van Montfrans, J. M., van Hooff, M. H., Martens, F., & Lambalk, C. B. (2002). Basal FSH, estradiol and inhibin B concentrations in women with a previous Down's syndrome affected pregnancy. Hum Reprod , 17, 44-47.

[90] Verger, P. (1997). Down syndrome and ionizing radiation. Health Phys , 73, 882-893.

[91] Wang, X., Thomas, P., Xue, J., & Fenech, M. (2004). Folate deficiency induces aneuploidy in human lymphocytes in vitro- evidence using cytokinesis-blocked cells and probes specific for chromosomes 17 and 21. Mutation Research , 551, 167-180.

[92] Warburton, D. (1989). The effect of maternal age on the frequency of trisomy: change in meiosis or in utero selection? Prog Clin Biol Res , 311, 165-181.

[93] Warburton, D. (2005). Biological aging and etiology of aneuploidy. Cytogenetics and Genome Res , 111, 266-272.

[94] Warren, A. C., Chakravarti, A., Wong, C., Slaugenhaupt, S. A., Halloran, S. L., Watkins, P. C., Metaxotou, C., & Antonarakis, S. E. (1987). Evidence for reduced recombination on the nondisjoined chromosomes 21 in Down syndrome. Science , 237, 652-654.

[95] Yang, Q., Sherman, S. L., Hassold, T. J., Allran, K., Taft, L., Pettay, D., Khoury, M. J., Erickson, J. D., & Freeman, S. B. (1999). Risk factors for trisomy 21: maternal cigarette smoking and oral contraceptive use in a population-based case-control study. Genet Med , 1, 80-88.

[96] Zetka, M., Rose, A., & (1995, . (1995). The genetics of meiosis in Caenorhabditis elegans. Trends Genet , 11, 27-31.

[97] Zlotogora, J. (1997). Genetic disorders among Palestinian Arabs: 1. Effects of consanguinity. Am J Med Genet , 68, 472-475.

Chapter 10

RCAN1 and Its Potential Contribution to the Down Syndrome Phenotype

Melanie A. Pritchard and Katherine R. Martin

Additional information is available at the end of the chapter

http://dx.doi.org/10.5772/52977

1. Introduction

Down Syndrome (DS) is caused by trisomy of *Hsa21* in humans [1]. It is the most common autosomal aneuploidy, occurring in about 1 in 700 live births [2]. The clinical features of DS are variable and affect many different aspects of development. In any given individual, there may be over 80 different clinical traits [3]. Major clinical features associated with DS include the distinctive craniofacial appearance, reduced size and altered morphology of the brain, cognitive impairments, hearing loss and defects of the gastrointestinal, immune and endocrine systems [3]. Whilst this constellation of anomalies has been described we are still far from understanding their cause. How does an extra set of normal *Hsa21* genes result in whole body system disturbances and what are the molecular genetics bases for these disturbances?

A large number of genes are simultaneously expressed at abnormal levels in DS, therefore, it is a challenge to determine which genes contribute to specific abnormalities, and then identify the key molecular pathways involved. We are advocates of the approach articulated by Nadel [4] - that a careful and detailed analysis of the clinical defects in humans be followed by the creation of mouse models that over-express only some of the genes triplicated on *Hsa21*, so that the genes responsible for specific features of the DS phenotype can be identified. We generated mice in which the *RCAN1* gene is over-expressed (RCAN1-TG) to study the consequences of excess RCAN1 and thus investigate its potential contribution to the DS phenotype. Our research adds to the growing body of work assigning specific functions to particular *Hsa21* genes. Other examples under study with a particular focus on brain function include, *DYRK1A* [5], *SOD1* [6], *APP* [7] [8] [9], *SNYJ1* [10] and *ITSN1* [11]. Once we understand the abnormalities caused by subtle over-expression of single genes, we can embark on a programme to generate mice expressing combinations of genes to examine potential additive effects. This sort of approach is consistent with the idea that the DS phenotype results from disturbances in biological pathways due to an accumulation of subtle changes brought about by the effects of the over-expression of many single genes. Indeed, such an approach is bearing fruit already - *RCAN1* and *DYRK1A* have been shown to act cooperatively to destabilise a calcineurin regulatory circuit when the genes are over-expressed in a combinatorial fashion [12].

The focus of this chapter will be to provide insight into *RCAN1* and its functions, and examine the evidence to suggest that this gene plays a role in the neurological, immune and vascular systems. We will firstly give an overview of the gene family to which *RCAN1* belongs; followed by a description of the functional domains of the protein product, including post translational modification domains; its tissue expression pattern; cellular pathways involving RCAN1; and finally, how its over-expression may contribute to the neurological, immune and cancer phenotypes associated with DS.

2. The RCAN gene family

DSCR1, renamed *RCAN1*, was first described by our group in 1995 after a search for genes located on *Hsa21* with the potential to be involved in DS [13]. *RCAN1* is a member of a family of calcineurin binding proteins and is conserved across species, from lower unicellular eukaryotes such as yeast to complex organisms including humans [14]. The high level of interspecies homology of this protein has been taken to indicate a conserved role during evolution [15] [16]. A number of different genes belonging to this family have now been identified in humans, including, *RCAN1, RCAN1L2, RCAN2* and *RCAN3* [15, 17]. The family was identified based on the presence of a short "signature" polypeptide FLISPPxSPP (part of the so called SP motif) [18] but there is a high degree of similarity across the entire protein in all RCAN family members. All members perform similar functions. For example, RCAN2 interacts with calcineurin with similar efficiency to RCAN1 [19] and the human gene can functionally replace the yeast gene [18]. Interestingly, while RCAN family members are all expressed in similar tissues, each family member displays a distinct expression profile. For instance, while all family members were expressed in the brain, each displayed different levels of expression, depending on the region and developmental stage examined [20]. Within these regions there were also differences in the cellular and subcellular location of the family members. RCAN1 was highly expressed in neurones and in the neutropil, while RCAN1L2 was expressed in scattered neurones and was the only RCAN family member detected in glial cells [20, 21]. The differential expression pattern of the RCAN family members in the brain indicates that they are all likely to be important in brain development and function, yet each member may be functionally distinct [20].

3. General tissue and cellular expression of RCAN1

The *RCAN1* gene spans about 100 kb of genomic DNA and consists of seven exons and six introns. Of the seven exons, the first four are alternative first exons (*RCAN1-1* to *RCAN1-4* containing exons 1 to 4, respectively). *RCAN1* encodes two major protein isoforms, RCAN1-1 and RCAN1-4. RCAN1-1 protein consists of 252 amino acids, while RCAN1-4 is a shorter, 197 amino acid protein [22, 23]. Using Northern blot analysis, *RCAN1-1* and *RCAN1-4* were found to be similarly distributed throughout the body [22]. *RCAN1-1* was highly expressed in the foetal brain and in the adult brain, heart and skeletal muscle. Lower levels were detected in the foetal lung, liver and kidney and in the adult pancreas, lung, liver and placenta. High levels of *RCAN1-4* were detected in the foetal kidney and in adult heart, skeletal muscle and placental tissues, with lower levels in the foetal brain, lung and liver and adult lung, liver, kidney and pancreas. While both isoforms exhibited a similar expression pattern, only very low levels of *RCAN1-4* were found in the adult brain and *RCAN1-1* expression could not be detected in the adult kidney [13, 22]. Northern blot and RT-PCR failed to detect exon 3 in any of the foetal or adult tissue studied, while isoform 2 was found only in the foetal brain and liver [22].

RCAN1-1 and RCAN1-4, the most predominantly expressed isoforms, are under the control of different promoters and are therefore likely to have different regulatory mechanisms and possibly even different functions. For example, *RCAN1-4* expression is regulated by calcium signalling. Experiments in PC-12 cells (a neuronal like cell line) found that when intracellular calcium levels increased through membrane depolarisation, *RCAN1-4* gene expression was rapidly induced [24] and this was mediated by the calcineurin/Nuclear factor activated T cells (NFAT) signalling pathway [24]. Studies on the *RCAN1-4* promoter identified the presence of putative NFAT binding sites. No study published to date has demonstrated Ca^{2+}/calcineurin-mediated expression of *RCAN1-1*. Interestingly, RCAN1 is able to function in an autoinhibitory manner as over-expression of any RCAN1 isoform resulted in an inhibition of *RCAN1-4* gene expression [24].

The subcellular location of RCAN1 protein was initially determined using tranfection of a RCAN1-GFP protein construct in C2C12 cells, a mouse myoblast cell line. RCAN1 protein was located in both the nuclear and cytosolic compartments and in the absence of treatments to activate the calcineurin signalling pathway, resided predominantly in the nucleus [25]. Various physiological and biochemical stresses have been demonstrated to influence the location of RCAN1 within a cell. For example, under normal circumstances RCAN1 was located within the nuclear compartment in various cell lines, including HT-1080 fibrosarcoma and I251 astroglioma cells. However, when these cells were subjected to oxidative stress, RCAN1 protein was redistributed to the cytoplasm [26]. The same observation was made following activation of the calcineurin signalling pathway, which resulted in the translocation of RCAN1 from the nucleus into the cytosolic compartment [27].

4. Functional domains of the RCAN1 protein

Initial studies found that both RCAN1 isoforms encode a proline rich protein consisting of a putative acidic domain, a serine proline motif, a putative DNA binding domain and a proline rich region typical of a SH3 domain ligand [22, 28]. These structural motifs are typically seen in proteins involved in transcriptional regulation and signal transduction. A more recent study on RCAN1 proteins in dozens of species revealed 4 highly conserved regions separated by other regions that are less well conserved. These four regions consist of: a region at the amino terminus capable of forming an RNA recognition motif; the gene family signature domain consisting of the highly conserved SP motif; a PxIxIT-like domain (x represents any amino acid) and a C-terminal TxxP motif [29] (see Figure 1). The functions of these highly conserved regions in RCAN1 proteins are yet to be fully explored.

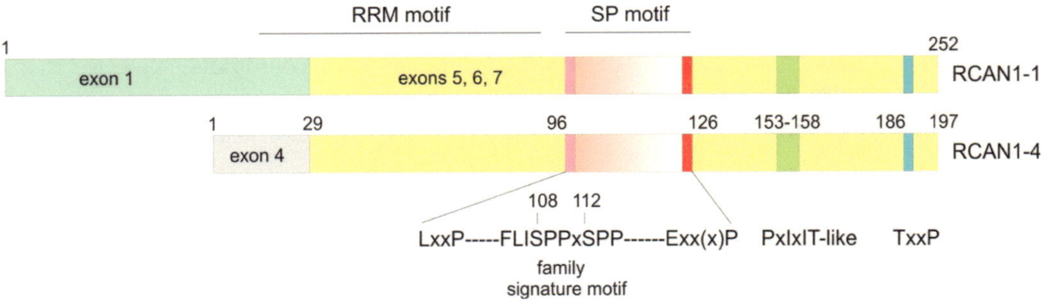

Figure 1. Schematic representation of the major RCAN1 protein isoforms. Protein motifs are shown: the RRM (RNA recognition motif); the SP (serine / proline) motif incorporating the LxxP, family signature and ExxP domains; the PxIxIT-like domain; and the TxxP motif. Serines 108 and 112 in RCAN1-4 are also indicated.

The most highly conserved region in the RCAN1 protein is the SP motif. This motif is similar to that present in NFAT proteins [30]. *In vitro,* the SP motif is able to bind to and inhibit calcineurin activity, however studies in cell lines have suggested that it is not necessary or sufficient to achieve this. By generating various deletion-constructs of the RCAN1 coding sequence it was found that RCAN1 was able to inhibit calcineurin in C2C12 myoblasts even when the SP domain was absent [31]. This study determined that two additional domains, one at the N-terminus, the other in the distal C-terminal region, were required to inhibit calcineurin activity [31]. Use of a truncated version of the RCAN1 protein also demonstrated that the last 33 amino acids were essential for nuclear localisation. In the absence of this 33 amino acid domain (which contains the SP motif and a region identified as a SH2 domain) RCAN1 protein accumulated in the cytoplasm [25].

Site-directed mutagenesis studies have shown that phosphorylation of the RCAN1 protein regulates its function, subcellular location and stability. Indeed, RCAN1 can be phosphorylated by various kinases at a number of different sites to change its activity towards calcineurin. For example, the serine residue within the SP domain at position 112 (Ser^{112}) (Ser^{167} in RCAN1-1) is variously phosphorylated by BMK1 [32], NIK [33] and DYRK1 [34] and acts as a priming site for subsequent phosphorylation at Ser^{108} (Ser^{163} in RCAN1-1) by GSK-3 [35] [31] [34]. Phosphorylation by TAK1 at Ser^{94} and Ser^{136} [36] and by DYRK1A at Thr^{193} [34] also change the activity of RCAN1 towards calcineurin (see later). NIK-mediated phosphorylation [33] or phosphorylation by PKA [37] augmented the half-life of RCAN1 protein. And, phosphorylation of a threonine residue (Thr^{166} in RCAN1-4) in the SH2 domain controlled its subcellular localisation since exchanging the threonine for an alanine resulted in an accumulation of RCAN1 protein within the cytoplasm [25]. Thus, nuclear localisation of RCAN1 is controlled, at least in part, by phosphorylation.

Other studies have shown that RCAN1 is cleaved by calpain and this cleavage appears to increase the stability of the protein by decreasing its proteasome-dependent degradation [38]. Further, the cleavage of RCAN1 by calpain also affects its interactions with other proteins. For example, cleavage of RCAN1-4 by calpain abolished its ability to bind to Raf-1 [38]. Yet another pathway involved in the post translational regulation of RCAN1 is the ubiquitin-proteasome system (UPS). The UPS is important in the regulation of protein turnover in response to changing cellular conditions and facilitates the degradation of defective proteins [39]. Ubiquitin is a polypeptide able to bind to lysine residues on proteins targeted for degradation. This binding occurs through sequential steps mediated by ubiquitin-activating enzyme (E1), ubiquitin-conjugating enzyme (E2) and ubiquitin-protein ligase (E3) [40]. Following this sequence of events, the 26s proteasome is able to recognise and degrade the poly-ubiquinated protein. The first evidence to suggest that RCAN1 was degraded by the ubiquitin pathway came from yeast two hybrid and co-immunoprecipitation experiments which found that RCAN1-4 interacted with ubiquitin [41]. More recent studies demonstrated that RCAN1 interacts with other members of the UPS, including, Skp1, Cullin/Cdc53, F-box protein Cdc4 (SCF^{Cdc4}) [42] and $SCF^{\beta\ TrCP1/2}$ [40]. The interaction between RCAN1 and the UPS is not only important in regulating turnover of the RCAN1 protein but may also influence its function. For example, increased degradation of RCAN1 by SCF^{Cdc4} diminished its ability to inhibit calcineurin signalling [42].

5. RCAN1 function—Signal transduction pathways

Interest in *RCAN1* surged after the discovery that it encoded a protein capable of inhibiting the protein serine/threonine phosphatase calcineurin (PP2B/PPP3C) [19] [27] [31] [43] [44]. RCAN1 has since been implicated in a variety of cellular processes, including oxidative stress [45] [46] [47] [48], angiogenesis [49], mitochondrial function [50] and immune responses and inflammation [44] [51]. Participation of RCAN1 in these processes has been mostly attributed to its interaction with the calcineurin pathway. Nonetheless, calcineurin-independent activities have been demonstrated [51] [52] [53] [54] [55]. Recently, RCAN1 mRNA and protein was found to increase in the peri-infarct region following middle cerebral artery occlusion (MCAO) in mice [56] and its up regulation was found to be protective [57].

5.1. The calcineurin pathway

The calcineurin pathway plays an integral role in the development and homeostatic regulation of a number of different cell types, including immune cells and neurones. The pathway is activated by increases in intracellular calcium (Ca^{2+}) due to oxidative stresses, chemical-mediated calcium increases and in response to biomechanical strain [58]. An increase in intracellular Ca^{2+} leads to the activation of calmodulin, which forms a complex with calcineurin to activate its phosphatase function. Activated calcineurin then dephosphorylates cytosolic NFAT leading to its translocation to the nucleus where it complexes with GATA-4 [59] allowing DNA binding and facilitation of the transcription of numerous gene targets [60].

RCAN1 interacts directly with calcineurin [19] [27]. Calcineurin is a heterodimer, consisting of a catalytic A subunit and a calcium binding regulatory B subunit [61]. RCAN1 is able to bind to the A subunit in a linker region between the calcineurin A catalytic domain and the calcineurin B binding region [19]. Deletion of the carboxyl-terminal half of the catalytic domain of calcineurin A abolished binding with RCAN1, indicating that this region was critical for the interaction [27]. Studies with RCAN1 have shown that exon 7 is able to bind to and regulate the activity of calcineurin and this binding occurs with a very high affinity [62]. While binding of RCAN1 to calcineurin did not interfere with the interaction between calcineurin and calmodulin, it is believed to interfere with the ability of calcineurin to bind NFAT by competing with the NFAT binding site [31]. Indeed, when *RCAN1* was over-expressed, it inhibited the activity of an exogenously added constitutively active calcineurin and transcription of a number of calcineurin-dependent genes including *IL-2* and *MEF2* was prevented [27]. *RCAN1* over-expression was found to inhibit NFAT translocation to the nucleus, thus inhibiting calcineurin-dependent gene transcription [19] but was unable to inhibit a constitutively active form of NFAT demonstrating that the inhibition of calcineurin signalling was through calcineurin, rather than interference with downstream components of the pathway [27].

Interestingly, activation of calcineurin signalling induces *RCAN1-4* expression [18, 19]. This occurs through a 900 base pair sequence located between exons 3 and 4 in an intragenic promoter region for *RCAN1-4*, which contains a dense cluster of consensus binding sites for the NFAT transcription factor [61]. The existence of such a site suggested that RCAN1 participates in a negative feedback loop, presumed to exist to prevent the adverse effects of unrestrained calcineurin activity following prolonged Ca^{2+} stimulation [27]. Indeed, following induction of the calcineurin pathway, levels of *RCAN1-4* mRNA increased within 1.5 hours and peaked 6 hours after treatment with a calcium stressor [45].

As more and more studies have emerged on RCAN1 and the propagation of calcium signals in the cell, it has become clear that the role of RCAN1 is not always to inhibit the calcineurin pathway. While the earliest studies found RCAN1 to negatively regulate the pathway, in other circumstances it seems to facilitate calcineurin activity. Indeed, contrary to expectations it was found that the absence of *Rcan1* diminished calcineurin signalling in yeast [18]. Similar results were found when *Rcan1* expression was disrupted in mice. *Rcan1*-null mice exhibited an unexpected decrease in calcineurin activity in the heart under normal physiological conditions and after stress [63] and a reduction of calcineurin activity was concomitant with reduced nuclear distribution of NFAT and a loss of NFAT-dependent gene transcription [64].

These apparently paradoxical actions of RCAN1 may be explained, at least in part, by its cellular concentration, its nuclear or cytosolic localisation and/or its phosphorylation status [64] [35] [32] [65] [25]. For example, the abundance of RCAN1 in the cell may determine its ability to either enhance or inhibit calcineurin signalling. Low or intermediate levels of RCAN1 were shown to facilitate calcineurin signalling while very high levels of over-expression were inhibitory, suggesting that RCAN1 oscillates between stimulatory and inhibitory forms depending on its concentration [35] [138]. In contrast, in another study, the functional role of RCAN1 was found to change in a dose-dependent fashion, but in the opposite direction to the aforementioned studies – RCAN1 was an inhibitor at low levels but a facilitator when levels were high [66]. Another study indicated that 4 highly conserved domains in the RCAN1 protein were important in determining its activity towards calcineurin. Specifically, that preferential binding of RCAN1 to calcineurin prevented NFAT binding resulting in inhibition of calcineurin signal transduction due to competition between RCAN1 and NFAT for calcineurin docking sites [29]. This preferential binding occurred in the presence of high levels of Rcan1 and required the LxxP domain within the SP motif and the PxIxIT domain [29]. Conversely, when Rcan1 was expressed at lower levels, the protein was able to stimulate calcineurin signalling. This stimulatory effect required the LxxP and ExxP domains within the SP motif as mutations within both of these domains prevented stimulation.

Other studies have suggested that it is the phosphorylation status of RCAN1 that determines its action as either an inhibitor or facilitator of calcineurin activity. A study in yeast found that for Rcan1 to facilitate calcineurin signalling it required phosphorylation of both serine residues located within the SP motif by a priming kinase (in this case MAPK) and Mck1, a member of the glycogen synthase kinase 3 (GSK-3) protein family. When the serines were mutated to alanines or in the absence of Mck1, Rcan1 was no longer able to stimulate calcineurin signalling resulting in inhibition [35]. Phosphorylation by TAK1, DYRK1A and NIK all switch RCAN1 from an inhibitor to a calcineurin facilitator [33] [32] [34]. At odds with most studies, phosphorylation of the serine residues within the SP motif of RCAN1 was reported to enhance its ability to inhibit calcineurin [23].

In summary, although the mechanisms responsible for the dual role of RCAN1 in the calcineurin signalling pathway is still under investigation, the results so far indicate that the primary function of RCAN1 is to facilitate calcineurin activity and this occurs when RCAN1 is expressed at lower or physiological levels. On the other hand, when RCAN1 is highly expressed, it has a secondary role of inhibiting calcineurin signalling by interfering with the interaction between calcineurin and NFAT.

5.2. GSK–3 signalling

Numerous studies outlined above have shown that GSK-3 phosphorylates RCAN1 to regulate its function. Interestingly, GSK-3 activity can also be regulated by RCAN1. PC-12 cells overexpressing RCAN1 displayed an increase in the absolute levels of GSK-3β protein, which in turn increased its kinase activity towards Tau [67]. Tau protein is a known target of GSK-3 which in its hyperphosphorylated form has been implicated in the aetiology of Alzheimer's disease [67]. Exactly how RCAN1 regulates the abundance of GSK-3 remains undetermined, but it seems that RCAN1 is acting at a post-transcriptional level as the amount of *GSK-3β* mRNA did not change upon increasing RCAN1 expression [67].

5.3. The MAPK/ERK signalling pathway

The MAPK/ERK signalling pathway mediates signal transduction from cell surface receptors to downstream transcription factors. This pathway plays a role in a number of cellular processes including proliferation, growth, motility, survival and apoptosis [68]. As indicated above, MAPK was able to phosphorylate RCAN1 at S^{112} within the SP motif to prime its subsequent phosphorylation by GSK-3. Moreover, the same study demonstrated that phosphorylation of RCAN1 by MAPK allowed RCAN1 to become a substrate for calcineurin [31], thus introducing a further level of control to keep the pathway operating at an optimal level.

5.4. The NFκβ inflammatory pathway

RCAN1 is also able to regulate the Nuclear factor κβ (NFκB) signalling pathway. NFκB is a transcription factor that regulates target genes involved in many physiological processes, including immunity, inflammation, cancer, synaptic plasticity and memory. Under normal circumstances, NFκB exists as a dimer and is sequestered in the cytoplasm through its interaction with an inhibitory molecule known as Inhibitor of κB (IκB). Upon stimulation of the NFκB signalling pathway, IκB is degraded by the ubiquitin/proteasome pathway releasing its inhibitory action on NFκB [69]. Degradation of IκB allows NFκB to translocate to the nucleus where it acts to induce the expression of various target genes including the inflammatory genes cyclooxygenase-2 (*Cox-2*) and interleukin 1 (*IL-1*) [69]. RCAN1 is able to negatively regulate the NFκB signalling pathway by attenuating NFκB activation. When RCAN1 was over-expressed in a glioblastoma cell line, it resulted in a decrease in the expression of a number of NFκB target genes including COX-2, IL-8, monocyte chemoattractant protein 1 (MCP-1), ICAM1 and VCAM1 [51]. This study demonstrated that RCAN1 inhibited NFκB signalling through a mechanism that reduced the basal turnover rate of IκBα thereby enhancing its stability [51]. By increasing the level of steady state IκBα, RCAN1 was able to exert anti-inflammatory effects by preventing NFκB activation following stimulation with inflammatory mediators such as TNFα and IL-1β.

Studies have also linked RCAN1 to NFκB signalling via other members of the pathway. For example, RCAN1 is able to negatively regulate the mRNA expression of NFκB inducing kinase (*NIK*) in PC-12 cells [70]. NIK is a member of the MAP kinase family which acts to phosphorylate and activate IκB kinase α (IKKα). Once active, IKKα phosphorylates IκBα, which in turn causes it to dissociate from NFκB, allowing the transcription factor to migrate into the nucleus and activate target genes. If RCAN1 negatively regulates the expression of *NIK*, IκB would remain bound to NFκB and inhibit NFκB signalling [33]. Interestingly, while RCAN1 regulates *NIK* expression, NIK also acts on RCAN1. As mentioned above, NIK phosphorylates the C-terminal region of RCAN1, the end result of which is to reduce RCAN1 proteasomal-dependent degradation and increase the stability of RCAN1 protein [33]. The functional consequences of this increased stability of RCAN1 on NFκB signalling have yet to be determined; however consistent with the study described above [51] it seems likely that elevated levels of RCAN1 would increase the stability of Iκβ which would in turn inhibit the NFκB signalling pathway.

5.5. Angiogenesis

Angiogenesis is a physiological process involving the growth of new blood vessels essential for embryonic development as well as growth and development throughout life. This process has also been associated with disease states including inflammation, tumourigenesis and cardiovascular disease [71]. Angiogenesis is orchestrated by a balance between pro-angiogenic factors and angiogenic inhibitors [72]. A critical mediator of angiogenesis is Vascular endothelial growth factor (VEGF) which acts to stimulate angiogenesis and vascular permeability [73-75]. VEGF stimulation of cells causes the rapid activation and translocation of NFAT into the nucleus which in turn results in the up regulation of numerous genes associated with angiogenesis [76]. A number of studies have implicated RCAN1 in angiogenesis. Early studies found that *RCAN1* mRNA increased by 6-fold when endothelial cell lines were treated with VEGF [77, 78] and RCAN1 protein increased in human aortic endothelial cells (HUVECs) similarly treated [49, 79]. RCAN1 gene expression was also up regulated by other mediators of angiogenesis including thrombin [80].

Both major RCAN1 isoforms are involved in angiogenesis and appear to be regulated by different mechanisms. When human endothelial cells were treated with VEGF, there was an induction of *RCAN1-4* mRNA after 30 min, with the highest levels observed after 1 hour. Expression returned to basal levels by 24 hours after treatment [79, 81]. Others reported that up regulation of *RCAN1-4* during angiogenesis was mediated by calcium and calcineurin signalling, because treatment with cyclosporine A (CsA), a calcineurin inhibitor, or intracellular calcium chelators prevented its up regulation [80, 82]. Further evidence to suggest that *RCAN1-4* was regulated by calcineurin signalling came from studies demonstrating that *RCAN1-4* expression following VEGF and thrombin treatment was dependent upon the cooperative binding of transcription factors NFAT and GATA to the *RCAN1-4* promoter [80]. RCAN1-1 expression also appears to be modulated during angiogenesis. While initial studies found that *RCAN1-1* was not induced following VEGF treatment [79, 81], more recent reports have indicated that RCAN1-1 is up regulated in cultured endothelial cells treated with VEGF and during angiogenesis *in vivo* [49, 83]. However, unlike expression of *RCAN1-4* during angiogenesis, *RCAN1-1* expression does not appear to be regulated by the calcineurin signalling pathway as its expression was unaffected by treatment with either CsA or intracellular calcium chelators [80, 82].

A number of reports have suggested that RCAN1-1 and RCAN1-4 may play opposing roles in angiogenesis, where RCAN1-1 appears to be pro-angiogenic and is capable of inducing the formation of new blood vessels, while RCAN1-4 inhibits angiogenesis and vessel formation. For example, siRNA-mediated silencing of *RCAN1-1* in HUVECs inhibited VEGF-induced endothelial cell proliferation and angiogenic responses [49]. Further, when *RCAN1-1* was over-expressed in these cells it induced angiogenesis even in the absence of VEGF. This effect was also observed *in vivo* when human skin melanoma (SK-MEL-2) cells, which over-express VEGF-A, were transfected with *RCAN1-1*, implanted into a matrigel and transplanted into mice. In this situation, exogenous expression of *RCAN1-1* in SK-MEL-2 cells induced angiogenesis and vessel formation [49]. In contrast, RCAN1-4 appears to be anti-angiogenic as over-expression of *RCAN1-4* in SK-MEL-2 cells inhibited angiogenesis and siRNA-mediated silencing of *RCAN1-4* enhanced VEGF-induced proliferation [49]. Another study [80] found that forced up regulation of *RCAN1-4* in primary endothelial cells resulted in a reduction in the expression of many pro-angiogenic genes, including cell cycle inhibitors and growth factors and cytokines involved in the formation of new blood vessels, and moreover, the formation of tube structures (as a model for blood vessel development) formed from primary human endothelial cells *in vitro* was inhibited. Consistent with this, B16 melanoma cells engineered to over-express *RCAN1-4* and implanted subcutaneously into C57BL6 mice displayed a reduction in tumour growth due to a decrease in blood vessel density [80]. Interestingly, RCAN1-4 is thought to exert its anti-angiogenic effects by providing a negative feedback loop to inactivate calcineurin, preventing nuclear translocation and transcriptional activity of NFAT after VEGF stimulation. In support of this, ablation of *RCAN1-4* expression in endothelial cells increased NFAT activity and was associated with increased transcription of NFAT-regulated genes, such as *E-selectin* and *VCAM1* [78]. Intriguingly, RCAN1-1 was found to activate NFAT activity and enhance is pro-angiogenic functions [49]. Thus, RCAN1-4 inhibits the calcineurin/NFAT pathway while RCAN1-1 activates it.

6. The consequences of RCAN1 over-expression in the DS brain

6.1. Down syndrome and the neural system

DS is the leading genetic cause of intellectual impairment in the general population and is thought to contribute to around 30% of all cases of moderate to severe mental retardation [84]. Mental retardation in DS is characterised by behavioural and cognitive impairments which include low IQ, language deficits and defects in both short and long term memory. Later these deficits are compounded by the early onset of dementia [85].

People with DS exhibit a reduced performance on a number of different tests designed to demonstrate short term or working memory, including visual perception, visual imagery and spatial imagery tasks [86]. Long term memory is also affected by DS with both implicit (defined as improvement in perceptual, cognitive or motor tasks without any conscious reference to previous experience) and explicit (intentional recall or recognition of experiences or information) memory impaired [87]. In addition to the cognitive defects observed throughout life, neuropsychological tests showed that there is a cognitive decline in DS individuals with age and these cognitive changes equate to those observed following the onset of dementia [88]. DS participants with early stage dementia displayed severely diminished long term memory as well as a decreased ability to retrieve stored information compared with the non-demented DS controls [88]. The decline in these forms of cognition, particularly the ability to form new long term memories, is analogues to the cognitive deterioration seen in early to moderate Alzheimer's disease (AD) [89]. Interestingly, the cognitive defects that characterise DS are associated with hippocampal-based learning and memory while prefrontal-mediated executive function and cognition remain relatively unaffected [85].

The cognitive impairments in DS are accompanied by many neuro-morphological changes. Individuals with DS have a significant reduction in brain weight and volume [90], despite brain weight falling within the normal range at birth [91]. DS brains have a shorter anterior-posterior diameter, a reduction in the size of the frontal lobes, a flatter occipital lobe and a smaller brain stem and cerebellum [91]. The anterior and posterior corpus callosum regions and hippocampus are also smaller [92-95]. The hippocampus is a key brain structure involved in learning

http://dx.doi.org/10.5772/52977

and memory and many of the behavioural and cognitive defects seen in DS are hippocampal-dependent [85]. The difference in hippocampal volume is most likely due to various structural abnormalities, including a decrease in the mean area of the dentate gyrus (DG) and inadequate migration of cells into the pyramidal cell layer [96]. Notably, in adults there is an additional age-related decrease in the volume of the hippocampus, most likely due to some degree of neurodegeneration [95].

Smaller brains in DS individuals probably result from a reduction in the total number of neurones, with certain regions preferentially affected. DS brains exhibit a decrease in neuronal density by adulthood of between 10-50% [91]. The cortex of DS adults exhibits decreases in neuronal number and density in addition to abnormal distribution of neurones [97]. This same pattern of neuronal loss was also observed in the hippocampus and visual cortex. Interestingly, DS foetuses exhibited the same pattern of neuronal development as normal foetuses, with similar neuronal morphology, dendritic spine number and density [98]. However shortly after birth defects were evident and became more pronounced with age [99]. This indicates that something happens after birth which results in alterations in neuronal number and morphology. Using Golgi staining which allows for the visualisation of neurones including their cell bodies, axons, dendrites and spines, the brains of DS infants exhibited shorter basilar dendrites with a significant decrease in the absolute number of spines [100], which was postulated to correlate with a 20-35% decrease in surface area per synaptic contact [91]. Why and how this decline in neuronal development occurs is currently undetermined. These same defects were observed in adults with DS, who exhibited decreased dendritic branching, dendrite length and spine density [101]. Biochemical examination of adult DS brains also revealed a significant reduction in the concentrations of various neurotransmitter markers including, noradrenaline, serotonin or 5-hydroxytraptamine (5-HT) and choline acetyltransferase (ChAT) [102, 103], again signifying neuro-functional deficits in the brain.

On top of the neurodevelopmental problems associated with DS, all individuals with the disorder develop the neuropathological and neurochemical changes associated with AD by the third decade of life [89]. This includes the accumulation of amyloid β (Aβ), formation of hyperphosphorylated Tau-containing neurofibrillary tangles (NFT) and senile plaques. The progression of AD-neuropathology is analogous in both DS and AD, despite occurring decades earlier in DS [104].

6.2. RCAN1 in the brain

RCAN1 has been implicated in development and function of the brain. *Rcan1* is expressed in the developing mouse neural tube from embryonic day (E) E9.5 onwards and at E11.5-E12.5 was detected in the telencephalic vesicles, the caudal hypothalamus, the pretectum and the basal plate of the hindbrain and spinal cord. In later stages of embryonic development, *Rcan1* was highly expressed in the neural proliferative and differentiation zones within the brain with lower expression observed in other regions, including the telecephalon, hypothalamus, pretectum, cortical plate, striatum, amygdala, midbrain, hindbrain and spinal cord. In the post natal brain *Rcan1* gene expression was widely distributed throughout, with the highest levels in the olfactory bulb, the cerebral cortex, hippocampus and dentate gyrus, striatum and septum, amygdala, hypothalamus and the habenula. Within the hippocampus and dentate gyrus, highest levels of expression were observed in the pyramidal and granular cell layers [105].

Western blot analysis using an antibody designed to detect both RCAN1-1 and RCAN1-4 proteins found that the two isoforms were differentially expressed in the adult mouse brain. RCAN1-1 was abundant throughout the brain, with the highest levels of expression detected in the cortex and hippocampus [20, 54, 106]. RCAN1-4 was generally found at lower levels in the hippocampus, striatum, cortex and prefrontal cortex [54]. Similar results have been observed in the adult human brain where RCAN1-1 was most highly expressed in the cerebral cortex, hippocampus, substantia nigra, thalamus and medulla oblongata [21]. It is worth noting that while one study indicated that both isoforms of RCAN1 were located exclusively within neurones and not in astrocytes or microglial cells [107], another study found a wider distribution pattern [106], with RCAN1-1 and RCAN1-4 detected in multiple cell types including astrocytes and microglia. The highest levels of expression were observed in neurones [106]. Moreover, RCAN1-1 was also detected in primary glial-like cell cultures containing microglial cells and expression of RCAN1-4 was strongly induced following calcium stress [106].

Experimental evidence suggests that RCAN1 has a role in brain function. For example, studies on the RCAN1 orthologue in *Drosophila* known as *nebula*, demonstrated that a loss-of-function mutation of *nebula* displayed a decrease in learning and memory acquisition and performed significantly worse on learning and memory tests after a single trial compared with WT controls. Testing after 1 hour found no difference in the short term memory performance, however tests of long term memory (after 24 hours) found that *nebula*-deficient flies displayed virtually no long term memory [108]. This defect was apparent despite the normal presence of mushroom bodies (the learning and memory centres in *Drosophila*). The decrease in learning and memory observed was attributed to abnormal calcineurin signalling, as *nebula* loss-of-function mutants exhibited a 40% increase in calcineurin activity [108]. Interestingly, over-expression of *nebula* resulted in a similar phenotype. When *Drosophila* over-expressing *nebula* were generated and tested, they displayed virtually no ability to learn. This study also found that transient over-expression of *nebula* was sufficient to cause learning and memory deficits, indicating that a biochemical defect was responsible for learning and memory rather than a pre-existing developmental abnormality [108], a finding that may have implications for DS treatment options.

Similar behavioural abnormalities were observed in RCAN1-KO mice. While the absence of *Rcan1* did not result in any gross anatomical changes within the brain, RCAN1-KO mice exhibited various behavioural and synaptic deficiencies. For example, RCAN1-KO mice were shown to have impaired learning and memory in the Morris Water Maze (MWM), a well-established paradigm of hippocampal-dependent learning and memory. During the acquisition phase of the trial, RCAN1-KO mice displayed a decreased ability to learn the location of the platform compared with WT controls. This indicated that RCAN1-KO mice had a spatial learning impairment. These mice also displayed a poor spatial memory because when the escape platform was removed, RCAN1-KO mice did not demonstrate a specific preference for the target quadrant. On the other hand, a passive avoidance test using electric shock found that long- and short-term contextual fear memory was normal in these mice [54]. Taken together results from this study suggested that the absence of *Rcan1* selectively affects some, but not all, types of memory.

These behavioural deficits in RCAN1-KO mice were accompanied by abnormal synaptic transmissions and impaired long term potentiation (LTP). LTP is a form of synaptic plasticity hypothesised to be a biological substrate for some forms of memory [109]. Two forms of LTP can be examined: early-component LTP (E-LTP), a weak and short-lived enhancement of synaptic transmission; and late-component LTP (L-LTP) which is a robust enhancement of synaptic transmission lasting many hours [110, 111]. Paired-pulse facilitation (PPF) is also a component of LTP and is a measure of pre-synaptic short-term plasticity and neurotransmitter release [112]. Absence of RCAN1 did not affect the basal level of synaptic transmission but did result in a reduction in PPF compared with the WT controls, suggesting that pre-synaptic short term plasticity was affected by the lack of *Rcan1*. While there was no difference in the E-LTP, L-LTP was adversely affected by the ablation of *Rcan1*, with RCAN1-KO mice exhibiting a reduction in initial amplitude of L-LTP as well as a reduction in duration of the potentiation [54]. This is significant because the amplitude and duration are the biological correlates of synaptic strength required to reinforce the laying down of memory.

The strongest evidence to suggest a role for RCAN1 in the neurological defects observed in DS comes from a recent study by our group examining *RCAN1* transgenic (RCAN1-TG) mice. Using mice engineered to over-express *RCAN1-1* at a level analogous to that observed in DS, we found up regulation of RCAN1 contributed to some of the neurological defects characteristic of DS. For example, RCAN1 over-expression resulted in multiple defects in the formation, structure and function of the hippocampus [55]. Specifically, there was a significant reduction in the overall size of the hippocampus and analysis of the various structures within the hippocampal formation revealed a decrease in the absolute volume and cellularity of the dentate gyrus [55], mirroring the structural hippocampal defects and marked neuronal loss observed in DS. Our study suggested that the decrease in neuronal cellularity within the hippocampus of RCAN1-TG mice was the result of defective neurogenesis because fewer terminally differentiated neurones within the dentate gyrus formed and progenitor cells isolated and cultured from the sub ventricular zone had diminished ability to differentiate into neurones. This also reflects changes observed in DS [113]. RCAN1 transgenic mice also exhibited neuro-physiological impairments. In particular, over-expression of RCAN1 resulted in a defect in the maintenance phase of LTP which may be explained in part, by the reduction in post-synaptic spine density observed in the brains of these mice. Failure to maintain LTP in hippocampal slices was accompanied by deficits in hippocampal-dependent spatial learning and in short and long term memory. At a molecular level, in response to LTP induction, we observed diminished calcium transients and decreased phosphorylation of CaMKII and ERK1/2, signifying that the processes essential for the maintenance of LTP and formation of memory [55] are defective in mice with an excess of RCAN1.

RCAN1 has also been shown by our group to be involved in neurotransmission. Using chromaffin cells cultured from the adrenal gland as a model for the neuronal system, cells from both RCAN1-TG and RCAN1-KO mice displayed a reduction in neurotransmitter release. Our study demonstrated that the normal function of RCAN1 was to regulate the number of synaptic vesicles fusing with the plasma membrane and undergoing exocytosis, and the speed at which the vesicle pore opens and closes [53]. Although our study showed that the final outcome was the same whether RCAN1 was in excess or deficit, increased expression of *RCAN1* had the opposite effect to *Rcan1* ablation on vesicle fusion kinetics - ablation slowed fusion pore kinetics while over-expression accelerated fusion pore kinetics.

6.3. RCAN1 in neurodegeneration

Although it has not been proven, there is circumstantial evidence to suggest that RCAN1 plays a role in neurodegenerative conditions (other than DS). For example, Northern blot analysis of human brain samples found that *RCAN1* expression was increased about 2-fold in brains of AD patients [21, 107]. This increased gene expression was confined to the regions of the brain affected by AD, such as the hippocampus and cerebral cortex. This study also found that regions of the brain containing NFT had up to 3 times more *RCAN1* mRNA compared with the same regions of the brain without tangles [21]. Immunohistochemistry on human brain tissue using a RCAN1-specific antibody, found that RCAN1 protein levels increased in abundance with normal ageing in pyramidal neurones with further increases observed in brains affected by moderate to severe AD [65, 107]. In addition to increased protein levels, there was an alteration in the subcellular location of RCAN1 in AD-affected neurones, with a significant increase in the amount of RCAN1 within the nucleus compared with non-diseased tissue [65]. Interestingly, there was an up regulation of RCAN1-1 mRNA and protein in the hippocampus of AD patients, with no changes observed in the abundance of RCAN1-4 [65, 107], suggesting divergent functions of the major isoforms.

While these observations are intriguing, the question remains, what effect does increased RCAN1 expression have on the ageing brain and does it play a role in AD-like neuropathology? While this question remains unanswered, there are a number of possible reasons as to why increased RCAN1 expression might lead to neurodegeneration. One proposed explanation invokes a possible relationship between elevated RCAN1 expression, AD-like neurodegeneration and Tau protein. Tau is involved in the stabilisation of the microtubule networks within neurones and its hyperphosphorylation has been linked to the pathogenesis of AD. Tau can be phosphorylated by a number of different kinases, including GSK-3β and Ca^{2+}/calmodulin-dependent protein kinases (CaMK). Hyperphosphorylation of Tau is detrimental and can lead to AD neuropathology, including formation of NFT [114-116]. During normal cellular processes, there is a proteasome-dependent degradation of Tau protein but when Tau becomes hyperphosphorylated, it is resistant to this degradation and accumulates within the cell [117]. Some studies have found that increased levels of RCAN1 result in a concomitant increase in the phosphorylation of Tau and thus may contribute to its neuronal accumulation [67, 117] and we showed an accumulation of hyperphosphorylated Tau in the brains of aged RCAN1-TG mice [118]. This observed enhancement in Tau phosphorylation may be due to the effect of RCAN1 on GSK-3 activity, since increased RCAN1 expression in PC-12 cells resulted in an increase in the absolute level of GSK-3β, which in turn enhanced its ability to phosphorylate Tau [67]. There have also been suggestions that excess RCAN1 can exacerbate AD-like neuropathology by inhibiting calcineurin. Calcineurin activity is decreased in AD [119] and hyperphosphorylated tau protein and cytoskeletal changes in the brain similar to those observed in AD accumulate when the phosphatase activity of calcineurin is reduced [120]. Thus, if RCAN1 is behaving as a calcineurin inhibitor it is possible that increased levels of RCAN1, as occurs in DS and AD, promote the development of AD [21] [121].

RCAN1, via its role as an inhibitor of calcineurin, has also been implicated in the pathogenesis of Huntington's disease (HD). In a mouse model of HD, phosphorylation of huntingtin at serine residue 421 was protective and treatment of HD neuronal cells with calcineurin inhibitors prevented their death by maintaining their phosphorylation status at Ser^{421} [122]. RCAN1-1L protein was significantly down regulated in human HD post mortem brains and exogenous expression of RCAN1-1L in a cell culture model of HD protected the cells against toxicity caused by mutant huntingtin [123]. This protection was attributed to the ability of excess RCAN1 to inhibit calcineurin phosphatase activity, indicating that in this circumstance RCAN1 over-expression is advantageous.

Another connection between RCAN1 and neurodegeneration may be through the formation of aggregates. When proteins accumulate within a cell a mitrotubule-based apparatus known as an aggresome acts to sequester proteins within the cytoplasm. The formation of aggresomes within cells is most likely a defence mechanism against the presence of misfolded or abnormal proteins. However if these misfolded proteins are not cleared appropriately it can lead to abnormal protein accumulation and eventual neurotoxicity [124]. The formation of aggresomes is believed to contribute to many neurodegenerative disorders including AD, Huntington's disease and cerebral ataxia [125]. When RCAN1 was over-expressed in various neuronal cell lines and in primary neurones, formation of aggregates occurred [124] and the aggregates were associated with microtubules, indicating that they had formed inclusion bodies within the cells. When RCAN1 was aggregated within neurones, neuronal abnormalities characterised by a decreased number and density of synapses were observed, which in turn altered synaptic function [124]. This constitutes another example of the damaging effects of excess RCAN1.

Finally, two polymorphisms located in the *RCAN1-4* promoter region have been associated with AD in the Chinese Han population [126]. One of these, rs71324311, in the heterozygous-deletion genotype confers protection while the other, rs10550296, also in the heterozygous-deletion configuration, is a risk factor. The functional consequences of these sequence variants are yet to be determined.

7. The consequences of RCAN1 over-expression in the DS immune system

7.1. The Down syndrome immune system

DS is associated with a multitude of immune system defects. People with DS are more susceptible to infections, particularly respiratory tract infections with pneumonia one of the major causes of early death [127]. The incidence of viral hepatitis and haematopoietic malignancies is also increased in people with DS as is their tendency to develop certain types of autoimmune disorders such as autoimmune thyroid disease (AITD) (Hashimoto type), coeliac disease and diabetes [127] [128]. Thus, DS appears to include a combination of immunodeficiency and immune dysfunction. Although the precise cause of this immune dysfunction is unclear, the DS immune system is characterised by a number of abnormalities thought to originate from defective innate and adaptive immunity.

7.2. Impairments in innate immunity

Innate immunity is the body's first line of defence against invasion. This arm of the immune system either prevents the entry of pathogens into the body, or upon entry, eliminates them before they can cause any damage or disease. If a pathogen is able to gain entry into the body, innate immunity includes various non-specific mechanisms which can eliminate and destroy foreign invaders. These mechanisms include phagocytosis and inflammation. DS is associated with defects in the innate immune system. For example, natural killer (NK) cells, components of the innate immune system involved in the recognition and elimination of bacteria, viruses and tumour cells, are defective in DS individuals [129]. Also, neutrophils from DS people exhibited a decreased ability to phagocytose [130] and the ability of DS-derived neutrophils and monocytes to migrate towards a site of injury or infection in response to chemokine release was reduced [131].

7.3. Impairments in adaptive immunity

T cell development and maturation occurs within the thymus. Bone marrow (BM) derived precursor cells migrate into the thymus where they receive developmental cues from the thymic microenvironment. Here they progress through a number of different stages of development broadly defined by the expression of CD4 and CD8 on the cell surface. Once cells become fully mature, expressing only CD4 or CD8 on the surface, they are able to migrate to the periphery and populate the immune system. The DS immune system is characterised by a number of abnormalities thought to originate from defective T cell development in the thymus. Typically, the DS thymus is small and morphologically abnormal. It exhibits cortical atrophy, loss of cortico-medullary demarcation and lymphopenia due to a defect in the development of thymocytes [114]. The number of cells expressing high levels of the TCR α-β-CD3 complex is reduced [132] as are the numbers of helper ($CD4^+$) T (Th) cells resulting in the inversion of the normal $CD4^+/CD8^+$ ratio in favour of the $CD8^+$ population. Th cells can be further subcategorised into either Th1 or Th2 cells where Th1 cells participate in the elimination of intra-vesicular pathogens, including bacteria and parasites via the activation of macrophages, while Th2 cells clear extracellular pathogens and toxins by assisting antibody production in B cells. There is an imbalance in the T helper responses of DS individuals, although there is some disagreement as to whether it is an alteration in the Th1 or Th2 phenotype. Some studies have suggested that Th2 responses are augmented in DS based on the observation that there is an increased number of circulating $CD3^+$/CD30 Th2 lymphocytes [133]. Others report an increase in the Th1 population in DS and this has been attributed to increased IFNγ production [134] because IFNγ polarises Th0 cells towards the Th1 phenotype. While there is no doubt that a defect in T cell development and maturation within the DS thymus exists, altered apoptosis of lymphocytes may also contribute to the decrease in overall numbers of T cells in the periphery, as well as to the alterations observed in the abundance of the various T cell subsets. For example, DS $CD3^+$ T cells and $CD19^+$ B cells expressed significantly higher levels of early apoptotic markers compared with control cells [135].

T lymphocytes isolated from DS people are also functionally compromised. Under conditions designed to simulate an infection using anti-CD3 antibodies or the non-specific mitogen, phytohemagglutinin to activate T cells, DS lymphocytes were diminished in their proliferative capacity [136, 137]. Not only did the DS-derived T cells have a proliferative defect, they showed increased expression of apoptotic markers including APO-I/Fas (CD95) antigen, a T cell death marker, and increased apoptosis was demonstrated in cultured T cells using Annexin V [138]. $CD8^+$ or cytotoxic T lymphocytes (CTLs) isolated from DS individuals were also compromised in their ability to kill target cells [139], indicating a functional defect in this cell type also. DS-derived T cells also produce abnormal levels of cytokines, the small proteins produced by immune cells that are involved in signalling and controlling immune responses. IL-2 is central to the proliferation and differentiation of T cells and is produced by T lymphocytes once activated. Inhibition or reduction in IL-2 results in suppression of the immune system. One study on adults with DS found that the levels of IL-2 secreted from cultured stimulated T cells were significantly reduced compared with T cells cultured from normal individuals [140]. Other studies have suggested that IL-2 is produced at comparable levels in both DS and normal individuals, but in DS the response to IL-2 may be defective [141]. Levels of IFN-γ and TNF α are also altered in DS and although the number of DS studies is small, the consensus is that IFN- γ and TNF α levels are increased [142] [134].

In addition to T cell lymphopenia, DS individuals have marked B lymphopenia [143-145]. As well as a reduction in the number and proportions of B lymphocytes, there is a skewing of the B cell subpopulations, suggesting that maturation of B cells is defective in DS [146] akin to the situation with T cells, although the exact nature of this defect has not been explored. Immunoglobulin levels in DS are also abnormal, with DS B lymphocytes producing lower levels of IgM, IgG_2 and IgG_4 and higher levels of IgG_1 [146, 147]. IgG_3 and IgA levels were unchanged. Also suggesting a B cell functional deficit is the finding that antibody responses to a variety of antigens are low in DS, including the responses to pneumococcal and bacteriophage ØX174 antigens and to vaccine antigens such as tetanus, influenza A and polio [148-150].

7.4. RCAN1 in innate immunity

There is evidence to indicate that RCAN1 has a role in innate immunity and inflammation. For example, when human mononuclear cells were activated with *Candida albicans,* a pathogen capable of eliciting an innate immune response, RCAN1 gene expression was rapidly induced [151]. RCAN1 expression was also induced in response to various pro-inflammatory cytokines involved in the innate immune system such as TNFα [78]. Other studies have found that RCAN1 regulates inflammatory mediators and cytokines that have previously been identified as components of the innate immune system. For example, forced over-expression of RCAN1 in endothelial cells using adenoviral vectors resulted in a decrease in the expression of inflammatory markers such as E-selectin, VCAM1, TNF and COX-2 mRNA [78]. This suggested that increased expression of RCAN1 may dampen inflammation and inhibit induction of the innate immune system. Conversely, knockdown of RCAN1 using siRNA resulted in an increase in the expression of inflammatory mediators [78].

Importantly, RCAN1 also mediates inflammatory responses *in vivo*. When mice were administered with lipopolysaccharide (LPS), a component of gram negative bacteria cell wall used experimentally to activate innate immune responses, *Rcan1* gene expression was induced [152]. Interestingly, RCAN1-KO mice had lower survival following LPS-induced endotoxaemia compared with their WT littermates [152]. Knockout mice had an accentuated response to LPS treatment, including lower heart rate, blood pressure and body temperature. An increase in the concentration of circulating IL-6 protein, a pro-inflammatory cytokine believed to be detrimental during infection was also found, along with a significant increase in the mRNA expression of inflammatory mediators such as *E-selectin*, *ICAM1* and *VCAM1* in organs including the heart and lung. There was a concomitant increase in the number of infiltrating leukocytes within these organs [152]. On the other hand, over-expression of *RCAN1-4* achieved by the intravenous injection of mice with a *RCAN1-4*-containing adenovirus, conferred a survival advantage upon LPS administration. A decrease in the levels of circulating IL-6 and an attenuation of the physiological responses to systemic LPS treatment were evident [152]. Induction of inflammatory mediators was also reduced and there was a marked reduction in leukocyte infiltrate in the heart, liver and lungs [152]. Another study found that following infection with the bacteria *Fransicella tularensis*, induction of pro-inflammatory cytokines including MCP1, IL6, IFNγ, and TNFα was significantly higher in *Rcan1*-deficient spleen and lung [153]. All this suggests that over-expression of RCAN1 is protective.

Other studies on the role of RCAN1 in innate immunity have focussed on identifying the mechanisms by which RCAN1 regulates inflammation. One plausible means is by modulation of the NFκB signal transduction pathway. As described earlier, RCAN1 is able to inhibit NFκB signalling by increasing the stability of IκB protein [51]. Given that NFκB is a transcription factor that controls the expression of pro-inflammatory genes and the subsequent activation of innate immune cells, negative regulation of this pathway by RCAN1 would result in inhibition of inflammation. Such a proposition is consistent with published *in vitro* and *in vivo* data. However, another study investigating the potential involvement of RCAN1 in the Toll-like receptor (TLR) pathway arrived at the opposite conclusion [154]. The TLR pathway is activated as a first line defence mechanism during microbial infection and culminates in the induction of interleukins and other pro-inflammatory mediators [155]. When RCAN1-4 (DSCR1-1S) was exogenously expressed in HEK293 cells, the end result was activation of NFκB-mediated inflammatory responses [154], not suppression. Here, RCAN1 was found to regulate the TLR pathway through a direct interaction with the adaptor protein known as Toll-interacting protein (Tollip). The normal cellular role of Tollip is to suppress TLR signalling by sequestering IL-1 receptor associated kinase 1 (IRAK-1). Exogenously added RCAN1 bound Tollip, causing the release of IRAK-1 from the complex thereby removing the block on IRAK-1 activity [154]. The end result was an enhancement of the inflammatory response and thus represents yet another example of the sometimes contradictory actions of RCAN1.

http://dx.doi.org/10.5772/52977

7.5. RCAN1 in adaptive immunity

The first evidence to suggest that RCAN1 functions in adaptive immunity came from experiments investigating T cell responses in human Jurkat cells, an immortalised T lymphocyte cell line. When these cells were stimulated with the T cell mitogens, CD3 and CD28, expression of *RCAN1-4* mRNA was induced [26]. This result was confirmed by stimulating primary T cells cultured from humans [156]. A more definitive role for RCAN1 in the adaptive immune system came from examining RCAN1-KO mice [44]. While these mice displayed normal T cell development and maturation with comparable numbers of mature thymocytes and equivalent numbers of $CD4^+$, $CD8^+$, $CD3^+$ T cells in the periphery, these cells exhibited functional deficits. When the T cells were isolated from the spleen and cultured *ex vivo*, the RCAN1-KO cells were functionally defective. Specifically, these T cells exhibited a 50% reduction in proliferation in response to mitogenic stimulation as well as a decrease in the production of IFNγ. This loss of IFNγ indicated that the Th1 population was especially affected by the lack of *Rcan1* expression. Indeed, these mice exhibited defective Th1 responses due to the premature death of this population of cells as a result of an up regulation of FasL and a loss of viability. Antibody class switching was also altered in RCAN1-KO mice, with a decrease in IgG_2 production. Notably, the T cell defect in RCAN1-KO mice could be rescued by treatment with the calcineurin inhibitor, CsA, suggesting that the defect was calcineurin/NFAT-dependent and presumably due to hyperactivation of the calcineurin signal transduction pathway [44]. However, despite restoration of T cell function in RCAN1-KO mice following CsA treatment, genetic loss of calcineurin Aβ superimposed on the *Rcan1* deficiency by crossing RCAN1-KO mice with CnAβ knockout mice, could not rescue the T cell defects [64]. In fact, loss of calcineurin Aβ in addition to the loss of *Rcan1* resulted in an increase in the severity of the T cell defect. This observation suggests that in these mice RCAN1 is acting to facilitate calcineurin activity rather than inhibit it as the use of CsA treatment had suggested. Our group also has evidence of RCAN1's involvement in adaptive immunity; our RCAN1-TG mice have T and B cell defects (unpublished data and manuscript in preparation).

In addition to its function in T cells, RCAN1 is involved in the normal function of mast cells. Mast cells are specialised immune cells that contain granules rich in histamine and heparin and are known to play a role in wound healing, defence against pathogens and the pathology of IgE-dependent allergic disease and anaphylaxis [157]. Mast cells are activated through the high affinity IgE receptor (FcεRI) on their cell surface and this activation is controlled by a number of activating and inhibitory molecules. The down regulation of mast cell activity by inhibitory signals is essential in preventing allergic disease and anaphylaxis [157]. RCAN1 is believed to be one of these inhibitory signals. Evidence to suggest this comes from experiments conducted on RCAN1-KO mice, which displayed an exaggerated mast cell response. While RCAN1-KO mice displayed normal mast cell maturation, many of the signalling pathways following mast cell activation were perturbed. For example, mast cells isolated from RCAN1-KO mice and stimulated with FcεRI had an increase in the activation of both the NFAT and NFκB signalling pathways. As expected, there was also an increase in the expression of many pro-inflammatory genes regulated by these two pathways including *IL-6*, *IL-13* and *TNFα* [158]. Further, when mice lacking *Rcan1* were sensitised with an intravenous injection of anti-IgE antibody and then later treated with an agent designed to elicit an anaphylactic reaction, *Rcan1* deficiency led to enhanced mast cell activation, degranulation and passive cutaneous anaphylaxis [158]. These results indicate that RCAN1 may be an inhibitor molecule that negatively controls mast cell function.

Eosinophils, another immune cell type, are predominant effector cells in allergic asthma and their presence in the lungs of asthma sufferers is regarded as a defining feature of this inflammatory disease. Absence of *Rcan1* was shown to prevent experimentally-induced allergic asthma in a mouse model due to an almost complete absence of eosinophils infiltrating the lungs [159]. Although the exact mechanism for this protection is not fully understood, it seems that a lack of *Rcan1* blocks the development and migration of eosinophil progenitors from the bone marrow and selectively lowers their production of the inflammatory mediator IL-4. This study implies that over-expression of RCAN1 would exacerbate the allergic response and in this regard it is interesting to note that a recent study reported an increased incidence of allergic asthma in people with DS [160]. Therefore, it would be very informative to test allergic asthma responses in RCAN1-TG mice.

8. The consequences of RCAN1 over–expression on the incidence of solid tumours in DS

8.1. Down syndrome and cancer

Individuals with DS are more likely to develop certain malignancies, especially of the immune system. There is a well-established link between leukaemia and DS, with an increased incidence in DS compared with the general population. Large population based studies conducted in different countries around the world have consistently found that the rates of leukaemia were between 10- to 19-fold higher in people with DS in comparison with the average population and there was an increased incidence of both lymphoid and myeloid leukaemias [140, 161-163]. While the incidence of both acute myeloid leukaemia (AML) and acute lymphatic leukaemia (ALL) was significantly higher in DS subjects than expected in the general population, there were significantly more cases of AML compared to ALL in DS [163]. This increased risk is most evident at a younger age, however remained throughout life. There is also a significant increase in the incidence of neoplastic disorders such as megakaryoblastic leukaemia, where the incidence is increased about 500-fold in DS [164, 165]. In males, there is also a link between DS and testicular cancer, possibly due to higher levels of follicular stimulating hormone, hypogonadism or cryptorchidism [166, 167]. Notably, those with DS are less likely to develop other solid tumours such as neuroblastomas and breast and lung cancers [162, 163, 168]. Indeed, DS individuals had a 50% reduction in the incidence of solid tumours compared to the number of cases expected in the general population and this was observed over all age groups examined [162]. Thus it seems likely that a number of tumour suppressor genes reside on *Hsa21*.

8.2. RCAN1 and tumourigenesis

While the identities of the *Hsa21* genes responsible for the reduction in solid tumour formation in DS remain unknown, there is evidence to suggest that up regulation of RCAN1 may afford

http://dx.doi.org/10.5772/52977

some protection. Firstly, a number of cancers display abnormal expression of RCAN1 and this expression varies depending on the stage of the cancer. For example, studies have shown that RCAN1 is up regulated in most primary papillary thyroid tumours but this expression is lost in the metastatic tissue of thyroid tumours [169]. This is interesting given that RCAN1 has been identified as a target gene for metastatin, a protein that functions to suppress metastatic tumour growth. It is possible that loss of metastatin in tumour cells leads to a loss of RCAN1 expression which may in turn contribute to tumour metastasis [169]. RCAN1 has also been linked to other cancers including colorectal cancer. Peroxisome proliferator-activated receptor γ (PPARγ) is a member the nuclear hormone receptor family of transcription factors and has been identified as a tumour suppressor gene in colon cancer. This gene is important in a number of cellular processes including inflammation, proliferation, apoptosis as well as adipocyte and intestinal epithelial cell differentiation and has been shown to suppress experimental colon carcinogenesis in mice (reviewed in [170]). Loss of *RCAN1-4* in *MOSER colon carcinoma cells* resulted in an inhibition of PPARγ-mediated tumour suppression and increased tissue invasion [171]. While not conclusive, these results indicate that RCAN1 may be required for PPARγ suppression of colorectal cancers [171]. Again this is consistent with the idea that RCAN1 can act as a tumour suppressor.

The strongest genetic evidence to suggest a role for *RCAN1* in tumourigenesis comes from experiments conducted on RCAN1-KO and RCAN1-TG mice. When RCAN1-KO mice were injected subcutaneously with renal carcinoma or colon carcinoma tumour cells, there was a significant suppression of tumour growth [172]. Tumour growth was suppressed due to an inability to form and maintain tumour vasculature within the solid tumours. Further investigation showed that RCAN1-KO mice had hyperactive VEGF-calcineurin-NFAT signalling, which resulted in a suppression of endothelial cell proliferation and an increase in apoptosis [172]. Tumour growth in the RCAN1-KO mice could be restored following treatment with CsA, suggesting that suppression of tumour cell growth in RCAN1-KO mice was dependent on hyperactive calcineurin signalling. Perhaps counterintuitively, but similar to the situation with the RCAN1-KO, mice over-expressing *RCAN1-4* were also resistant to tumour growth when injected subcutaneously with Lewis lung or B16F10 tumour cells [173]. Tumours isolated from these mice also displayed a decrease in the density of microvessels and the vessels lacked a functional lumen. Moreover, it appeared that *RCAN1-4* mediated tumour growth through the calcineurin pathway as *RCAN1-4* transgenic tumour cells had a decrease in both calcineurin and NFAT activity [173]. The exact mechanisms by which RCAN1 suppresses solid tumour growth remain unknown, but both studies strongly suggest that regulation of angiogenesis by RCAN1 underpins the inhibition of tumour growth by reducing the formation of blood vessels throughout the tumour. It is interesting to note that RCAN1-KO and RCAN1-TG mice displayed a similar phenotype, with both exhibiting a decrease in tumour formation due to an inhibition of angiogenesis preventing the formation of microvessels required to support tumour growth. Perhaps more intriguing is that opposite effects on the calcineurin pathway produced the same end result. Also intriguing is that microvessel formation was also decreased in teratomas generated from human DS-derived pluripotent stem cells transplanted into WT mice, indicating that decreased angiogenesis may be responsible for tumour suppression in DS [173].

Finally, the significance of RCAN1 in tumour suppression in DS was elegantly demonstrated using yet another DS genetic model. TS65Dn mice that harbour a third copy of many *Hsa21*-orthologous genes, including *Rcan1*, were bred with RCAN1-KO mice, thereby returning the gene dosage of *Rcan1* to normal. When tumour cells were injected into these mice, there was a significant increase in the formation of microvessels within solid tumours compared with their TS65Dn littermates expressing 3 copies of *Rcan1* [173]. This is more evidence to support the idea that elevated levels of *RCAN1* are responsible, at least in part, for the decrease in the incidence of solid tumour formation in DS.

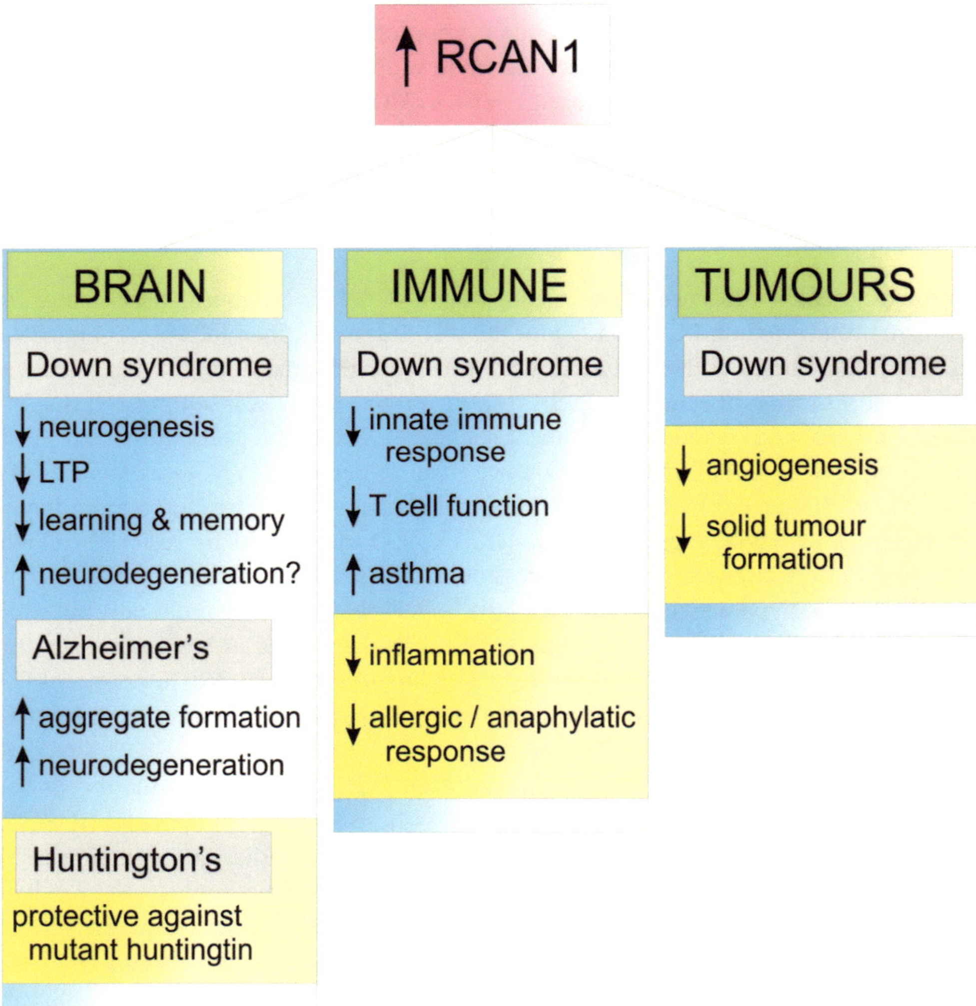

Figure 2. Summary of the positive and negative effects of excess RCAN1. Effects on the brain, immune system and solid tumour formation in Down syndrome are shown. The putative contributions of an over abundance of RCAN1 have either been demonstrated in mouse models or in cell lines or implied from *Rcan1*-KO studies where, in the absence of data to the contrary, the assumption is that over-expression will produce the opposite effect to the deficiency. Detrimental effects are shown in blue and protective effects in yellow.

9. Conclusion

In this review we have attempted to summarise what is currently known about the function of the *RCAN1* gene and its pleiotropic actions in three areas of relevance to DS (see Figure 2). No matter which system you look at, the reports on RCAN1 function are often contradictory – we still have much to learn. Researchers with a passionate interest in DS and its molecular genetic aetiology have suggested that specific down regulation of a few of the genes produced in excess in DS tissues may provide an avenue for therapies. We and others have suggested that inhibition of RCAN1 signalling may have pharmacological potential for reducing neuronal loss and treating cognitive decline in DS and AD, but we still have much to learn about the molecular function and physiological role of RCAN1 and how we can manipulate its activity to ameliorate/treat pathology.

Author details

Melanie A. Pritchard and Katherine R. Martin

Department Biochemistry & Molecular Biology, Monash University, Clayton, Victoria, Australia

References

[1] Lejeune, J, Turpin, R, & Gautier, M. *Chromosomic diagnosis of mongolism].* Arch Fr Pediatr, (1959). , 962-963.

[2] Sherman, S. L, et al. *Epidemiology of Down syndrome.* Ment Retard Dev Disabil Res Rev, (2007). , 221-227.

[3] Reeves, R, Baxter, L, & Richtsmeier, J. *Too much of a good thing: mechanisms of gene action in Down syndrome.* TRENDS in Genetics, (2001). , 83-88.

[4] Nadel, L. *Down's syndrome: a genetic disorder in biobehavioral perspective.* Genes Brain Behav, (2003). , 156-166.

[5] Smith, D. J, et al. *Functional screening of 2 Mb of human chromosome 21q22.2 in transgenic mice implicates minibrain in learning defects associated with Down syndrome.* Nat Genet, (1997). , 28-36.

[6] Gahtan, E, et al. *Reversible impairment of long-term potentiation in transgenic Cu/Zn-SOD mice.* Eur J Neurosci, (1998). , 538-544.

[7] Cataldo, A. M, et al. *App gene dosage modulates endosomal abnormalities of Alzheimer's disease in a segmental trisomy 16 mouse model of down syndrome.* J Neurosci, (2003). , 6788-6792.

[8] Salehi, A, et al. *Increased App expression in a mouse model of Down's syndrome disrupts NGF transport and causes cholinergic neuron degeneration.* Neuron, (2006). , 29-42.

[9] Lamb, B. T, et al. *Introduction and expression of the 400 kilobase amyloid precursor protein gene in transgenic mice [corrected].* Nat Genet, (1993). , 22-30.

[10] Kim, W. T, et al. *Delayed reentry of recycling vesicles into the fusion-competent synaptic vesicle pool in synaptojanin 1 knockout mice.* Proc Natl Acad Sci U S A, (2002). , 17143-17148.

[11] Yu, Y, et al. *Mice deficient for the chromosome 21 ortholog Itsn1 exhibit vesicle-trafficking abnormalities.* Hum Mol Genet, (2008). , 3281-3290.

[12] Arron, J. R, et al. *NFAT dysregulation by increased dosage of DSCR1 and DYRK1A on chromosome 21.* Nature, (2006). , 595-600.

[13] Fuentes, J. J, et al. *A new human gene from the Down syndrome critical region encodes a proline-rich protein highly expressed in fetal brain and heart.* Hum Mol Genet, (1995). , 1935-1944.

[14] Strippoli, P, et al. *The murine DSCR1-like (Down syndrome candidate region 1) gene family: conserved synteny with the human orthologous genes.* Gene, (2000). , 223-232.

[15] Strippoli, P, et al. *A new gene family including DSCR1 (Down Syndrome Candidate Region 1) and ZAKI-4: characterization from yeast to human and identification of DSCR1-like 2, a novel human member (DSCR1L2).* Genomics, (2000). , 252-263.

[16] Lee, J. I, et al. *The Caenorhabditis elegans homologue of Down syndrome critical region 1, RCN-1, inhibits multiple functions of the phosphatase calcineurin.* J Mol Biol, (2003). , 147-156.

[17] Mulero, M. C, et al. *Inhibiting the calcineurin-NFAT (nuclear factor of activated T cells) signaling pathway with a regulator of calcineurin-derived peptide without affecting general calcineurin phosphatase activity.* J Biol Chem, (2009). , 9394-9401.

[18] Kingsbury, T. J, & Cunningham, K. W. *A conserved family of calcineurin regulators.* Genes Dev, (2000). , 1595-1604.

[19] Fuentes, J. J, et al. *DSCR1, overexpressed in Down syndrome, is an inhibitor of calcineurin-mediated signaling pathways.* Hum Mol Genet, (2000). , 1681-1690.

[20] Porta, S, et al. *Differential expression of members of the RCAN family of calcineurin regulators suggests selective functions for these proteins in the brain.* Eur J Neurosci, (2007). , 1213-1226.

[21] Ermak, G, Morgan, T. E, & Davies, K. J. *Chronic overexpression of the calcineurin inhibitory gene DSCR1 (Adapt78) is associated with Alzheimer's disease.* J Biol Chem, (2001). , 38787-38794.

[22] Fuentes, J. J, Pritchard, M. A, & Estivill, X. *Genomic organization, alternative splicing, and expression patterns of the DSCR1 (Down syndrome candidate region 1) gene.* Genomics, (1997). , 358-361.

[23] Genesca, L, et al. *Phosphorylation of calcipressin 1 increases its ability to inhibit calcineurin and decreases calcipressin half-life.* Biochem J, (2003). Pt 2): , 567-575.

[24] Cano, E, et al. *Depolarization of neural cells induces transcription of the Down syndrome critical region 1 isoform 4 via a calcineurin/nuclear factor of activated T cells-dependent pathway.* J Biol Chem, (2005). , 29435-29443.

[25] Pfister, S. C, et al. *Mutational analyses of the signals involved in the subcellular location of DSCR1.* BMC Cell Biol, (2002). , 24.

[26] Narayan, A. V, et al. *Redox response of the endogenous calcineurin inhibitor Adapt 78.* Free Radic Biol Med, (2005). , 719-727.

[27] Rothermel, B, et al. *A protein encoded within the Down syndrome critical region is enriched in striated muscles and inhibits calcineurin signaling.* J Biol Chem, (2000). , 8719-8725.

[28] Strippoli, P, et al. *Segmental paralogy in the human genome: a large-scale triplication on 1p, 6p and 21q.* Mamm Genome, (2002). p. 456-62.

[29] Mehta, S, et al. *Domain architecture of the Regulators of Calcineurin (RCANs) and identification of a divergent RCAN in yeast.* Mol Cell Biol, (2009).

[30] Crabtree, G. R. *Generic signals and specific outcomes: signaling through Ca2+, calcineurin, and NF-AT.* Cell, (1999). , 611-614.

[31] Vega, R. B, et al. *Multiple domains of MCIP1 contribute to inhibition of calcineurin activity.* J Biol Chem, (2002). , 30401-30407.

[32] Abbasi, S, et al. *Protein kinase-mediated regulation of calcineurin through the phosphorylation of modulatory calcineurin-interacting protein 1.* J Biol Chem, (2006). , 7717-7726.

[33] Lee, E. J, et al. *NF-kappaB-inducing kinase phosphorylates and blocks the degradation of Down syndrome candidate region 1.* J Biol Chem, (2008). , 3392-3400.

[34] Jung, M. S, et al. *Regulation of RCAN1 protein activity by Dyrk1A protein-mediated phosphorylation.* J Biol Chem, (2011). , 40401-40412.

[35] Hilioti, Z, et al. *GSK-3 kinases enhance calcineurin signaling by phosphorylation of RCNs.* Genes Dev, (2004). , 35-47.

[36] Liu, Q, Busby, J. C, & Molkentin, J. D. *Interaction between TAK1-TAB1-TAB2 and RCAN1-calcineurin defines a signalling nodal control point.* Nat Cell Biol, (2009). , 154-161.

[37] Kim, S. S, et al. *Protein kinase A phosphorylates Down syndrome critical region 1 (RCAN1).* Biochem Biophys Res Commun, (2012)., 657-661.

[38] Cho, Y. J, et al. *Raf-1 is a binding partner of DSCR1.* Arch Biochem Biophys, (2005)., 121-128.

[39] Ciechanover, A. *The ubiquitin-proteasome pathway: on protein death and cell life.* EMBO J, (1998)., 7151-7160.

[40] Asada, S, et al. *Oxidative stress-induced ubiquitination of RCAN1 mediated by SCFbeta-TrCP ubiquitin ligase.* Int J Mol Med, (2008)., 95-104.

[41] Silveira, H. C, et al. *A calcineurin inhibitory protein overexpressed in Down's syndrome interacts with the product of a ubiquitously expressed transcript.* Braz J Med Biol Res, (2004)., 785-789.

[42] Kishi, T, et al. *The SCFCdc4 ubiquitin ligase regulates calcineurin signaling through degradation of phosphorylated Rcn1, an inhibitor of calcineurin.* Proc Natl Acad Sci U S A, (2007)., 17418-17423.

[43] Rothermel, B. A, et al. *Myocyte-enriched calcineurin-interacting protein, MCIP1, inhibits cardiac hypertrophy in vivo.* Proc Natl Acad Sci U S A, (2001)., 3328-3333.

[44] Ryeom, S, et al. *The threshold pattern of calcineurin-dependent gene expression is altered by loss of the endogenous inhibitor calcipressin.* Nat Immunol, (2003)., 874-881.

[45] Crawford, D. R, et al. *Hamster adapt78 mRNA is a Down syndrome critical region homologue that is inducible by oxidative stress.* Arch Biochem Biophys, (1997)., 6-12.

[46] Davies, K. J, Harris, C. D, & Ermak, G. *The essential role of calcium in induction of the DSCR1 (ADAPT78) gene.* Biofactors, (2001)., 91-93.

[47] Leahy, K. P, et al. *adapt78, a stress-inducible mRNA, is related to the glucose-regulated protein family of genes.* Arch Biochem Biophys, (1999)., 67-74.

[48] Porta, S, et al. *RCAN1 (DSCR1) increases neuronal susceptibility to oxidative stress: a potential pathogenic process in neurodegeneration.* Hum Mol Genet, (2007)., 1039-1050.

[49] Qin, L, et al. *Down syndrome candidate region 1 isoform 1 mediates angiogenesis through the calcineurin-NFAT pathway.* Mol Cancer Res, (2006)., 811-820.

[50] Chang, K. T, & Min, K. T. *Drosophila melanogaster homolog of Down syndrome critical region 1 is critical for mitochondrial function.* Nat Neurosci, (2005)., 1577-1585.

[51] Kim, Y. S, et al. *Down syndrome candidate region 1 increases the stability of the IkappaBalpha protein: implications for its anti-inflammatory effects.* J Biol Chem, (2006)., 39051-39061.

[52] Lee, J. E, et al. *Down syndrome critical region 1 enhances the proteolytic cleavage of calcineurin.* Exp Mol Med, (2009).

[53] Keating, D. J, et al. *DSCR1/RCAN1 regulates vesicle exocytosis and fusion pore kinetics: implications for Down syndrome and Alzheimer's disease.* Hum Mol Genet, (2008). , 1020-1030.

[54] Hoeffer, C. A, et al. *The Down syndrome critical region protein RCAN1 regulates long-term potentiation and memory via inhibition of phosphatase signaling.* J Neurosci, (2007). , 13161-13172.

[55] Martin, K. R, et al. *Over-expression of RCAN1 causes Down syndrome-like hippocampal deficits that alter learning and memory.* Hum Mol Genet, (2012). , 3025-3041.

[56] Cho, K. O, et al. *Upregulation of DSCR1 (RCAN1 or Adapt78) in the peri-infarct cortex after experimental stroke.* Exp Neurol, (2008). , 85-92.

[57] Sobrado, M, et al. *Regulator of calcineurin 1 (Rcan1) has a protective role in brain ischemia/reperfusion injury.* J Neuroinflammation, (2012). , 48.

[58] Wang, Y, et al. *Direct biomechanical induction of endogenous calcineurin inhibitor Down Syndrome Critical Region-1 in cardiac myocytes.* Am J Physiol Heart Circ Physiol, (2002). , H533-H539.

[59] Molkentin, J. D, et al. *A calcineurin-dependent transcriptional pathway for cardiac hypertrophy.* Cell, (1998). , 215-228.

[60] Wilkins, B. J, & Molkentin, J. D. *Calcineurin and cardiac hypertrophy: where have we been? Where are we going?* J Physiol, (2002). Pt 1): , 1-8.

[61] Yang, J, et al. *Independent signals control expression of the calcineurin inhibitory proteins MCIP1 and MCIP2 in striated muscles.* Circ Res, (2000). , E61-E68.

[62] Chan, B, et al. *Identification of a peptide fragment of DSCR1 that competitively inhibits calcineurin activity in vitro and in vivo.* Proc Natl Acad Sci U S A, (2005). , 13075-13080.

[63] Vega, R. B, et al. *Dual roles of modulatory calcineurin-interacting protein 1 in cardiac hypertrophy.* Proc Natl Acad Sci U S A, (2003). , 669-674.

[64] Sanna, B, et al. *Modulatory calcineurin-interacting proteins 1 and 2 function as calcineurin facilitators in vivo.* Proc Natl Acad Sci U S A, (2006). , 7327-7332.

[65] Cook, C. N, et al. *Expression of calcipressin1, an inhibitor of the phosphatase calcineurin, is altered with aging and Alzheimer's disease.* J Alzheimers Dis, (2005). , 63-73.

[66] Shin, S. Y, et al. *A hidden incoherent switch regulates RCAN1 in the calcineurin-NFAT signaling network.* J Cell Sci, (2011). Pt 1): , 82-90.

[67] Ermak, G, et al. *RCAN1 (DSCR1 or Adapt78) stimulates expression of GSK-3beta.* FEBS J, (2006). , 2100-2109.

[68] Shaul, Y. D, & Seger, R. *The MEK/ERK cascade: from signaling specificity to diverse functions.* Biochim Biophys Acta, (2007). , 1213-1226.

[69] Yates, L. L, & Gorecki, D. C. *The nuclear factor-kappaB (NF-kappaB): from a versatile transcription factor to a ubiquitous therapeutic target.* Acta Biochim Pol, (2006). , 651-662.

[70] Ermak, G, et al. *DSCR1(Adapt78) modulates expression of SOD1.* FASEB J, (2004). , 62-69.

[71] Carmeliet, P. *Angiogenesis in life, disease and medicine.* Nature, (2005). , 932-936.

[72] Liekens, S, De Clercq, E, & Neyts, J. *Angiogenesis: regulators and clinical applications.* Biochem Pharmacol, (2001). , 253-270.

[73] Dvorak, H. F, et al. *Induction of a fibrin-gel investment: an early event in line 10 hepatocarcinoma growth mediated by tumor-secreted products.* J Immunol, (1979). , 166-174.

[74] Ferrara, N. *Molecular and biological properties of vascular endothelial growth factor.* J Mol Med (Berl), (1999). , 527-543.

[75] Nissen, N. N, et al. *Vascular endothelial growth factor mediates angiogenic activity during the proliferative phase of wound healing.* Am J Pathol, (1998). , 1445-1452.

[76] Armesilla, A. L, et al. *Vascular endothelial growth factor activates nuclear factor of activated T cells in human endothelial cells: a role for tissue factor gene expression.* Mol Cell Biol, (1999). , 2032-2043.

[77] Abe, M, & Sato, Y. *cDNA microarray analysis of the gene expression profile of VEGF-activated human umbilical vein endothelial cells.* Angiogenesis, (2001). , 289-298.

[78] Hesser, B. A, et al. *Down syndrome critical region protein 1 (DSCR1), a novel VEGF target gene that regulates expression of inflammatory markers on activated endothelial cells.* Blood, (2004). , 149-158.

[79] Iizuka, M, et al. *Down syndrome candidate region 1,a downstream target of VEGF, participates in endothelial cell migration and angiogenesis.* J Vasc Res, (2004). , 334-344.

[80] Minami, T, et al. *Vascular endothelial growth factor- and thrombin-induced termination factor, Down syndrome critical region-1, attenuates endothelial cell proliferation and angiogenesis.* J Biol Chem, (2004). , 50537-50554.

[81] Yao, Y. G, & Duh, E. J. *VEGF selectively induces Down syndrome critical region 1 gene expression in endothelial cells: a mechanism for feedback regulation of angiogenesis?* Biochem Biophys Res Commun, (2004). , 648-656.

[82] Riper, D. V, et al. *Regulation of vascular function by RCAN1 (ADAPT78).* Arch Biochem Biophys, (2008). , 43-50.

[83] Liu, X, et al. *Transcription enhancer factor 3 (TEF3) mediates the expression of Down syndrome candidate region 1 isoform 1 (DSCR1-1L) in endothelial cells.* J Biol Chem, (2008). , 34159-34167.

[84] Epstein, C. J. *Epilogue: toward the twenty-first century with Down syndrome--a personal view of how far we have come and of how far we can reasonably expect to go.* Prog Clin Biol Res, (1995). , 241-246.

[85] Pennington, B. F, et al. *The neuropsychology of Down syndrome: evidence for hippocampal dysfunction.* Child Dev, (2003). , 75-93.

[86] Vicari, S. *Motor development and neuropsychological patterns in persons with Down syndrome.* Behav Genet, (2006). , 355-364.

[87] Vicari, S. *Implicit versus explicit memory function in children with Down and Williams syndrome.* Downs Syndr Res Pract, (2001). , 35-40.

[88] Krinsky-McHaleS.J., D.A. Devenny, and W.P. Silverman, *Changes in explicit memory associated with early dementia in adults with Down's syndrome.* J Intellect Disabil Res, (2002). Pt 3): , 198-208.

[89] Schapiro, M. B, Haxby, J. V, & Grady, C. L. *Nature of mental retardation and dementia in Down syndrome: study with PET, CT, and neuropsychology.* Neurobiol Aging, (1992). , 723-734.

[90] Solitare, G. B, & Lamarche, J. B. *Brain weight in the adult mongol.* J Ment Defic Res, (1967). , 79-84.

[91] Wisniewski, K. E. *Down syndrome children often have brain with maturation delay, retardation of growth, and cortical dysgenesis.* Am J Med Genet Suppl, (1990). , 274-281.

[92] Kesslak, J. P, et al. *Magnetic resonance imaging analysis of age-related changes in the brains of individuals with Down's syndrome.* Neurology, (1994). , 1039-1045.

[93] Raz, N, et al. *Selective neuroanatomic abnormalities in Down's syndrome and their cognitive correlates: evidence from MRI morphometry.* Neurology, (1995). , 356-366.

[94] Teipel, S. J, et al. *Age-related cortical grey matter reductions in non-demented Down's syndrome adults determined by MRI with voxel-based morphometry.* Brain, (2004). Pt 4): , 811-824.

[95] Teipel, S. J, et al. *Relation of corpus callosum and hippocampal size to age in nondemented adults with Down's syndrome.* Am J Psychiatry, (2003). , 1870-1878.

[96] Sylvester, P. E. *The hippocampus in Down's syndrome.* J Ment Defic Res, (1983). Pt 3): , 227-236.

[97] Marin-padilla, M. *Structural abnormalities of the cerebral cortex in human chromosomal aberrations: a Golgi study.* Brain Res, (1972). , 625-629.

[98] Becker, L. E, Armstrong, D. L, & Chan, F. *Dendritic atrophy in children with Down's syndrome.* Ann Neurol, (1986). , 520-526.

[99] Schmidt-sidor, B, et al. *Brain growth in Down syndrome subjects 15 to 22 weeks of gestational age and birth to 60 months.* Clin Neuropathol, (1990). , 181-190.

[100] Takashima, S, et al. *Abnormal neuronal development in the visual cortex of the human fetus and infant with down's syndrome. A quantitative and qualitative Golgi study.* Brain Res, (1981). , 1-21.

[101] Takashima, S, et al. *Dendrites, dementia and the Down syndrome.* Brain Dev, (1989). , 131-133.

[102] Godridge, H, et al. *Alzheimer-like neurotransmitter deficits in adult Down's syndrome brain tissue.* J Neurol Neurosurg Psychiatry, (1987). , 775-778.

[103] Nyberg, P, Carlsson, A, & Winblad, B. (1982). *Brain monoamines in cases with Down's syndrome with and without dementia.*, 289-299.

[104] Hof, P. R, et al. *Age-related distribution of neuropathologic changes in the cerebral cortex of patients with Down's syndrome. Quantitative regional analysis and comparison with Alzheimer's disease.* Arch Neurol, (1995). , 379-391.

[105] Casas, C, et al. *Dscr1, a novel endogenous inhibitor of calcineurin signaling, is expressed in the primitive ventricle of the heart and during neurogenesis.* Mech Dev, (2001). , 289-292.

[106] Mitchell, A. N, et al. *Brain expression of the calcineurin inhibitor RCAN1 (Adapt78).* Arch Biochem Biophys, (2007). , 185-192.

[107] Harris, C. D, Ermak, G, & Davies, K. J. *RCAN1-1L is overexpressed in neurons of Alzheimer's disease patients.* FEBS J, (2007). , 1715-1724.

[108] Chang, K. T, Shi, Y. J, & Min, K. T. *The Drosophila homolog of Down's syndrome critical region 1 gene regulates learning: implications for mental retardation.* Proc Natl Acad Sci U S A, (2003). , 15794-15799.

[109] Lynch, M. A. *Long-term potentiation and memory.* Physiol Rev, (2004). , 87-136.

[110] Huang, Y. Y, & Kandel, E. R. *Modulation of both the early and the late phase of mossy fiber LTP by the activation of beta-adrenergic receptors.* Neuron, (1996). , 611-617.

[111] and A biochemist's view of long-term potentiation. Learn Mem, (1996). , 1-24.

[112] Zucker, R. S. *Short-term synaptic plasticity.* Annu Rev Neurosci, (1989). , 13-31.

[113] Ishihara, K, et al. *Enlarged brain ventricles and impaired neurogenesis in the Ts1Cje and Ts2Cje mouse models of Down syndrome.* Cereb Cortex, (2010). , 1131-1143.

[114] Luna-munoz, J, et al. *Earliest stages of tau conformational changes are related to the appearance of a sequence of specific phospho-dependent tau epitopes in Alzheimer's disease.* J Alzheimers Dis, (2007). , 365-375.

[115] Rapoport, M, et al. *Tau is essential to beta-amyloid-induced neurotoxicity.* Proc Natl Acad Sci U S A, (2002). , 6364-6369.

[116] Santacruz, K, et al. *Tau suppression in a neurodegenerative mouse model improves memory function.* Science, (2005). , 476-481.

[117] Poppek, D, et al. *Phosphorylation inhibits turnover of the tau protein by the proteasome: influence of RCAN1 and oxidative stress.* Biochem J, (2006). , 511-520.

[118] Ermak, G, et al. *Do RCAN1 proteins link chronic stress with neurodegeneration?* FASEB J, (2011). , 3306-3311.

[119] Ladner, C. J, et al. *Reduction of calcineurin enzymatic activity in Alzheimer's disease: correlation with neuropathologic changes.* J Neuropathol Exp Neurol, (1996). , 924-931.

[120] Kayyali, U. S, et al. *Cytoskeletal changes in the brains of mice lacking calcineurin A alpha.* J Neurochem, (1997). , 1668-1678.

[121] Keating, D. J, Chen, C, & Pritchard, M. A. *Alzheimer's disease and endocytic dysfunction: clues from the Down syndrome-related proteins, DSCR1 and ITSN1.* Ageing Res Rev, (2006). , 388-401.

[122] Pardo, R, et al. *Inhibition of calcineurin by FK506 protects against polyglutamine-huntingtin toxicity through an increase of huntingtin phosphorylation at S421.* J Neurosci, (2006). , 1635-1645.

[123] Ermak, G, et al. *Regulator of calcineurin (RCAN1-1L) is deficient in Huntington disease and protective against mutant huntingtin toxicity in vitro.* J Biol Chem, (2009). , 11845-11853.

[124] Ma, H, et al. *Aggregate formation and synaptic abnormality induced by DSCR1.* J Neurochem, (2004). , 1485-1496.

[125] Olzmann, J. A, Li, L, & Chin, L. S. *Aggresome formation and neurodegenerative diseases: therapeutic implications.* Curr Med Chem, (2008). , 47-60.

[126] Lin, K. G, et al. *Two polymorphisms of RCAN1 gene associated with Alzheimer's disease in the Chinese Han population.* East Asian Arch Psychiatry, (2011). , 79-84.

[127] Kusters, M. A, et al. *Intrinsic defect of the immune system in children with Down syndrome: a review.* Clin Exp Immunol, (2009). , 189-193.

[128] da Rosa UtiyamaS.R., et al., *Autoantibodies in patients with Down syndrome: early senescence of the immune system or precocious markers for immunological diseases?* J Paediatr Child Health, (2008). , 182-186.

[129] Nurmi, T, et al. *Natural killer cell function in trisomy-21 (Down's syndrome).* Clin Exp Immunol, (1982). , 735-741.

[130] Licastro, F, et al. *Derangement of non-specific immunity in Down syndrome subjects: low leukocyte chemiluminescence activity after phagocytic activation.* Am J Med Genet Suppl, (1990). , 242-246.

[131] Barkin, R. M, et al. *Phagocytic function in Down syndrome--I. Chemotaxis.* J Ment Defic Res, (1980). Pt 4: , 243-249.

[132] Murphy, M, & Epstein, L. B. *Down syndrome (trisomy 21) thymuses have a decreased proportion of cells expressing high levels of TCR alpha, beta and CD3. A possible mechanism for*

diminished T cell function in Down syndrome. Clin Immunol Immunopathol, (1990). , 453-467.

[133] Bertotto, A, et al. *CD3+/CD30+ circulating T lymphocytes are markedly increased in older subjects with Down's syndrome (Trisomy 21).* Pathobiology, (1999). , 108-110.

[134] Franciotta, D, et al. *Interferon-gamma- and interleukin-4-producing T cells in Down's syndrome.* Neurosci Lett, (2006). , 67-70.

[135] Elsayed, S. M, & Elsayed, G. M. *Phenotype of apoptotic lymphocytes in children with Down syndrome.* Immun Ageing, (2009). , 2.

[136] Bertotto, A, et al. *T cell response to anti-CD3 antibody in Down's syndrome.* Arch Dis Child, (1987). , 1148-1151.

[137] Burgio, G. R, et al. *Derangements of immunoglobulin levels, phytohemagglutinin responsiveness and T and B cell markers in Down's syndrome at different ages.* Eur J Immunol, (1975). , 600-603.

[138] Corsi, M. M, et al. *Proapoptotic activated T-cells in the blood of children with Down's syndrome: relationship with dietary antigens and intestinal alterations.* Int J Tissue React, (2003). , 117-125.

[139] Nair, M. P, & Schwartz, S. A. *Association of decreased T-cell-mediated natural cytotoxicity and interferon production in Down's syndrome.* Clin Immunol Immunopathol, (1984). , 412-424.

[140] Park, E, et al. *Partial impairment of immune functions in peripheral blood leukocytes from aged men with Down's syndrome.* Clin Immunol, (2000). Pt 1): , 62-69.

[141] Scotese, I, et al. *T cell activation deficiency associated with an aberrant pattern of protein tyrosine phosphorylation after CD3 perturbation in Down's syndrome.* Pediatr Res, (1998). , 252-258.

[142] Murphy, M, et al. *Tumor necrosis factor-alpha and IFN-gamma expression in human thymus. Localization and overexpression in Down syndrome (trisomy 21).* J Immunol, (1992). , 2506-2512.

[143] Cossarizza, A, et al. *Precocious aging of the immune system in Down syndrome: alteration of B lymphocytes, T-lymphocyte subsets, and cells with natural killer markers.* Am J Med Genet Suppl, (1990). , 213-218.

[144] De Hingh, Y. C, et al. *Intrinsic abnormalities of lymphocyte counts in children with down syndrome.* J Pediatr, (2005). , 744-747.

[145] Spina, C. A, et al. *Altered cellular immune functions in patients with Down's syndrome.* Am J Dis Child, (1981). , 251-255.

[146] Verstegen, R. H, et al. *Down syndrome B-lymphocyte subpopulations, intrinsic defect or decreased T-lymphocyte help.* Pediatr Res, (2010). , 563-569.

[147] Lockitch, G, et al. *Age-related changes in humoral and cell-mediated immunity in Down syndrome children living at home.* Pediatr Res, (1987)., 536-540.

[148] Costa-carvalho, B. T, et al. *Antibody response to pneumococcal capsular polysaccharide vaccine in Down syndrome patients.* Braz J Med Biol Res, (2006)., 1587-1592.

[149] Lopez, V, et al. *Defective antibody response to bacteriophage phichi 174 in Down syndrome.* J Pediatr, (1975)., 207-211.

[150] Philip, R, et al. *Abnormalities of the in vitro cellular and humoral responses to tetanus and influenza antigens with concomitant numerical alterations in lymphocyte subsets in Down syndrome (trisomy 21).* J Immunol, (1986)., 1661-1667.

[151] Barker, K. S, Liu, T, & Rogers, P. D. *Coculture of THP-1 human mononuclear cells with Candida albicans results in pronounced changes in host gene expression.* J Infect Dis, (2005)., 901-912.

[152] Minami, T, et al. *The Down syndrome critical region gene 1 short variant promoters direct vascular bed-specific gene expression during inflammation in mice.* J Clin Invest, (2009)., 2257-2270.

[153] Bhoiwala, D. L, et al. *The calcineurin inhibitor RCAN1 is involved in cultured macrophage and in vivo immune response.* FEMS Immunol Med Microbiol, (2010)., 103-113.

[154] Lee, J. Y, et al. *Down syndrome candidate region-1 protein interacts with Tollip and positively modulates interleukin-1 receptor-mediated signaling.* Biochim Biophys Acta, (2009)., 1673-1680.

[155] Takeda, K, & Akira, S. *TLR signaling pathways.* Semin Immunol, (2004)., 3-9.

[156] Aubareda, A, Mulero, M. C, & Perez-riba, M. *Functional characterization of the calcipressin 1 motif that suppresses calcineurin-mediated NFAT-dependent cytokine gene expression in human T cells.* Cell Signal, (2006)., 1430-1438.

[157] Bischoff, S. C. *Role of mast cells in allergic and non-allergic immune responses: comparison of human and murine data.* Nat Rev Immunol, (2007)., 93-104.

[158] Yang, Y. J, et al. *Rcan1 negatively regulates Fc epsilonRI-mediated signaling and mast cell function.* J Exp Med, (2009)., 195-207.

[159] Yang, Y. J, et al. *Regulator of calcineurin 1 (Rcan1) is required for the development of pulmonary eosinophilia in allergic inflammation in mice.* Am J Pathol, (2011)., 1199-1210.

[160] Schieve, L. A, et al. *Health of children 3 to 17 years of age with Down syndrome in the 1997-2005 national health interview survey.* Pediatrics, (2009)., e253-e260.

[161] Goldacre, M. J, et al. *Cancers and immune related diseases associated with Down's syndrome: a record linkage study.* Arch Dis Child, (2004)., 1014-1017.

[162] Hasle, H, Clemmensen, I. H, & Mikkelsen, M. *Risks of leukaemia and solid tumours in individuals with Down's syndrome.* Lancet, (2000)., 165-169.

[163] Patja, K, et al. *Cancer incidence of persons with Down syndrome in Finland: a population-based study.* Int J Cancer, (2006). , 1769-1772.

[164] Zipursky, A. *Transient leukaemia--a benign form of leukaemia in newborn infants with trisomy 21.* Br J Haematol, (2003). , 930-938.

[165] Zipursky, A, Peeters, M, & Poon, A. *Megakaryoblastic leukemia and Down's syndrome: a review.* Pediatr Hematol Oncol, (1987). , 211-230.

[166] Dieckmann, K. P, Rube, C, & Henke, R. P. *Association of Down's syndrome and testicular cancer.* J Urol, (1997). , 1701-1704.

[167] Horan, R. F, Beitins, I. Z, & Bode, H. H. *LH-RH testing in men with Down's syndrome.* Acta Endocrinol (Copenh), (1978). , 594-600.

[168] Yang, Q, Rasmussen, S. A, & Friedman, J. M. *Mortality associated with Down's syndrome in the USA from 1983 to 1997: a population-based study.* Lancet, (2002). , 1019-1025.

[169] Stathatos, N, et al. *KiSS-1/G protein-coupled receptor 54 metastasis suppressor pathway increases myocyte-enriched calcineurin interacting protein 1 expression and chronically inhibits calcineurin activity.* J Clin Endocrinol Metab, (2005). , 5432-5440.

[170] Zou, B, Qiao, L, & Wong, B. C. *Current Understanding of the Role of PPARgamma in Gastrointestinal Cancers.* PPAR Res, 2009. (2009). , 816957.

[171] Bush, C. R, et al. *Functional genomic analysis reveals cross-talk between peroxisome proliferator-activated receptor gamma and calcium signaling in human colorectal cancer cells.* J Biol Chem, (2007). , 23387-23401.

[172] Ryeom, S, et al. *Targeted deletion of the calcineurin inhibitor DSCR1 suppresses tumor growth.* Cancer Cell, (2008). , 420-431.

[173] Baek, K. H, et al. *Down's syndrome suppression of tumour growth and the role of the calcineurin inhibitor DSCR1.* Nature, (2009). , 1126-1130.

Section 4

Neural Development in Down Syndrome

Chapter 11

Laterality Explored: Atypical Hemispheric Dominance in Down Syndrome

George Grouios, Antonia Ypsilanti and Irene Koidou

Additional information is available at the end of the chapter

http://dx.doi.org/10.5772/53829

1. Introduction

Down syndrome (DS) is a genetic disorder caused by an extra copy of chromosome 21 (trisomy 21), with an incidence in 1 in 700 live births. The third chromosome causes a series of physical, biological and behavioural characteristics that are syndrome-specific including intellectual disability, heart defects, problems in the endocrine and immune system and other medical conditions (Epstein et al., 1991). Moreover, there is established evidence for the language difficulties in people with DS particularly in expressive vocabulary and grammar. Research on language has documented a specific pattern of cerebral lateralization that commonly characterizes these individuals, that is unique to the syndrome compared to typically developing individuals and individuals with intellectual disability (ID) non-DS. This realization has triggered the interest of neuropsychologists to investigate atypical hemispheric dominance in DS.

Atypical hemispheric Dominance, or otherwise termed "anomalous dominance" or "anomalous cerebral organization", refers to the atypical lateralization of language areas within the brain (Geschwind & Galaburda, 1985). Usually, most right-handed individuals (97%) exhibit left-hemisphere lateralization for language. The remaining 3% of right-handed individuals exhibit bilateral or right hemisphere lateralization for language (Bishop, 1990). In left-handed individuals this distribution is very different. About 60% of left-handed individuals exhibit left-hemisphere lateralization for language, 30% bilateral lateralization and 10% right-hemisphere lateralization for language (Bishop, 1990). Geschwind and Behan (1982) termed anomalous dominance that in which the pattern of language laterality differed from the "... standard dominance pattern" (pp. 70). Bryden, McManus and Bulman-Fleming (1994) criticized this definition, highlighting that if one accepts this description "... we run the risk of defining the majority of the population as being anomalous" (pp. 111). According to Geschwind and Galaburda (1985a; 1985b), atypical dominance may involve the inverse or weak dominance of three features; hand dominance, language dominance and visuospatial dominance. Previc (1994) distinguished the term atypical laterality into anatomical atypical asymmetry, which involves the decreased volume of the left hemisphere compared to the right hemisphere, particularly in the temporal region, and is observed in approximately 30-35% of the normal population, and functional atypical asymmetry, which relates to the bilateral or right hemisphere language dominance.

During the past decades atypical laterality has been studied in a number of pathological conditions, including individuals with intellectual disability (ID) (e.g., Grouios, Sakadami, Poderi, & Alevriadou, 1999), DS (e.g., Heath & Elliott, 1999), autism (Cornish & McManus, 1996), Turner syndrome (Ganou & Grouios, 2008), Klinefelter syndrome (Ganou, Grouios, koidou, & Alevriadou, 2010), Williams syndrome (Järvinen-Pasley, Pollak, Yam, Hill, Grichanik et al., 2010), fragile-X syndrome (Cornish, Pigram, & Shaw, 1997), developmental stuttering (Foundas, Corey, Angeles, Bollich, Crabtree-Hartman et al., 2003), developmental dyslexia (Illingworth & Bishop, 2009), disabled reading (Dalby & Gibson, 1981), attention-deficit/hyperactivity disorder (Hale, Zaidel, McGough, Phillips, & McCracken, 2006), depression (Pinea, Kentgena, Bruderb, Leiteb, Bearmana et al., 2000), schizophrenia (Giotakos, 1999) and epilepsy (Slezicki, Cho, Brock, Pfeiffer, McVearry et al., 2009). The aim of the present review is to present and discuss research on atypical cerebral laterality in DS.

2. Laterality measures

There are several techniques with which one can assess the laterality of cognitive functions. A broad division of these techniques is that between invasive and non-invasive laterality measures.

An invasive technique is one, which penetrates or breaks the skin or enters a body cavity. The only available invasive technique for the assessment of lateralization of cognitive functions is the intracarotid amobarbital procedure (IAP) or Wada test. The IAP is a procedure first described by Wada (1949) and Wada and Rasmussen (1960) for anaesthetizing cerebral hemispheres for the purpose of lateralizing language and memory functions. The procedure consists of unilateral injection of sodium amobarbital into the internal carotid, which temporarily anaesthetizes the hemisphere ipsilateral to the injection site. While one hemisphere is anaesthetized, language and memory functions of the hemisphere contralateral to the injection site can be tested. After the effect of the anaesthesia has dissipated, the process is repeated with the other hemisphere. Determining the lateralization of language and memory functions is of both theoretical and practical interest, establishing cerebral language lateralization, predicting patients who are at risk for developing a post-surgical amnestic syndrome and identifying lateralized dysfunction to help confirm seizure onset laterality (Loring & Meador, 2000). Scientific investigation of cerebral lateralization in individuals with ID using the IAP is generally hampered for obvious moral and ethical reasons.

http://dx.doi.org/10.5772/53829

A scientific procedure is strictly defined as non-invasive when no break in the skin is created and there is no contact with the mucosa, or skin break, or internal body cavity, beyond a natural or artificial body orifice. Non-invasive techniques for the assessment of cerebral lateralization can be further subdivided into neuroimaging techniques and behavioural techniques.

Neuroimaging techniques include both anatomical techniques, which create "constructed" images of brain structure, and functional techniques, which generate a series of dynamic brain images reflecting ongoing brain activity (Ganou, Kollias, Koidou, & Grouios, 2012). The anatomical techniques, which are the classical methods to image the brain, comprise computed tomography and structural magnetic resonance imaging. The functional techniques contain both direct (electroencephalography and magnetoencephalography) and indirect (positron-emissiontomography, single photon emission computed tomography and functional magnetic resonance imaging) measures of neural activity, which basically measure haemodynamic responses or differences in metabolic concentrations to cognitive stimulation (for more information see Cohen & Sweet, 2011; Hüsing, Jäncke, & Tag, 2006).

Neuroimaging have offered a broad range of investigative tools to basic (e.g., Aziz-Zadeh, Koski, Zaidel, Mazziotta, & Iacoboni, 2006; Jansen, Menke, Sommer, Forster, Bruchmann et al., 2006; Tomasi & Volkow, 2012) and clinical (e.g., Desmond, Sum, Wagner, Demb, Shear et al., 1995; khondi-Asi, Jafari-Khouzani, Elisevich, & Soltanian-Zadeh, 2011; Oertel, Knöchel, Rotarska-Jagiela, Schönmeyer, Lindner et al., 2010) laterality research that fulfill the popular fantasy of being able to "read the mind," albeit in the form of "seeing the brain" both structurally and functionally (Kerr & Denk, 2008).

Over the past 20 years, evidence for atypical cerebral lateralization in individuals with DS has been adduced using various neuroimaging techniques (Azari, Horwitz, Pettigrew, Grady, Haxby, et al., 1994; Menghini, Costanzo, & Vicari, 2011; Pinter, Eliez, Schmitt, Capone, & Reiss, 2001). However, despite the large and growing literature describing patterns of brain structure and function in the healthy and diseased human brain, scientific research on Down syndrome has not been well integrated into the mainstream of human neuroimaging research. Nevertheless, a few investigators have demonstrated success in applying digital imaging technology in individuals with DS.

For example, Uecker, Mangan, Obrzut and Nadel (1993) argued that diffuse language lateralization in individuals with DS is likely to be a contributor to their poor visuospatial performance. Frangou, Aylward, Warren, Sharma, Barta et al. (1997) investigated whether the anatomic substrate for language are abnormal in DS. They examined volumetric Magnetic Resonance Imaging (MRI) measures of the superior temporal gyrus and the planum temporale for community-dwelling individuals with DS and matched healthy comparison subjects. It was found that brain abnormalities in DS were not uniform. Specifically, the planum temporale volume of the individuals with DS was smaller than that of the healthy subjects. The volume of the superior temporal gyrus in the DS individuals was proportionally similar to that of the comparison group. For the subjects with DS, neither superior temporal gyrus nor planum temporale volume was significantly correlated with performance on language tests. Losin, Rivera, O'Hare, Sowell, and Pinter (2009) compared functional Magnetic Resonance Imaging (fMRI) activation patterns during passive story listening in young adults with DS and approximately age-matched, typically developing controls. They found that individuals with DS exhibited differences in blood oxygen level dependant activation patterns compared to a typically developing group during the fMRI story-listening task. In particular, their results indicated that the DS group showed almost no difference in activation patterns between the language (forward speech) and non-language (backward speech) conditions. Menghini, Costanzo and Vicari (2011) investigated regional grey matter density in adolescents with DS compared to age-matched controls and correlated MRI data with neuropsychological measures in the DS group. Their findings revealed that a number of brain regions subserved the neuropsychological abilities of participants with DS. Although adolescents with DS showed typical organization of brain structures related to some cognitive abilities, in particular spatial memory and visuoperception, they presented abnormal brain organization related to other cognitive domains, such as linguistic and verbal memory. Jacola, Byars, Chalfonte-Evans, Schmithorst, Hickey et al. (2011) used fMRI to investigate neural activation during a semantic-classification/object-recognition task in individuals with DS and typically developing control participants. A comparison between groups suggested atypical patterns of brain activation for the individuals with DS.

Behavioural techniques that have frequently been used to assess cerebral lateralization include those that involve measurement of perceptual asymmetries, those that engage evaluation of sensory asymmetries and those that implicate determination of motor (or manual) asymmetries.

Studies of perceptual asymmetries have been utilized to explore lateral dominance of brain function and comprise dichotic, dichoptic and dichaptic stimulation. The rationale underlying the dichotic listening technique is that contralateral projections from each ear override ipsilateral projections when both ears are simultaneously presented with an auditory stimulus (e.g. a speech sound, digit or a musical tone) and the subject has to report what he/she has heard (Kimura 1967). Individuals with left hemisphere dominance for speech generally show a right-ear advantage for verbal stimuli. The stimuli, most commonly consonant vowel syllables or monosyllabic words, are presented to the participant via ear-phones. Right-handers commonly exhibit a right ear advantage for verbal stimuli (e.g., Elliot & Weeks, 1993; Hugdahl, 2005), although individual differences seem to affect performance (e.g., gender, age) (Cowell & Hugdahl 2000). Empirical research, using dichotic listening techniques, has stressed asymmetry at the perceptual level in individuals with DS (e.g., Bowler, Cufflin, & Kiernan, 1985; Bunn, Welsh, Simon, Howarth, & Elliott, 2003; Hartley, 1981).

In the dichoptic presentation technique (or divided visual field technique), the subject is asked to report verbal stimuli (letters, words) that are rapidly flashed tachistoscopically into one visual half-field, thereby, limiting visual input to the contralateral hemisphere (Banich, 2003). The very short tachistoscopic presentation time prevents possible eye movements and, thus, bilateral cortical projection of the stimuli. Speech stimuli presented in the right visual field and, thus, transmitted primarily to the left hemisphere are recognized and named more rapidly and certainly than stimuli presented in the left visual field (McKeever & Huling, 1970; Hines, 1972). The dominance of the left hemisphere is shown more distinct-

http://dx.doi.org/10.5772/53829

ly in recognition of abstract rather than concrete nouns (Ellis & Shepard, 1974, Hines, 1978) and also of words that only elicit a visual imagination with difficulty (Day, 1979). Right-handers usually show a right visual field advantage for verbal stimuli, as determined by the speed and correctness of the responses (Belin, Jullien, Perrier, & Larmande, 1990). A limited body of literature, using dichoptic presentation techniques, has documented the existence of perceptual asymmetries in individuals with DS (e.g., Chua, Weeks, & Elliott, 1996; Weeks, Chua, Elliot, Lyons, & Pollock, 1995).

The dichaptic stimulation technique requires the subject to feel two different objects with meaningless shapes presented one to each hidden hand at the same time (Witelson, 1974). Upon dichaptic examination, the subject is asked to identify the two shapes from among a collection of six visually displayed shapes (Springer & Deutsch, 1981). Thus, hemispheric differences in haptic perception might be uncovered because of the complexity of the task, by making verbal mediation impossible, or by interfering with the interhemispheric transfer of information through the activation of homologous cortical areas. It has been shown that when meaningless stimuli are used, perceptual asymmetries are usually found in favor of the left hand for right-handed individuals (Benton, Harvey, & Varney, 1973; Dodds, 1978; Verjat, 1988), which reflects a better treatment of spatial information by the right hemisphere. Experimental data, using dichaptic stimulation techniques, have supported the existence of perceptual asymmetries in individuals with DS (e.g., Chua, Weeks, & Elliott, 1996; Elliott, Pollock, Chua, & Weeks, 1995; Weeks, Chua, Elliot, Lyons, & Pollock, 1995).

Laterality researchers have increasingly come to recognize the importance of sensory asymmetries in determining observed patterns of cerebral dominance (Dittmar, 2002). Lateral asymmetries in the use of sensory organs, based on their preferential use or/and functional primacy in a specific situation, are among the most obvious functional lateral preferences (Hellige, 1993), and they figure prominently in explanations of our evolutionary past (Corballis, 1989), of ontogenetic development (Best, 1988; Levy, 1981), and of various abnormalities (Geschwind & Galaburda, 1985). The rationale for using the sensory asymmetries paradigm in the n the context of brain laterality is based on the presumption that difference in sensory performance between sensory stimuli presented to a sensory organ contralateral or ipsilateral to the dominant hemisphere would reflect a hemispheric bias in their attribution strategy (Porac, Coren, Steiger, & Duncan, 1980). Sensory asymmetries are most prominent with respect to the auditory (e.g., Reiss & Reiss, 1998), visual (e.g., Porac & Coren, 1976), tactile (e.g., Harada, Saito, Kashikura, Sato, Yonekura et al., 2004) and chemical senses [taste (e.g., Faurion, Cerf, Van De Moortele, Lobel, MacLeod et al., 1999) and smell (e.g., Royet & Plailly, 2004)]. As far as we know, no study to date has examined sensory asymmetries in DS individuals.

Motor indices of laterality, namely hand and foot preference and performance, have been used extensively to explore fundamental properties of the human brain, such as lateralization of brain functions, both in typically developing individuals (e.g., De Agostini & Dellatolas, 2001; Reiss, Tymnik, Kogler, Kogler, & Reiss 1999) and individuals with DS (e.g., Porac, Coren & Duncan, 1980; Grouios, Sakadami, Poderi & Aleuriadou, 1999). The most commonly used index of laterality is handedness. The main consideration in the assessment of handedness is the use of different handedness measures, which produce different types of handedness. For example, hand preference can be assessed using questionnaires (e.g., Briggs & Nebes, 1972; Oldfield, 1971) on a five-scale continuum ranging from strong left-handers to strong right-handers. Alternatively, researchers have used preference measures to distinguish between left and right-handers (2 categories), excluding intermittent hand preferences (e.g., Coren & Porac, 1980), or right and non-right handers (2 categories) (e.g., Ypsilanti, 2009) or right-handers, left handers and ambiguous (or mixed) handers (3 categories) (e.g., Cornish & McManus, 1996).

In attempting to clarify both the conceptual and theoretical issues surrounding handedness assessment methodology, it is important to discriminate between "direction of hand preference", "degree of hand preference" and "consistency of hand preference" (Cornish & McManus, 1996). Direction of hand preference refers to the degree of dexterity or sinistrality that an individual exhibits (Bishop, 1990). Degree of hand preference is determined by whether an individual consistently exhibits a specific hand preference *across* several tasks or behaviours (Cornish & McManus, 1996). Consistency of hand preference is ascertained by whether an individual exhibits a specific hand preference for the same task on several occasions (Cornish & McManus, 1996). Consistency of hand preference was previously described by Palmer (1964), which he termed "variable hand preference" and postulated to be increased in left-handers. Moreover, the degree of hand preference was also previously described by Palmer (1964) which he termed "ambidexterity or mixed motor preference" referring to the degree of hand differentiation across different tasks.

Classification of handedness is further complicated by the fact that a researcher may assess hand preference (be that the direction, degree, or consistency) by a self-reported questionnaire (e.g., Briggs & Nebes, 1972) or a behavioural measure of hand preference (e.g., Bryden, Pryde, & Roy, 2000) or observation of hand preference (Porac & Coren, 1981) and/or hand performance or hand skill, which evaluates the proficiency of one hand over the other in performing a specific task (e.g., pegboard). The advantage of accessing hand preference is that one can evaluate several tasks (e.g., writing, throwing, cutting and dealing cards), rather than assessing hand performance on one task. However, assessing hand performance assists in the more qualitative understanding of handedness by allowing individuals to document their relative proficiency of one hand over the other. Most researchers (e.g., Porac & Coren, 1981; Bishop, 1990) agree that the assessments of hand preference and hand skill are two qualitatively different measures (i.e., they measure different things) of handedness. The mechanisms that mediate preference and performance are different representing two dimensions of laterality. In essence hand preference is mediated more by cognitive mechanisms that support the choice of hand-use, while hand skill may be less mediated by cognitive mechanisms and more supported by motoric systems. Annett, Hudson and Turner (1974) have supported the use of performance measures, suggesting that the relative proficiency of one hand over the other would most likely lead to increased preference of the more skilled hand.

The assessment of preference in populations with DS using questionnaires has been scarce since most clinical groups document ID, which may interfere with the process of answering questionnaires (even if those are read to them). It has become very common during the pasts decades to use behavioural measures of hand preference (e.g., Bryden, Pryde, & Roy, 2000; Bishop, Ross, Daniel, & Bright, 1996) or observation of hand preference on a number of tasks (Porac & Coren, 1981). These tasks are comprised of 10-12 preference measures (to assess degree of hand preference), which are examined twice (to assess hand consistency) and handedness is usually evaluated on a three point scale of preference; left, right, mixed. However, studies have used the demonstration of hand preference based on the items of an inventory and a five-point scale has been used classifying individuals as strongly left, weak left, ambitexter, weak right, strongly right (Van Strein, Lagers, van Haselen, van Hagen, de Coo, Frens, & van der Geest, 2005). An alternative example of such a task is the WatHand Box Test (Bryden, Pryde, & Roy, 2000), which assesses direction and consistency of hand preference using a variety of unimanual tasks (e.g., lifting a cupboard door, using a toy hammer, placing rings on hooks and tossing a ball). In addition, Bishop's card reaching task (Bishop, Ross, Daniel, & Bright, 1996) that provides a measure of the degree and the direction of hand preference has commonly been used in individuals with neurodevelopmental disorders (see Desplanches, Deruelle, Stefanini, Ayoun, Volterra, Vicari et al, 2006).

Performance measures of handedness are used less often to assess the relative proficiency of on hand over the other in individuals with neurodevelopmental disorders. Tasks that have commonly been utilized to assess hand skill are finger tapping (Elliott, Edwards, Weeks, Lindley, & Carnahan, 1987; Elliott, Weeks, & Jones 1986) and the pegboard (e.g., Cornish & McManus, 1996; Cornish, Pigram, & Paw, 1997).

Other laterality indexes, such as ear, eye and foot, are also assessed both as preference and as performance. For example, foot preference can be assessed using a questionnaire or using a demonstration of foot preference across a number of tasks (e.g., Porac & Coren, 1981). Moreover, foot performance can also be examined by assessing the relative proficiency of one foot over the other. Up until now, no study that we know has specifically addressed relative foot performance in individuals with DS.

3. Atypical laterality in individuals with Down syndrome (Dichotic listening studies)

In dichotic listening studies the participants selectively attend one of the two messages presented simultaneously in both ears indicating a left or right ear advantage for linguistic material. Most evidence agrees that right-handed individuals with DS exhibit a unique pattern of ear dominance that is syndrome-specific and cannot be attributed to the mental retardation per se (Heath & Elliot, 1999). Support for this dissociation in ear preference comes from various studies assessing individual with DS, individuals with mental retardation (non-DS) and typically developing participants (e.g., Hartley, 1981; Pipe, 1983; Elliot & Weeks, 1993; Heath & Elliot, 1999; Giencke & Lewandowski, 1989). There is increased evidence for left ear/right hemisphere dominance for language in right-handed individuals with DS, which is indicative of a reversed cerebral specialization for speech perception (see Elliot, Weeks &

Chua, 1994 for a meta-analysis). This reversed pattern has been linked to the poor linguistic abilities of these individuals although dissociation between laterality for speech perception and speech production that involves oral motor systems has also been suggested (Elliot, Weeks, & Elliot, 1987; Giencke & Lewandowski, 1989; Heath & Elliot, 1999). During the past decade, studies explored the issue of the dissociation of lateralized systems for speech perception and speech production in individuals with DS using a verbal-motor task that tapped interhemispheric integration (Welsh, Elliot, & Simon, 2003). Their results supported their model of functional dissociation between perception and oral-motor production for speech stimuli that are typically supported by the same cerebral hemisphere in typically developing individuals. Moreover, this atypical pattern of cerebral specialization is specific to DS and is not observed in other populations with mental retardation (non-DS) of unknown etiology.

Unlike typically developing individuals, DS people exhibit right hemisphere lateralization for receptive language and a left hemisphere lateralization for the production of simple and complex movement. This separation of speech perception and motor movement in addition to the morphological callosal deficiencies (causing poor intrahemispheric communication) may be responsible for the verbal difficulties of DS individuals (Heath, Grierson, Binsted, & Elliott, 2007).

Pipe (1983) used dichotic listening tasks to assess language laterality in young children with DS, individuals with mental retardation (non-DS) and typically developing individuals. Their results indicated an atypical left-ear right-hemisphere advantage for speech stimuli in individuals with DS a pattern that was only observed in this clinical group. Non-DS individuals with mental retardation exhibited a right-ear left-hemisphere advantage for speech stimuli a pattern that was similar to typically developing individuals. In accordance with With Elliott, Edwards, Weeks, Lindley and Carnahan's (1987) study, Pipe (1983) observed the unique pattern of ear preference in individuals with DS, which seems to be expressed over and above the degree of mental retardation and may be described as syndrome-specific. It should be noted here that most researchers (e.g., Pipe, 1983; Elliott, Edwards, Weeks, Lindley, & Carnahan, 1987 Heath & Elliot, 1999) have linked this unique pattern of cerebral laterality for language in individuals with DS with the weak linguistic abilities that they exhibit. However, further research assessing different clinical syndromes that also exhibit linguistic deficits (e.g., Williams syndrome) using dichotic listening tasks is needed to support this hypothesis.

On the other hand, Paquette, Bourassa and Peretz (1996) documented a left ear advantage in individuals with ID of unknown etiology. Their results indicated a left ear/ right hemisphere advantage for speech stimuli in both impaired groups and the opposite pattern in typically developing individuals. This pattern of ear preference supports the notion of atypical cerebral laterality in individuals with mental retardation as a consequence of the early brain damage that affects intellectual functioning and cerebral specialization.

The importance of studies using non-invasive techniques, such as dichotic listening and handedness, to assess cerebral laterality in individuals with mental retardation is of vast importance. Firstly, non-invasive measures are easy and safe to administer to such populations and produce significant information to researchers in this field. Secondly, such

http://dx.doi.org/10.5772/53829

studies provide insight into the functioning of the brain and its lateralization. They also provide evidence for the representation of cognitive systems within the brain. For example, it may be suggested that the brains of individuals with DS may represent processing centers bilaterally causing a delay in the production of relevant cognitive and motor material. In addition, by combining neuroimaging with behavioral laterality techniques one can infer that certain brain areas are predominately involved in specific processes, while other areas are unable to execute their intended function. For instance, perhaps the weak collaboration of the two hemispheres is due to the thinner corpus callosum in individuals with DS (Wang, Doherti, Hesselink, & Bellugi, 1992) that may cause the isolation of the functions of the hemispheres enhancing weak intra-hemispheric integration at least for verbal-motor stimuli (Welsh, Elliot, & Simon, 2003).

4. Atypical laterality and Down syndrome (handedness studies)

Ear preference using dichotic listening tasks indicates a syndrome- specific pattern of cerebral laterality in individuals with DS. This pattern can perhaps be documented using other laterality indexes, such as hand, foot and eye preference. To date there has not been a study assessing individuals with DS on various laterality indexes using preference and performance measures and controlling for the effect of age, gender and degree of mental retardation. Such studies are currently been undertaken in our laboratory to assist further in the understanding of atypical laterality in individuals with DS.

However, handedness studies in individuals with DS have been reported since the 70's. Pickersgill and Pank (1970) assessed the prevalence of left handedness in individuals with DS, individuals with mental retardation non-DS and typically developing individuals. They found a higher prevalence of left-handedness in individuals with mental retardation non-DS compared to individuals with DS and typically developing adults. More specifically, the prevalence of left-handedness in typically developing individuals in their sample was 15.6% and that of individuals with DS 18.7%, while individuals with mental retardation non-DS exhibited an almost twofold increased prevalence of left-handedness (31%).

In a later study, Batheja and Mc Manus (1985) explored the prevalence of left-handedness in individuals with DS, individuals with mental retardation (non-DS) and typically developing Individuals, matched for age, and found no difference between the two clinical groups (DS=27% left-handers, non-DS= 29% left-handers), although there was a marked difference in the non-clinical groups (age matched controls=11% left-handers).

In a similar study, Pipe (1987) assessed hand preference in individuals with DS, individuals with mental retardation non-DS and age-matched controls including her families to determine whether familial sinistrality is documented in these populations. Their results indicated that the two clinical groups, regardless of their etiology (DS or non-DS) exhibited 35-36% of non-right handedness (i.e., left and mixed handedness) and increased familial sinistrality compared to the non-clinical population. The authors explained that the increased prevalence of mixed handedness and familial sinistrality in individuals with mental retardation couldn't support Satz's (1973) model of pathological left-handedness. If non-right handedness is caused by early brain insult, as the model suggests, then there should not be an increased prevalence of familial sinistrality in these populations. Rather as Batheja and McManus (1985) suggested non-right handedness may be the result of any biological disturbance causing variability in cerebral asymmetry. Alternatively, specific hormones such as testosterone, delays the development of left-hemisphere functions resulting in increased prevalence of non-right handedness in clinical populations.

Lewin, Kohen and Mathew (1993) investigated handedness in individuals with DS, epilepsy and autism. Their results indicated a significantly increased prevalence of non-right handers in all three populations with no differences between the three groups and no differences associated with the level of mental retardation as reported elsewhere (e.g., Hicks & Barton, 1975). It was proposed that the theory of left-handedness (Satz, 1972) may explain the increased incidence of non-right handers in individuals with epilepsy in which focal brain damage may be assumed, however, it may not hold true for individuals with DS or autism. The theory of increased randomness (Palmer, 1964) may explain this pattern in individuals with learning disabilities, since the arrested development of the nervous system may lead to the undifferentiation of the two hemispheres documented by the increased prevalence of non-right handers in these populations. Table 1 below presents research using laterality indexes in DS and ID.

Findings from our laboratory confirm the existence of an atypical pattern of handedness preference in individuals with DS (n=50) and ID (n=50), compared to typically developing (TD) individuals (n=100) (Ypsilanti, 2009) (Figure 1). Specifically, our results demonstrate no significant differences between DS and ID individuals with similar level of intellectual functioning (mean IQ=43). However, they indicate statistically significant differences between both clinical groups and TD individuals (χ^2= 46.86, d.f.=2, p<0.01).

In reviewing studies of atypical laterality in individuals with DS, compared to individuals with ID (non-DS) and typically developing individuals, two conclusions can be drawn. Firstly, in the existing literature there seems to be inconsistent findings even when similar methodologies are employed. For example, Pickersgill and Pank (1970) found no significant differences in laterality in individuals with DS and typically developing individuals, while other studies have found such differences consistently (e.g., Batheja & McManus, 1985; Pipe, 1987). The reason for this discrepancy may be linked to various laterality measures that have been used to assess hand preference in individuals with neurodevelopmental disorders as well as the different age groups that have been selected in each case. Moreover, differences in the degree of mental retardation may have interfered with the results of different studies. Secondly, few studies have taken into account the fact that individuals with DS do not exhibit focal brain lesion during fetal development, which has converted them from natural right-handers to pathological left-handers as in the cases of individuals with focal brain injury in the left hemisphere (Satz, 1972). As Batheja and McManus (1985) proposed it is more likely that the difference in the prevalence of hand preference may be due to "... any form of biological noise" (pp. 66) (Batheja & McManus, 1985) that disrupts the development of typical asymmetry in these individuals at its genesis.

http://dx.doi.org/10.5772/53829

Study no.	Reference	Participants	N[1]	Preference/ performance	Indices	Results
1	Gordon (1921)	ID		Preference	Hand	LH 18% LH 7%
2	Merphy (1962)	ID, DS	64	Preference	Hand	LH 31% of ID LH 13% of DS
3	Lenneberg, Nickols and Rosenberger (1964)	DS	61	Preference	Hand	M 42.6%
4	Clausen (1966)	ID	276	Preference	Hand	LH 17%
5	Rengstroff (1967)	ID	395	Preference	Hand, eye	81.8% RH 18.2 LH - 48.5% RE 51.4 LE%
6	Peckersgill & Pank (1970)	ID, DS	32	Performance	Hand	LH 18% in Ds LH 31% in ID
7	Hicks & Barton (1975)	ID	550	Preference	Hand	LH 20.7% * Mild & Moderate: (13%) Severe & Profound: (28%)
8	Silva & Satz (1979)	ID	1409	Performance	Hand	LH 15.5 M 12.7%
9	Porac, Coren, & Duncan (1980)	ID	128	Preference	Hand, eye, ear, foot	LH 15.9 M 44.2%
10	Burns & Zeaman (1980)	ID	20	Preference	Hand, eye, ear, foot	Hand is more lateralized than foot, ear, eye in both groups.
11	Hartley (1981)	ID, DS		Performance	Ear	LEA in DS
12	McManus (1983)	ID	68	Preference (mother's report)	Hand	LH 13.2
13	Pipe (1983)	ID, DS		Performance	Ear	LEA in DS
14	Bradshaw, Hick & Kinsbourne (1984)	ID	232	Performance	Hand	More LH
15	Elliot, D (1985)	ID DS	38	Preference/ performance	Hand	
16	Batheja & McManus (1985)	ID, DS	130	Performance	Hand	LH 27% LH 29% LH 11%
17	Elliott, Weeks & Jones (1986).	DS		Performance	Hand	DS same asymmetry on finger-tapping

Study no.	Reference	Participants	N[1]	Preference/ performance	Indices	Results
18	Searleman, Cunningham & Goodwin (1987)	ID	90	Preference/ performance	Hand	LH 17.8 M 5.6
19	Soper et al., (1987)	ID	73	Preference	Hand	LH 9.6%, M 45.2%, RH 45.2%
20	Pipe (1987)	ID, DS	318	Preference	Hand	M 35%* LRH 36%* LRH 18%
21	Elliot et al. (1987)	DS	12	Preference/ performance	Hand	
22	Lucas et al., (1989)	ID	238	Preference	Hand	LH 17.4% mild LH 28.0% severe
23	Morris & Romski, (1993)	ID	50	Preference	Hand	LH 19%, LRH 32%, RH 49%
24	Paquatte et al (1996)	ID	16	Performance	Ear	LEA in ID
25	Mandal et al (1998)	ID	50	Preference	Hand	Mixed handedness.
26	Grouios et al. (1999)	ID	73	Preference	Hand	LH 17.8%, LRH 38.4%, RH 43.8% LH 9.6%, LRH 4.1%, RH 86.3%
27	Vlachos & Karapetsas, (1999)	DS	41	Preference	Hand	LH & LRH in DS
28	Heath & Elliot (1999)	DS	10	Performance	Ear	
29	Carlier et al., (2006)	DS, WS	79	Preference		
30	Leconte and Fagard (2006)	ID	30	Preference	Hand Eye Foot	Crossed Eye-hand
31	Desplanches et al, 2006			Preference		
32	Mulvey, Ringenbach & Jung, 2011	DS	25	Preference & perfromance	Hand	Reduced hand asymmetry in bimanual coordination
33	Carlier et al., 2011	DS, WS, DiGeorge syndrome		Preference	Hand Eye, Ear & Foot	Increased mixed handedness and footedness in all groups, related to degree of ID.

1Sorted by year of study

Table 1. Laterality indices in ID and DS

http://dx.doi.org/10.5772/53829

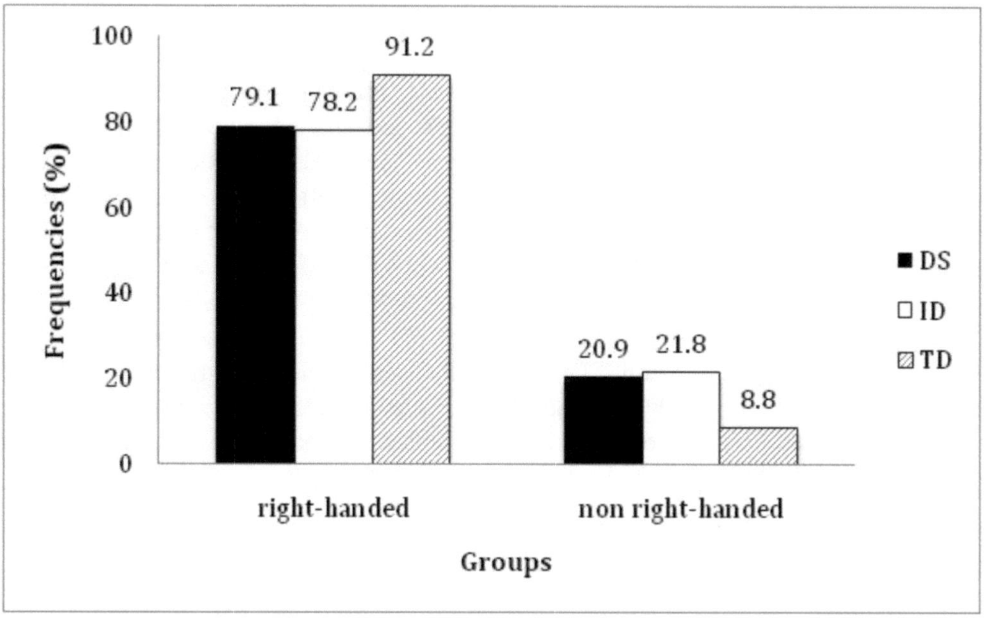

Figure 1. Frequencies of right and non-right handed individuals with DS, ID and TD.

5. Theoretical explanations of atypical laterality

Several accounts have been put forward to explain the increased incidence of atypical laterality in individuals with ID. It has been suggested that theories on atypical laterality fall into two categories; namely, pathological and natural (Satz, 1973). However, for the purposes of clarity this discrimination will not be adapted in the present paper. Rather a detailed analysis of all the theories will be presented including those that are scarcely discussed in the literature.

One of the most prominent theories has been put forward by Geschwind and Galaburda (1987), who implicated the levels of testosterone in the development of atypical laterality. According to the theory, several genetic factors, such as chromosomes and antigens, as well as environmental factors that affect fetal development, like the endocrine environment and the cyclic variation, alter the levels of testosterone to the fetus. This effect is directly linked to both the delayed growth of the left hemisphere and the increased growth of the right hemisphere particularly in the posterior regions. The decreased growth of the left hemisphere has been linked to mental retardation and poor verbal ability, which are some of the characteristics of individuals with neurodevelopmental disorders. In essence, the model predicts that the increased levels of testosterone will have an impact on the development of the left hemisphere, causing reduced language and visual-spatial dominance. Therefore, individuals with this condition will exhibit increased left and mixed handedness compared to the normal population. In support of their theory, Geschiwind and Galaburda (1985a, 1985b,

1985c) presented a series of studies associating atypical laterality (or "anomalous dominance") with developmental learning disorders, autism and immune disorders.

Although Geschwind's and Galaburda's (1987) theory has been considered one of the most prominent theories in the field of cognitive neuropsychology, it has been strongly criticized for its complexity and its arbitrary predictions (e.g., McManus & Bryden, 1991; McManus, Bryden, & Bulman-Fleming, 1994; Annett, 1994; Previc, 1994). Bryden McManus and Bulman-Fleming (1994) suggest that the relationship between language dominance and handedness, as discussed by Geschwind and Galaburda (1987), is weak and the conclusions drawn based on this assumption are poorly supported by empirical findings. Moreover, the predictions made by Geshwind and Galaburda (1987) are farfetched and the experimental data cannot support the numerous associations that are predicted by theory. On the other hand, the theory, although long and complex, contributed greatly to the understanding of the biological factors (i.e., hormones) that may be linked to atypical laterality and triggered a large number of studies in atypical laterality and neurodevelopmental disorders.

Genetic theories have also been put forward to explain atypical laterality (Annett & Alexander, 1996; Bryden & McManus, 1985). The main focus of these genetic theories was to explain the origin of left and right-handedness in normal populations (Annett 1972, 1985). More specifically, Annett's (1972) theory, referred to as "right-shift theory", explained the exhibition of right and left handedness as the outcome of left hemisphere speech induced by a single gene. In the case of atypical handedness Annett (1994) suggested that atypical developmental effects could trigger randomness in the absence of the right-shift gene and inhibit the "natural" cerebral asymmetry that is observed in typical development. Moreover, individuals lacking the gene for right hemisphere speech (rs+ gene) are at risk for various difficulties that affect language expression and phonology such as dyslexia. In other words, Annett (1985) proposed that atypical laterality may be a "... natural variation in cerebral asymmetry" (pp. 241) triggered by the absence of the right-shift gene (Annett, 1994).

Previc (1991) postulated that cerebral asymmetry derives from the asymmetric development of the vestibular system (left ear dominance in approximately 70% of the population), which is established during prenatal life and is directly linked to the postural position of the fetus and the pattern of maternal movements during the final trimester of the pregnancy. Moreover, the anatomy of the female uterus induces fetuses in the final trimester of pregnancy to be positioned "… with their head to the left side of the mother's midline and their right ear facing outward" (pp. 301) (Previc, 1991). This postural asymmetry of the fetus and the mother favours a sinistral vestibular dominance at birth, which is documented by the dextral lie preference of newborns and is correlated with the development of right hand preference later in life. The asymmetrical development of the two vestibular organs, the ear and the labyrinth, may be responsible for the asymmetry of the left and right hemisphere and the difference in ear preference documented in the literature using dichotic listening tasks (e.g., Heath & Elliott, 1999). Previc (1991) proposed a link between poor motoric lateralization (i.e., mixed or left handedness), the vestibular system and neurodevelopmental disorders that are associated with vestibular dysfunction; namely autism, dyslexia and deafness. In essence, Previc's (1991) theory predicted increased percentages of non-right handedness in

http://dx.doi.org/10.5772/53829

these disorders, in addition to other neurodevelopmental disorders, that exhibit abnormalities in the brain stem, the basal ganglia, the cerebellum and the temporal lobes, since these systems are directly affected or affect the vestibular system. Also, increased percentages of poor motoric dominance (i.e., non-right handedness) are likely to exist in pre-term infants, since they have not been exposed long enough to the right face position allowing for right handedness to be established. Previc's (1991) theory initiated a new era in the research of human laterality. The presence of prenatal factors that affect and essentially define motoric dominance in humans in combination with genetic, environmental and cultural theories could provide an important framework for the development of a stronger and more inclusive theory that encompasses strengths of all other theories.

An alternative model attempting to explain the increased incidence of atypical laterality in individuals with neurodevelopmental disorders is the theory of pathological left-handedness (Satz, 1973) According to this account, there is a subgroup of left-handed individuals which are described as pathological left handers. This subgroup was genetically natural right-handers, but suffered early brain insult to the left hemisphere causing a mild dysfunction of the contralateral hand for motor movements. The result of this dysfunction was a switch of hand dominance to the other hand (i.e., left hand) to perform complex motor tasks. Therefore, although these individuals were genetically programmed to become right-handers having left hemisphere dominance for language an early brain insult (before the age of six) caused a switch hand preference making them pathological left-handers. This subgroup is differentiated for natural left-handers who have no history of brain insult early in development and are naturally born with left hand dominance. In addition, the model describes a subgroup of pathological right-handers who were natural left-handers but an early brain injury in the right hemisphere caused them to switch hand preference to the opposite hand, thus becoming pathological right-handers. The account of pathological left-handedness can predict the increased incidence of left-handers in populations with ID and epilepsy, since both groups seem to have brain abnormalities exhibited early in development. Therefore, within a population of individuals with mental retardation, there will be an 8% of natural left-handers, as in the typical population, and approximately another 8-9% who are pathological left-handers. This model would explain the almost twofold percentage of manifest left-handers in individual with mental retardation.

Several studies have provided evidence for the model of pathological left-handedness, since the initial account was put forward (Satz, 1973). However, the theory has been tested in cross cultural studies (Satz, Baymure, & Van der Vlugt, 1979), in studies using EEG recordings (Silva & Satz, 1979), in studies with individuals with left or right congenital hemiplegia (Carlsson, Hugdahl, Uvenbrant, Wiklund, & Von Wentd, 1992), in relation to familial sinistrality (Orsini, Satz, Soper, & Light, 1985; Pipe 1987) and degree of ID (Bradshaw-McAnulty, Hicks, & Kinsbourne, 1984) and has been termed the pathological left handedness syndrome (Satz, Orsini, Saslow, & Henry, 1985). Since the original study (Satz, 1973) Soper and Satz (1984) incorporated one more type of pathological handedness in their model, termed ambiguous handedness, to explain the increased incidence of mixed handedness in individuals with early brain insult. The new explanatory model predicted increased incidence of ambiguous handedness in the more severe groups with neurodevelopmental disorders, such as infantile autism and severe ID (Soper & Satz, 1984), which has also been reported elsewhere (e.g., Tsai, 1982).

Although the above-mentioned theories contribute to the understanding of the increased incidence of non-right handers in individuals with neurodevelopmental disorders, the evidence for this link is far from conclusive. Satz's (1973) theory of pathological left handedness could account for the increased incidence of left handers in individual with focal brain injury, but in clinical populations with defuse brain damage (e.g., DS, Williams syndrome) and lack of hand preference (i.e., increased mixed handedness) the theory seems inadequate. Particularly in individuals with ID, it has long been recognized that ambiguous handedness rather than left-handedness is most commonly observed (e.g., Porac, Coren, Steiger, & Duncan, 1980). This lack of handedness would be documented by random hand preference in preference measures.

Palmer (1964) termed this observation "increased randomness" referring to the increased ambiguous hand preference in individuals with mental retardation. In particular, he postulated that handedness is a developmental process and could be utilized as an index of typical motor development. This developmental process progresses from a bilateral undifferentiated state early in infancy to a unilateral state that is viewed as a "… differentiation from a whole" (pp. 258) (Palmer, 1964), since it initiates from the trunks before the shoulders and then the hands. Therefore, Palmer (1964) proposed a maturational process that is linked to typical cerebral laterality and one-sidedness. If this maturational process is arrested or lagged it could cause increased randomness, which would be documented by lack of hand preference (i.e., ambiguous handedness). One of the main conclusions that could be drawn from Palmer's (1964) theory is that mixed and left-handedness has long been considered differentiated states and should be studied separately. Particularly in populations with neurodevelopmental disorders, "lack of hand preference" (i.e., mixed handedness) may be a more significant indicator of atypical cerebral laterality than left-handedness.

Along this vein, Bishop (1983, 1990) postulated that non right-handedness is an indicator of an immature development of the motor system, caused by diffuse brain abnormalities in individuals with mental retardation. In contrast to Satz's (1973) theory and other genetic theories, Bishop (1990) suggests that differentiated hand preference indicates mature motor development. According to Bishop (1990), studies assessing hand preference in individuals with mental retardation should utilize a control group matched for motor development rather than chronological or mental age. The question remains whether there is correspondence between motor and mental age and whether measuring motor age when assessing handedness can further contribute to the existing literature. To our knowledge, there are no published data on of handedness in neurodevelopmental disorders that utilises a control group matched for motor age. On the other hand, mental age as assessed using the WISC III (Wechsler, 1992) may also be problematic because the verbal subtests of the WISC III (Wechsler, 1992) may undermine the motor development of an individual with mental retardation. The link between mental retardation and motor retardation has not been widely investigated. Perhaps using the performance subscales of the WISC III (Wechsler, 1992), or

http://dx.doi.org/10.5772/53829

another measure of non-verbal intelligence (e.g., Raven, 1985), would be more appropriate for matching control groups. Further, research in the area of motor development and the assessment of handedness in relation to motor age are needed to clarify the issue.

A link has also been postulated between literacy and handedness, suggesting that cerebral organization may change as a result of schooling and literacy, although the evidence for this link is contradictory (Tzavaras, Kaprinis, & Gatzouas, 1981). In controversy with genetic theories, this approach suggests that literacy reinforces the left hemisphere dominance for language. According to the theory, there should be an increased number of individuals with atypical laterality among illiterate populations exhibiting right or bilateral dominance for language. Tzavaras, Kaprinis and Gatzouas (1981) examined this possibility using the dichotic listening technique as a measure of language dominance in an illiterate population and found an increased left-right ear difference in the illiterate population compared to the literate individuals. The authors suggested that this difference might be due to the poor strategic techniques used by illiterate subjects, which do not enhance bi-hemispheric participation for speech as in the educated brain. However, it has been found that aphasia is less severe and more provisional in illiterate patients suggesting a right hemisphere involvement of language in these individuals (Lecours, Mehler, Parente, Behrami, Tolipan, Cary, et al, 1988; Cameron, Currier, & Haerer, 1971). Castro-Caldas, Reis and Geurreiro (1997) in a review on literacy and laterality concluded that the empirical findings of studies from aphasic patients and dichotic listening tasks are inconclusive about the link between atypical laterality and literacy and further research is need to clarify this postulation. To the authors' knowledge, no studies have been reported linking the observed atypical laterality of individuals with neurodevelopmental disorders with literacy and schooling. However, a number of researchers propose that lateral preferences may be affected by the type of task used and may be related to the level of experience and practice that a group of individuals have (e.g., Bishop, 1983). If one accepts this notion, it is probable that individuals with mental retardation are less skilled than typically developing individuals with objects like pencils, scissors and playing cards, which are commonly used to assess hand preference in these populations. In this case, inconsistent hand preference when manipulating such objects may be affected by the immature behaviour exhibited by these individuals due to decreased experience. More specifically, the effect of limited schooling and skilfulness in individuals with mental retardation may have an indirect impact on lateral preferences particularly when the preference measures presented are school-related utilities.

Another line of research suggests that individuals with DS exhibit atypical neural activation in left/right hemisphere regions compared to typically developing individuals (Jacola, Byars, Chalfonte-Evans, Schmithorst, Hickey, Patterson, et al., 2011). In an fMRI study with 13 DS individuals, there was a positive association between visual-spatial ability and occipito-parietal and dorso-frontal activation exclusively in individuals with DS compared to control counterparts.

6. Epilogue

Research in laterality in individuals with DS has been fruitful. Findings from dichotic listening studies suggest that individuals with DS exhibit a unique pattern of lateralization of language, which is syndrome specific. Specifically, it has been repeatedly supported that there is a left-ear, right-hemisphere advantage for speech stimuli, unlike that observed in typical populations or individuals with ID of other aetiologies. Moreover, handedness studies demonstrate that lateralization of language may be pathological with increased incidence of left-handedness, left- footedness, left-eyedness and cross eye-hand preferences. Several theories have been put forward to explain this atypicality, including, hormonal, structural and neural anomalies related to the syndrome. This atypical pattern of functional lateralization, most likely contributes to the linguistic difficulties observed in individuals with DS, which are rather permanent. At the same time, limited educational and motor training leaves little space for improvement in linguistic and motor efficiency in individuals with DS. Other developmental milestones that are fundamentally delayed in individuals with DS obstruct the developmental transition from an undifferentiated state to a lateralized state.

Author details

George Grouios, Antonia Ypsilanti and Irene Koidou

Laboratory of Motor Control and Learning, Department of Physical Education and Sport Sciences, Aristotle University of Thessaloniki, Greece

References

[1] Annett, M. & Alexander, M. P. (1996). Atypical cerebral dominance: Predictions and tests of the right shift theory. *Neuropsychologia, 34,* 1215-1227.

[2] Annett, M. (1972). The distribution of manual asymmetry. *British Journal of Psychology, 65,* 343-358.

[3] Annett, M. (1972). The distribution of manual asymmetry. British Journal of Psychology, 63, 343-358.

[4] Annett, M. (1985). *Left, right hand and brain: The right shift theory*. London: Erlbaum.

[5] Annett, M. (1994). Commentary Geschwind's legacy. *Brain and Cognition, 26,* 236-242.

[6] Annett, M., Hudson, P. T. W., & Turner, A. (1974). The reliability of differences between the hands in motor skill. *Neuropsychologia,* 12, 527-531.

[7] Azari, N. P., Horwitz, B., Pettigrew, K. D., Grady, C. L., Haxby, J. V., Giacometti, K. R., & Schapiro, M. B. (1994). Abnormal pattern of cerebral glucose metabolic rates in-

volving language areas in young adults with Down syndrome. *Brain and Language*, 46, 1-20.

[8] Aziz-Zadeh, L., Koski, L., Zaidel, E., Mazziotta, J., & Iacoboni, M. (2006). Lateralization of the human mirror neuron system. *The Journal of Neuroscience*, 26, 2964-2970.

[9] Banich, M. T. (2003). The divided visual field technique in laterality and interhemispheric integration. In K. Hugdahl (ed.), *Experimental methods in neuropsychology* (pp. 47-63). New York, NY: Kluwer Publishers.

[10] Batheja, M. & McManus, I.C. (1985). Handedness in the mentally handicapped. *Developmental Medicine and Child Neurology, 27*, 63-68.

[11] Belin, C., Jullien, S., Perrier, D., & Larmande, P. (1990). La tachistoscopie: une méthode expérimentale d'étude de la specialisation hémisphérique. *Journal français d'ophtalmologie*, 13, 293-297.

[12] Benke, T., Koylu, B., Visani, P., Karner, E., Brenneis, C., Bartha, L., Trinka, E., Trieb, T., Felber, S., Bauer,G., Chemelli, A., & Willmes, K. (2006). Language lateralization in temporal lobe epilepsy: a comparison between fMRI and Wada Test. *Epilepsia, 47*, 1308-1319.

[13] Benton, A. L., Harvey, S. L., & Varney, N. R. (1973). Tactile perception of direction in normal subjects. *Neurology*, 23, 1248-1250.

[14] Best, C. T. (1988). The emergence of cerebral asymmetries in early human development: A literature review and a neuroembryological model. In D. L. Molfese and S. J. Segalowitz (eds.), *Brain lateralization in children. Developmental implications* (pp. 5-34). New York, NY: Guilford Press.

[15] Bishop, D. V. M. (1990). *Handedness and developmental disorders*. Hillsdale: Erlbaum.

[16] Bishop, D. V. M., Ross, V., Daniels, M. S., & Bright, P. (1996). The measurement of hand preference. A validation study comparing three groups of right-handers. *British Journal of Psychology, 87*, 269–285.

[17] Bourne, V. J. (2006). The divided visual filed paradigm: methodological considerations. *Laterality, 11*, 373-393.

[18] Bowler, D. M., Cufflin, J., & Kiernan, C. (1985). Dichotic listening of verbal and nonverbal material by Down syndrome children and children of normal intelligence. *Cortex*, 21, 637-644.

[19] Bradshaw- McAnulty, G., Hicks, R., & Kinsbourne, M. (1984). Pathological left-handedness and familial sinistrality in relation to degree of mental retardation. *Brain and Cognition*, 3, 349-356.

[20] Briggs, G. G. & Nebes, R. D. (1975) Patterns of hand preference in a student population. *Cortex 11*, 230-238.

[21] Bryden, M. P., McManus, I. C., & Bulman-Fleming, M. B. (1994). Evaluating the empirical support for the Geschwind-Behan-Galaburda model of cerebral lateralization. *Brain and Cognition, 26,* 103-167.

[22] Bryden, P. J., Pryde, K. M., & Roy, E. A. (2000). A performance measure of the degree of hand preference. Brain and Cognition, 44, 402–414.

[23] Bunn, L., Welsh, T. N., Simon, D. A., Howarth, K., & Elliott, D. (2003). Dichotic ear advantages in adults with Down's syndrome predict speech production errors. *Neuropsychology,* 17, 32-38.

[24] Burns, B., & Zeaman, D. (1980). A comparison of laterality indices in college and retarded subjects. Journal of Psychology, 104, 241-247.

[25] Camekon, R. F., Currier, R. D., & Haeker, A. F. (1971). Aphasia and literacy. *British Journal of Disorders of Communication, 6,* 161-163.

[26] Carlier, M., Desplanches, A. G., Philip, N., Stefanini, S., Vicari, S., Volterra, V., Deruelle, C., Fisch, G., Doyen, A. L., Swillen, A. (2011). Laterality preference and cognition: cross-syndrome comparison of patients with trisomy 21 (Down), del7q11.23 (Williams-Beuren) and del22q11.2 (DiGeorge or Velo-Cardio-Facial) syndromes. *Behavioral Genetics, 41,* 413-422.

[27] Carlier, M., Stefanini, S., Deruelle, C., Volterra, V., Doyen, A., Lamard, C., dePortzamparc, V., Vicari, S., & Fisch, G. (2006). Laterality in persons with intellectual disability. I-Do patients with trisomy 21 and Williams-Beuren syndrome differ from typically developing persons? *Behaviour Genetics, 36,* 365-376.

[28] Carlsson, R., Hugdahl, K., Uvebrant, P., Wiklund, L.M., & VonWendt, L. (1992). Pathological left-handeness revisited: Dichotic listening in children with left vs right congenital hemiplegia. *Neuropsychologia, 30,* 471-481.

[29] Castro-Caldas, A., Reis, A., & Guerreiro. M. (1997). Neuropsychological aspects of illiteracy. *Neuropsychological Rehabilitation, 7,* 327–338.

[30] Cherry, E. C. (1953). Some experiments on the recognition of speech, with one and two ears. *Journal of the Acoustical Society of America 25,* 975–979.

[31] Chua, R., Weeks, D. J, & Elliott, D. (1996). A functional systems approach to understanding verbal-motor integration in individuals with Down syndrome. *Down Syndrome Research and Practice, 4,* 25-36.

[32] Clausen, J. (1966). *Ability, structure and subgroups in mental retardation.* Washington DC: Spartan.

[33] Cohen, A., R. & Sweet, H. L. (2011). Brain imaging in behavioral medicine and clinical neuroscience. In R. A. Cohen and L. H. Sweet (eds), *Brain imaging in behavioral medicine and clinical neuroscience: an introduction* (pp. 1-9). New York: Springer Science.

[34] Corballis, M. C. (1989). Laterality and human evolution. *Psychological Review, 96,* 492-505.

[35] Cornish, K. M., & McManus, I. C. (1996). Hand preference and hand skill in children with autism. *Journal of Autism and Developmental Disorders, 26,* 597-609.

[36] Cornish, K. M., Pigram, J., & Shaw, K. (1997). Do anomalies of handedness with frazile -X. *Laterality, 2,* 91-101.

[37] Cowell, P. & Hugdahl, K. (2000). Individual differences in neurobehavioral measures of laterality and interhemispheric function as measured by dichotic listening studies. *Developmental Neuropsychology, 18,* 95-112.

[38] Dalby, J. T. & Gibson, D. (1981). Functional cerebral lateralization in subtypes of disabled readers. *Brain and Language, 14,* 34-48.

[39] Day, J. (1979). Visual half field word recognition as a function of syntactic class and imageability. *Neuropsychologia, 17,* 515-519.

[40] De Agostini, M. & Dellatolas, G. (2001). Lateralities in normal children ages 3 to 8 and their role in cognitive performances. *Developmental Neuropsychology, 20,* 429-444.

[41] Desmond, J. E., Sum, M., Wagner, A. D., Demb, J. B., Shear, P. K., lover, G. H., Gabrieli, J. D., & Morrell, M. J. (1995). Functional MRI measurement of language lateralization in Wada-tested patients. *Brain, 118,* 1411-1419

[42] Desplanches, A., Derualle, C., Stefanini, S., Ayoun, C., Volterra, V., Fisch, G., Carlier, M. (2006). Laterality in persons with intellectual disability II. Hand, foot, ear and eye laterality in persons with trisomy 21 and Williams-Beuren syndrome. *Developmental Psychobiology, 48,* 482-491.

[43] Dittmar, M. (2002). Functional and postural lateral preferences in humans: Interrelations and life-span age differences. *Human Biology, 74,* 569-585.

[44] Dodds, A. G. (1978). Hemispheric differences in tactuo-spatial processing. *Neuropsychologia, 16,* 247-254.

[45] Elliott, D., & Weeks, D. J. (1993). Cerebral specialization for speech perception and movement organization in adults with Down's syndrome. *Cortex, 29,* 103–113.

[46] Elliott, D., Edwards, J. M., Weeks, D. J., Lindley, S., & Carnahan, H. (1987). Cerebral specialization in young adults with Down syndrome. *American Journal of Mental Deficiency,* 91, 480-485

[47] Elliott, D., Pollock, B., Chua, R., & Weeks, D J. (1995). Cerebral specialization for spatial processing in adults with Down syndrome. American Journal on Mental Retardation, 99, 605-615.

[48] Elliott, D., Weeks, D. J., & Chua, R. (1994). Anomalous cerebral lateralization and Down syndrome. *Brain and Cognition, 26,* 191–195.

[49] Elliott, D., Weeks, D. J., & Elliott, C. L. (1987). Cerebral specialization in individuals with Down syndrome. *American Journal on Mental Retardation, 92,* 263–271.

[50] Elliott, D., Weeks, D. J., & Jones, R. (1986). Lateral asymmetries in finger-tapping by adolescents and young adults with Down syndrome. *American Journal of Mental Deficiency*, 90, 472-475.

[51] Ellis, H. D., & Shepard, J. W. (1974). Recognition of abstract and concrete words presented in left and right visual fields. *Journal of Experimental Psychology*, 103, 1035-1036.

[52] Faurion, A., Cerf, B., Van De Moortele, P. F., Lobel, E., MacLeod, P., & Le Bihan, D. (1999). Human taste cortical areas studied with functional magnetic resonance imaging: evidence of functional lateralization related to handedness. *Neuroscience Letters*, 277, 189-192.

[53] Foundas, A. L., Corey, D. M., Angeles, V., Bollich, A. M., Crabtree-Hartman, E., & Heilman, K. M. (2003). Atypical cerebral laterality in adults with persistent developmental stuttering. *Neurology*, 61, 1378-1385.

[54] Frangou, S., Aylward, E., Warren, A., Sharma, T., Barta, P., & Pearlson, G. (1997). Small planum temporale volume in Down's syndrome: A volumetric MRI study. *American Journal of Psychiatry*, 154, 1424-1429.

[55] Ganou, M., & Grouios, G. (2008). Cerebral laterality in Turner syndrome: a critical review of the literature. *Child Neuropsychology*, 14, 135-147.

[56] Ganou, M., Grouios, G., Koidou, I., & Alevriadou, A. (2010). The concept of abnormal cerebral lateralization in Klinefelter syndrome. *Applied Neuropsychology*, 17, 144-152.

[57] Ganou, M., Kollias, N., Koidou, I., & Grouios, G. (2012). Atypical cerebral laterality in autism: a review of current research. (Submitted for publication).

[58] Geschwind, N. & Behan, E. (1982). Left-handedness: Association with immune disease, migraine, and developmental learning disorder. *Proceedings of the National Academy of Science, 79*, 5097-5100.

[59] Geschwind, N. & Galaburda, A. M. (1985a). Cerebral lateralization: Biological mechanisms, associations, and pathology: I. A hypothesis and a program for research. *Archives of Neurology, 42*, 428-459.

[60] Geschwind, N. & Galaburda, A. M. (1985b). Cerebral lateralization: Biological mechanisms, associations, and pathology: II. A hypothesis and a program for research. *Archives of Neurology, 42*, 521-552.

[61] Giencke, S. & Lewandowski, L. (1989). Anomalous dominance in Down syndrome young adults. *Cortex, 25*, 93-102.

[62] Giotakos, O. (2002). Crossed hand-eye dominance in male psychiatric patients. *Perceptual and Motor Skills, 95*, 728-732.

[63] Goldstein, R. Z. & Volkow, N. D. (2011). Dysfunction of the prefrontal cortex in addiction: neuroimaging findings and clinical implications. *Nature Reviews Neuroscience, 12,* 652-669.

[64] Gordon, H. (1921). Left-handedness and mirror writing, especially among defective children. *Brain, 43,* 313-368.

[65] Grouios, G. & Ypsilanti, A. (2011). Language and visuospatial abilities in down syndrome phenotype: A cognitive neuroscience perspective. In S. K. Day (ed.), Genetics and etiology of Down syndrome (pp. 275-286). Rijeka, Croatia: InTech.

[66] Grouios, G., Sakadami, N., Poderi, A. & Alevriadou, A. (1999). Excess of non-right handedness among individuals with intellectual disability: Experimental evidence and possible explanations. *Journal of Intellectual Disability Research, 43,* 306–313.

[67] Hale, T. S., Zaidel, E., McGough, J. J., Phillips, J. M., & McCracken, J. T. (2006). Atypical brain laterality in adults with ADHD during dichotic listening for emotional intonation and words. *Neuropsychologia,* 44, 896-904.

[68] Harada, T., Saito, D. N., Kashikura, K., Sato, T., Yonekura, Y., Honda, M., & Sadato, N. (2004). Asymmetrical neural substrates of tactile discrimination in humans: a functional magnetic resonance imaging study. *The Journal of Neuroscience,* 24, 7524-7530.

[69] Hartley, X. Y. (1981). Lateralization of speech stimuli in young Down's syndrome children. *Cortex, 17,* 241–248.

[70] Heath, M. & Elliott, D. (1999). The cerebral specialization for speech production in persons with Down syndrome. *Brain and Language, 69,* 193–211.

[71] Heath, M., Grierson, L., Binsted, G., & Elliott, D. (2007). Hemispheric transmission time in persons with Down Syndrome. *Journal of Intellectual Disability Research,* 51, 972-981.

[72] Hellige, J. B. (1993). *Hemispheric asymmetry: What's right and what's left.* Cambridge, MA: Harvard University Press.

[73] Hicks, R. E. & Banton, K. A. (1975). A note on left-handedness and severity of mental retardation. *Journal of Generic Psychology, 127,* 323-324.

[74] Hines, D. (1972). Bilateral tachistoscopic recognition of verbal and nonverbal stimuli. *Corex,* 7, 313-322.

[75] Hines, D. 1978). Visual information processing in the left and right hemispheres. *Neuropsychologia,* 16, 593-600.

[76] Hugdahl, K. (2005). Symmetry and asymmetry in the human brain. *European Review,* 13, 119-133.

[77] Hüsing, B., Jäncke, L., & Tag, B. (2006). *Impact assessment of neuroimaging.* Amsterdam: IOS Press.

[78] Illingworth, S. & Bishop, D. V. M. (2009). Atypical cerebral lateralisation in adults with compensated developmental dyslexia demonstrated using functional transcranial Doppler ultrasound. *Brain and Language, 111*, 61-65.

[79] Jacola, L., Byars, A., Chalfonte-Evans, M., Schmithorst, V., Hickey, F., Patterson, B., Hotze, S., Vannest, J., Chiu, C., Holland, S, & Schapiro, M. (2011). Functional Magnetic Resonance Imaging of Cognitive Processing in Young Adults With Down Syndrome. *American Journal on Intellectual and Developmental Disabilities*, 116, 344-359.

[80] Jansen, A., Menke, R., Sommer, J., Forster, A. F., Bruchmann, S., Hempleman, J., Weber, B., & Knecht, S. (2006). The assessment of hemispheric lateralization in functional MRI: Robustness and reproducibility. *Neuroimage*, 33, 204-217.

[81] Järvinen-Pasley, A., Pollak, S. D., Yam, A., Hill, K. J., Grichanik, M., Mills, D., Reiss, A. L., Korenberg, J. R., & Bellugi, U. (2010). Atypical hemispheric asymmetry in the perception of negative human vocalizations in individuals with Williams syndrome. *Neuropsychologia*, 48, 1047-1052.

[82] Kerr, J. N. D. & Denk, W. (2008). Imaging in vivo: Watching the brain in action. *Nature Reviews Neuroscience*, 9, 195-205.

[83] khondi-Asi, A., Jafari-Khouzani, K., Elisevich, K., & Soltanian-Zadeh, H. (2011). Hippocampal volumetry for lateralization of temporal lobe epilepsy: Automated versus manual methods. *Neuroimage*, 54 (Supplement 1), S218-S226.

[84] Kimura, D. (1967). Functional asymmetry of the brain in dichotic listening. *Canadian Journal of Psychology*, 15, 156-65.

[85] Leconte, P. & Fagard, J. (2006). Lateral preferences in children with intellectual deficiency of idiopathic origin. *Developmental Psychobiology, 48*, 492-500.

[86] Lecours, A. R., Mehler, J., Parente, M. A., Behrami, M. C., Tolipan, L. C., Cary, L., Castro, M. J., Carrono, V., Chagastelles, L., Dehaut, F., Delgado, R., Evangelista, A., Faigenbaum, S., Fontoura, C., Karmann, D., Gurd, J., Torne, C. H., Jakybovicz, R., Kac, R., Lefevre, B., Lima, C., Maciel, J., Mansur, L., Martinez, R., Nobrega, M. C., Osorio, Z., Paciornik, J., Papaterram F., Penedo, M. A. J., Saboya, B., Scheuer, C., da Silva, A. B., Spinardi, M., Teixeira, M. (1988). Illiteracy and brain damage 3: contribution to the study of speech and language disorders in illiterates with unilateral brain damage (initial testing). *Neuropsychologia, 26*, 575-589.

[87] Lennenberg, E. H., Nichols, I. A., & Rosenberger, E. F. (1967). Primitive stages of language development in mongolism. In *Disorders of Communication*, Vol. XLII: Research Publications," A.R.N.M.D., pp. 119-37.

[88] Lewin, J., Kohen, D., & Mathew, G. (1993). Handedness in mental handicap: investigation into populations of Down's syndrome, epilepsy and autism. *British Journal of Psychiatry, 163*, 674-676.

[89] Loring, D. W. & Meador, K. J. (2000). Pre-surgical evaluation for epilepsy surgery. *Saudi Medical Journal*, 21, 609-616.

[90] Losin, E. A., Rivera, S. M., O'Hare, E. D., Sowell, E. R., & Pinter, J. D. (2009). Abnormal fMRI activation pattern during story listening in individuals with Down syndrome. *American Journal on Intellectual and Developmental Disabilities,* 11, 369-380.

[91] Lucas, J. A., Rosenstein, L. D., & Bigler, E. D. (1989). Handedness and language among the mentally retarded: implications for the model of pathological left handedness and gender differences in hemispheric specialization. Neuropsychologia, 27, 713-723.

[92] Mandal M. K., Pandey G., Tulsi Das C., & Bryden M. P. (1998). Handedness in mental retardation. Laterality 3, 221-225.

[93] McKeever,, W. F. & Huling, M. D. (1970). Lateral dominance in tachistoscopic word recognition as a function of hemisphere stimulation and interhemispheric transfer time. Neuropsychologia, 9, 291-299.

[94] McManus, I. C. (1983). The interpretation of laterality. *Cortex, 19,* 187-214

[95] Menghini, D., Costanzo, F., & Vicari, S. (2011). Relationship between brain and cognitive processes in Down syndrome. *Behavior Genetics,* 41, 381-393.

[96] Morris, C.A. & Mervis, C.B. (2000). Williams syndrome and related disorders. *Annual Review of Genomics and Human Genetics, 1,* 461-484.

[97] Mulvey, M., Ringenbach, S. D. R., & Jung, M. L. (2011). Reversal of handedness effects on bimanual coordination in adults with Down syndrome. *Journal of Intellectual Disability Research 55,* 998-1007.

[98] Murphy, M. M. (1962). Hand preference in three diagnostic groups of severely deficient males. *Perceptual and Motor Skills, 14,* 508.

[99] Oertel, V., Knöchel, C., Rotarska-Jagiela, A., Schönmeyer, R., Lindner., M., van de Ven, V., Haenschel, C., Uhlhaas, P., Maurer, K., & Linden, D. E. J. (2010). Reduced laterality as a trait marker of schizophrenia: Evidence from structural and functional neuroimaging. *The Journal of Neuroscience,* 30, 2289-2299.

[100] Oldfield, R. C. (1971). The assessment and analysis of handedness: The Edinburgh inventory. *Neuropsychologia, 9,* 97-113.

[101] Orsini, D. L., Sazt, P., Soper, H. V., & Light, R. K. (1985). The role of familial sinistrality in cerebral organization. *Neuropsychologia, 23,* 223-232.

[102] Palmer, R. D. (1964). Development of differentiated handedness. *Psychological Bulletin, 62,* 257-272.

[103] Paquette, C., Bourassa, M., & Peretz, I. (1996). Left-ear advantage in pitch perception of complex tones without energy at the fundamental frequency. *Neuropsychologia ,* 34, 153-157.

[104] Pickersgill, M. & Pank, P. (1970). Relation of age and mongolism to lateral preferences in severely subnormal subjects. *Nature, 228,* 1342-1344.

[105] Pinea, D. S., Kentgena, L. M., Bruderb, G. E., Leiteb, P., Bearmana, K., Maa, Y., & Kleinc, R. G. (2000) Cerebral laterality in adolescent major depression. *Psychiatry Research*, 93, 135-144.

[106] Pinter, J. D., Eliez, S., Schmitt, J. E., Capone, G. T., & Reiss, A. L. (2001). Neuroanatomy of Down's syndrome: a high-resolution MRI study. *American Journal of Psychiatry*, 158, 1659-1665.

[107] Pipe, M. E. (1983). Dichotic-listening performance following auditory discrimination training in Down's syndrome and developmentally retarded children. *Cortex, 19*, 481–491.

[108] Pipe, M. E. (1987). Pathological left-handedness: is it familial? Neuropsychologia, 25, 571-577.

[109] Porac, C. & Coren, S. (1976). The dominant eye. *Psychological Bulletin*, 83, 880-897.

[110] Porac, C. & Coren, S. (1981). *Lateral preferences and human behavior.* New York: Springer.

[111] Porac, C., Coren, S., & Duncan, P. (1980). Lateral preferences in retardates: Relationships between hand, eye foot and ear preference. *Journal of Clinical Neuropsychology, 2*, 173-188.

[112] Porac, C., Coren, S., Steiger, J. H., & Duncan, P. (1980). Human laterality: a multidimensional approach. *Canadian Journal of Psychology*, 34, 91-96.

[113] Previc, F. H. (1994). Assessing the legacy of the GBG model. *Brain and Cognition, 26*, 174-180.

[114] Raven, J. C., Court, J. H., Javen, J. (1985). *A manual for Raven's progressive matrices and vocabulary scales.* London: H. K. Lewis.

[115] Reiss, M. & Reiss, G. (1998). Ear preference: Association with other functional asymmetries of the ears. *Perceptual and Motor Skills*, 86, 399-402.

[116] Reiss, M., Tymnik, G., Kogler, P., Kogler, W., & Reiss, G. (1999). Laterality of hand, foot, eye, and ear in twins. *Laterality, 4*, 287-297.

[117] Rengstorff, R. H. (1967). The types and incidence of hand-eye preference and its relationship with certain reading abilities. *American Journal of Optometric Archives of the American Academy of Optometry*, 44, 233.

[118] Royet, J. P, & Plailly, J. (2004): Lateralization of olfactory processes. *Chemical Senses, 29*, 731-745.

[119] Salmaso, D. & Longoni, A.M. (1985). Problems in assessing hand preference. *Cortex, 21*, 533-549.

[120] Satz, P. (1973). Left-handedness and early brain insult: An explanation, *Neuropsychologia, 11*, 115-117.

[121] Satz, P., Baymur, L., & Van der Vlugt, H. (1979). Pathological left-handedness: Cross-cultural tests of a model. *Neuropsychologia, 17,* 77-81.

[122] Satz, P., Orsini, D.L., Saslow, E., & Henry, R. (1985). The pathological left-handedness syndrome, *Brain and Cognition, 4,* 27-46.

[123] Searleman, A., Cunningham, T. F., & Goodwin, W. (1988). Association between familial sinistrality and pathological left-handedness: A comparison of mentally retarded and nonretarded subjects. *Journal of Clinical and Experimental Neuropsychology, 10,* 132-138.

[124] Silva, D. A. & Satz, P. (1979). Pathological left-handedness: evaluation of model. *Brain and Language,* 7, 8-16.

[125] Slezicki, K. I., Cho, Y. W., Brock, M. S., Pfeiffer, M., McVearry, K., & Tractenberg, R. E., Motamedi, G. K. (2009). Incidence of atypical handedness in epilepsy and its association with clinical factors. *Epilepsy and Behavior,* 16, 330-334.

[126] Soper, H. V., Satz, P., Orsini, D. L., Henry, R. R., Zvi, R., & Sehulman, M. (1986). Handedness patterns in autism suggest subtypes. *Journal of Autism and Developmental Disorders, 16,* 155-167.

[127] Soper, H. V. & Satz, P. (1884). Pathological left-handedness and ambiguous handedness: A new explanatory model. *Neuropsychologia, 22,* 511-515.

[128] Soper, H. V., Satz, P., Orsini, D. L., Vangorp, W. G., & Green, M.F., (1987). Handedness distribution in a residential population with severe or profound mental-retardation. *American Journal of Mental Deficiency.* 92, 94– 102.

[129] Springer, S. & Deutsch, G. (1981). Left brain, right brain. San Francisco, CA: W. H. Freeman.

[130] Tomasi, D. & Volkow, N. D. (2012). Laterality patterns of brain functional connectivity: Gender effects *Cerebral Cortex,* 22, 1455-1454.

[131] Tzavaras , A., Kaprinis, G., & Gatzoyas, A. (1981). Literacy and hemispheric specialisation for language: Digit dichotic listening in illiterates. *Neuropsychologia, 19,* 565-570.

[132] Uecker, A., Mangan, P. A., Obrzut, J. E. & Nadel, L. (1993). Down syndrome in neurobiological perspective: An emphasis on spatial cognition. *Journal of Clinical Child and Adolescent Psychology,* 22, 2, 266-276.

[133] Van Strien, J. W., Lagers-van Haselen, G. C., van Hagen, J. M., de Coo, I. F. M., Frens, M. A., & van der Gest, J. N. (2005). Increased prevalences of left-handedness and left-eye sighting dominance individuals with Williams-Beuren syndrome. *Journal of Clinical and Experimental Neuropsychology, 27,* 967-976.

[134] Verjat, I. (1988). Dissymmetry in manual perception by children on form recognition tasks with tactually presented forms. *European Bulletin of Cognitive Psychology,* 8, 223-239.

[135] Vlachos, F. & Karapetsas, A. (1999). A developmental study of handedness in Down syndrome pupils. *Perceptual and Motor Skills,88*, 427-428.

[136] Wada, J. & Rasmussen, T. (1960). Intracarotid injection of sodium amytal for the lateralization of speech dominance. *Journal of Neurosurgery, 17*, 266-282.

[137] Wada, J. (1949). A new method for determination of the side of cerebral speech dominance: A preliminary report on the intracarotid injection of sodium amytal in man. *Igaku Seibutsugaku*, 4, 221-222.

[138] Wang, P. P., Doherty, S., Hesselink, J. R., & Bellugi, U. (1992). Callosal morphology concurs with neurobehavioral and neuropsychological findings in two neurodevelopmental disorders. *Archives of Neurology, 49*, 407–411.

[139] Wechsler D. (1992) *Wechsler intelligence scale for children (3rd ed).* Kent UK: The Psychological Corporation, Harcourt Brace & Co, Sidcup.

[140] Weeks, D. J., Chua, R, Elliot, D, Lyons, J, & Pollock, B. J. (1995). Cerebral specialisation for receptive language in individuals with Down syndrome. *Australian Journal of Psychology*, 47, 137-140.

[141] Welsh, T. N., Elliott, D., & Simon, D. (2003). Cerebral specialization and verbal-motor integration in adults with and without Down syndrome. *Brain and Language, 84*, 152-169.

[142] Witelson, S. F. (1974). Hemispheric specialization for linguistic and nonlinguistic tactual perception using dichotomous stimulation technique. Cortex, 10, 3-17.

[143] Ypsilanti, A. (2009). *Investigating functional cerebral asymmetry with preference and performance measures in individuals with intellectual disability*. Unpublished Doctoral Dissertation. Aristotle University of Thessaloniki. Thessalon;iki, Greece.

Chapter 12

Genetic and Epigenetic Mechanisms in Down Syndrome Brain

Jie Lu and Volney Sheen

Additional information is available at the end of the chapter

http://dx.doi.org/10.5772/52807

1. Introduction

Down syndrome (DS) is the most common congenital disorder in children, affecting one in 800 live births. While the large number of contiguous genes from a trisomy of chromosome 21 (HSA21) is expected to broadly affect various organ systems during development, significant advances in medicine have been made in this disorder such that those with DS live fairly long life spans. Individuals with DS, however, uniformly demonstrate some degree of mental retardation. Arguably, cognitive disabilities are the more devastating aspect of DS disorder. Part of the cognitive dysfunction lies not only in the progressive neuronal degeneration/cell death and impaired neurogenesis seen in this developmental and degenerative disorder, but also in the reduction in dendrite formation and spine density, resulting in a disruption of synaptic function. These neurological endophenotypes seen in DS may not be merely due to genomic imbalance from triplication of HSA21 genes, but also to additive influences on associated genes within a given network or pathway and modification of gene expressions caused by epigenetic factors including DNA methylation.

Epigenetic factors regulate gene expression largely through DNA modification. Histones are alkaline proteins that package and order DNA into structural nucleosomes. Acetylation and deacetylation, as well as methylation, of histones can modify the density of chromatin and thereby regulate gene transcription through chromatin remodeling. In a parallel manner, biochemical modification of DNA can occur through DNA methylation. This process involves the addition of a methyl group to the 5 position of the cytosine pyrimidine ring or the number 6 nitrogen of the adenine purine ring. DNA methylation at the 5 position of cytosine has the specific effect of reducing gene expression by physically impeding the binding of transcriptional proteins to the gene itself, or by recruiting protein complexes including methyl-CpG-binding domain proteins (MBDs), histone deacetylases (HDACs) and other chromatin remodeling proteins. Furthermore, environmental factors such as chemical toxins or oxidative stress can accumulate over time and effect gene transcription. Collectively, these processes modify DNA transcription and may affect many neurodevelopmental processes.

Recent advances in high throughput screening of both mRNA expression and DNA methylation have provided a means to examine changes in gene activation and expression, and to understand the integral relationship between gene clusters in effecting particular pathways. The following review begins by exploring the potential contribution of both genetic and epigenetic factors in regulation of various DS endophenotypes. More specifically, our prior work has examined changes in DS neural progenitor mRNA expression and has led us to identify several important pathways affected in this disorder, such as oxidative stress, mitochondrial dysfunction and gliogenesis. Ongoing studies suggest that changes in DNA methylation in DS may have an effect on oxidative phosphorylation, ubiquitin proteolysis and insulin signaling. The confirmation of mRNA and DNA methylation changes and the clarification of these possible causal pathways may have implications for impaired synaptic function and neurogenesis, which contribute to the cognitive impairment seen in DS. These ongoing studies may further provide informative targets for early pharmaceutical interference to ameliorate the symptoms of mental retardation (MR) in DS.

2. Genetic mechanisms underlying the DS phenotype

The triplication of genes on HSA21 causes a wide spectrum of neurological phenotypes in DS, including mental retardation. DS individual displays not only delayed linguistic skills and a relatively low IQ (Intelligent Quotient) but also behavioral issues such as attention-deficit disorder (sometimes with hyperactivity) and autism [1-5]. The cognitive impairments extend further after development, as individuals with DS are more prone to develop Alzheimer's type dementia [6]. In addition, individuals with DS are susceptible to epilepsy in the form of infantile spasms and tonic clonic seizures with myoclonus at early ages [7-9]. These pathological abnormalities in humans are, in part, replicated in DS animal models which show defects in learning, social interactions, memory, and seizures [10-14].

Several genes on HSA21 are implicated in the abnormal neurodevelopment in DS [15]. They can affect cellular function at every stage of neural development, such as proliferation and differentiation of neuroprogenitor cells, neuronal survival and death, synapse formation, maturation and plasticity, as well as myelination. Disruption of each of these pathways can conceptually contribute to the MR seen in DS. Moreover, HSA21 genes have global effects on other genes; a meta-analysis of heterogeneous DS data identified 324 genes with consistent dosage effects, 77 on HSA21 and 247 on non-HSA21 [16]. Therefore, the over-expression of a not so small group of genes on HSA21 may initiate cascades of other signaling pathways on other chromosomes thorough an interactive network. The combinatorial effects from activation of these processes may further contribute to the impairments seen during neurodevelopment in DS.

2.1. Genetic mechanisms underlying oxidative stress in DS

Increased levels of oxidative stress and reactive oxygen species (ROS) have commonly been associated with the DS brain. Free radicals are thought to disrupt the mitochondrial respiratory system, induce apoptosis of neurons and stimulate gliosis, which can further promote neuronal damage. This cyclical pathway may contribute to neuronal losses during neurogenesis as well as neuronal degeneration in adulthood. Several HSA21 genes have been implicated in generation of ROS including *DYRK1A, DSCR1, SOD1, ETS2, S100B, APP* and *BACH1* [15, 17]. Additionally, more recent studies would suggest a synergistic role for various HSA21 genes in induction of this pathological process. For example, over-expression of HSA21 genes *APP* and *S100B* synergistically increase hydrogen peroxide levels and decrease membrane potential in the mitochondria of human DS neuroprogenitor cells. The combination of a loss of mitochondrial integrity and an increase of oxidative stress promotes apoptosis (changes in caspase and respiratory chain protein expression) and gliosis (increase of GFAP). S100B induction can occur through RAGE (Receptor for Advanced Glycation Endproducts) with consequent activation of JNK/p38 and JAK/STAT signaling. These stress response pathways are known to serve as downstream effectors potentially relevant to reactive gliosis, induction of S100B and glial associated aquaporin 4 [18, 19]. Increased levels of S100B and APP further enhance this cyclical cascade by promoting RAGE activation and inflammation with reactive gliosis. Lastly, multiple HSA21 genes have demonstrated enhanced APP-dependent toxic effects on the mitochondria whereas network prediction analyses have shown that four HSA21 proteins are components of the JAK/STAT pathway. These studies imply that an additional 19 HSA21 (among 2004 in total) proteins interact with components in this pathway [20]. These findings reiterate the large cascade of molecules that can be perturbed in a pathway following over-expression of a single gene.

Although oxidative stress in DS patients is considered to be a primary contributor of neurodegeneration such as Alzheimer's Disease (AD) in adult patients, evidences from both human and animal models suggest that these same processes could also affect neurodevelopment and cognitive function at a much earlier age [19, 21-23]. Oxidative stress could therefore not only alter neuronal numbers through degeneration and changes in synaptic plasticity through impaired mitochondrial function, but also affect the generation of neurons during development. In this respect, ongoing effects from over-expression of HSA21 genes likely promote the cognitive dysfunction in DS throughout the lifetime of an individual with this disorder.

2.2. Genetics mechanisms underlying neurogenesis in DS

The observation of reduced cortical volume and decreased neuronal numbers in DS patients and animal models could in part be attributed to a reduction in the generation of neurons [24-27]. Over-expression of several HSA21 genes has been implicated in neurogenesis by either altering the rate or proliferation or by changing cell fate specification. By over-expressing HSA21-associated OLIG2, we observed a phenotypic shift in the neural progenitor pool toward glial progenitor phenotypes, accompanied by a corresponding decrease in the number of neuronal progenitors. This change can partly be explained by OLIG2-dependent inhibition of the expression and activity of KCNA3 outward rectifying potassium channels whose activation stimulates proliferation of neural progenitors [28]. With respect to proliferation, APP overexpression can antagonistically compete with APPBP1, a protein required for the cell cycle progression from G1 to S phase [29]. Similarly, increased S100B levels stimulate p53 nuclear accumulation and inhibit proliferation [30]. DYRK1A has alternatively been shown to phosphorylate p53, impair G1/S phase transition and inhibit proliferation [31]. Finally, many HSA21 genes regulate neurogenesis through their effects on NGF, hedgehog, WNT, Notch and insulin signaling pathways [20]. Changes in expression of various HSA21 genes can also regulate subpopulations of progenitors. For example, microarray profiling of DS human neuroprogenitors implicated a defect in interneuron neurogenesis through increased expression of glial progenitor genes such as *OLIG1, OLIG2, OMG* and *COUP-TF1/NR2F1* and downregulation of the interneuron related genes *DLX1, DLX2* and *DLX5* [32].

2.3. Genetics mechanisms underlying synaptic formation, maturation and plasticity in DS

A reduction in brain volume in DS has been attributed to impaired dendritic and synaptic maturation. Dendritic branching and spine number are dramatically reduced in pyramidal neurons in the hippocampus, visual cortex and motor cortex after 4 months postnatal age in individuals with DS [33-35]. The decreased number of spines is usually accompanied by aberrant spine morphology including enlarged or irregular spine heads, and sparse, small, short stalks intermingled with unusually long spines [34, 36]. In addition, DS brains also show changes in expression levels of various synaptic proteins such as decreased SEPT6, SYN1, SNAP-25, SYP and increased SYNJ1 levels [37-41]. Similar morphological changes have been observed in DS animal models and correlate on a molecular level with synaptic protein level changes and functionally with synaptic plasticity defects, observed through LTP, LTD and imbalance of excitatory-inhibitory neurotransmission [42-50]. Many genes on HSA21 (*TINM1, SYNJ1, ITSN1; KCNJ6, KCNJ15, KCNE1, KCNE2; NRIP1, ETS2, PCP4, DSCR1, DYRK1A, S100B, APP, OLIG1, OLIG2*) have been implicated in the synaptic pathology in DS, and the resulting phenotype likely involves a complex interrelationship between these various genes and their direct or indirect effect on various synaptic proteins [15, 48]. For instance, Dyrk1A overexpression could impair synaptic vesicle endocytosis, reduce dendrite branching and spine density of neurons; these phenotypes might be attributed to Dyrk1A induced hyperphosphorylation of Tau and APP, or other synaptic proteins such as SYNJ1, resulting in impaired hippocampal-dependent learning [51-53]. Moreover, the multiple genetic interactions can additively promote the pathological DS synaptic endophenotype, as more severe defects were observed in Ts65dn mice than in Ts1Cje mice, the former of which contain a larger number of HSA21 associated genes [54].

3. Epigenetic mechanisms underlying the DS phenotype

DNA methylation refers to a process of DNA modification that involves the enzymatic transfer of a methyl group from a methyl donor S-adenosylmethionine to carbon 5 of cytosine at 5′-CpG-3′ sites. The enzymes carrying out this reaction are called DNA methyltransferases (DNMTs). There are five members in this family: DNMT1, DNMT2, DNMT3A, DNMT3B and

http://dx.doi.org/10.5772/52807

DNMT3L. DNMT1 is responsible for DNA methylation maintenance while DNMT3A and DNMT3B are involved in *de novo* DNA methylation. DNMT2 is involved in RNA methylation. DNMT3L (DNA methyltransferase 3-like) does not have enzymatic activity but can stimulate DNMT3A and DNMT3B activation [55-57]. The addition of a methyl group to cytosine may physically impede the binding of transcriptional factors to the gene itself, or by recruiting protein complexes including methyl-CpG-binding protein 2 (MECP2), methyl-CpG-binding domain proteins (MBDs), HDACs and other chromatin remodeling proteins [58]. Alternatively, other enzymes involved in DNA demethylation can reverse this process. These molecules include cytidine deamination (AID, APOBEC) for deamination of cytosine and 5-methylcytosine and hydroxylation (TETs) for converting 5-methylcytosine to 5-hydroxymethylcytosine [59]. DNA modification, especially in the promoter region, by these various regulators may alter gene expression, and thereby affect many physiological processes [60]. In this context, proteins that affect the methylation machinery in DS are likely to alter gene expression and contribute to the DS phenotype.

Epigenetic modification is thought to be an important contributor to development and numerous diseases. Several disorders associated with cognitive impairment such as X-linked alpha-thalassemia mental retardation (ATRX) syndrome, Rett syndrome, and Rubinstein–Taybi Syndrome involve some level of disruption in gene regulation through epigenetic effects [61]. The pathology is medicated by different mechanisms including histone modification, chromosome remodeling, small RNAs (siRNA, miRNA and other non-coding RNA) regulation and DNA methylation. More directly, *DNMT3B* mutations are associated with Immunodeficiency, Centromere instability and Facial anomalies syndrome (ICF) with MR, suggesting that epigenetic alterations in the expression of genes regulating neurogenesis, axon branching, and neuronal migration such as IGF1 and ROBO1, contribute to cognitive impairment [62]. Certain features in DS may, in a similar fashion, be caused by epigenetic changes. For instance, HSA21 genes *DYRK1A*, *BRWD1* and *RUNX1* are associated with SWI/SNF complex, a chromatin remodeling complex that regulates the expression of subsets of genes such as *HDMTs*, *HMTs* and *HDACs*- histone modification proteins involved in controlling the expression of various interacting genes [63-65]. HSA21 genes *CHAF1B* and *HMGN1* express chromatin constitutive proteins involved in nucleosome assembly, which controls gene expression through DNA methylation and histone methylation or acetylation [66, 67]. Over-expression of HSA21 derived miRNA miR-155, miR802 in DS brain could also inhibit MECP2 expression, thereby mimicking *MECP2* loss of function in Rett syndrome with mental retardation. MECP2 transcriptionally activates and silences *CREB1* and *MEF2C*, genes that are critical in neurodevelopment [68-70]. DNA methylation is another extensively studied epigenetic regulator, being shown as impaired in many diseases. Although its importance has been recognized in cancers, its involvement in neurological disorders such as DS has not been well studied yet.

Several observations suggest that DNA methylation may play an important role in the DS endophenotype. Oxidative stress from over-expression of various HSA21 genes [15] could modulate DNA methylation directly through DNA damage or modification at the CpG sites, thereby preventing normal binding of DNMTs to DNA [71, 72]. DNMT3L is localized on

HSA21, and its triplication in DS suggests aberrant levels of expression. DNMT3L can form a heterotetramer with DNMT3A, and increased DNMT3L levels could potentially promote release of DNMT3A as well as increase its methylation activity [56]. DNMT3L can also stimulate DNMT3B activity directly [57, 73]. In addition, Dnmt3a modulates neurogenesis and synaptic plasticity in developing mouse neuroprogenitors and mature neurons by regulating related genes expression, such as *Bdnf, Reln, Dlx2, Gbx2, Sp8* and *Stat1* [74-77]. It remains to be seen whether other HSA21 genes in addition to DNMT3L can change the expression or activity of various epigenetic modifiers including the DNMTs, MBDs, HDACs or TETs. Overall, epigenetic modification provides an added layer of complexity to the interactive network established from over-expression of genes on HSA21. These modifiers also server as attractive candidates for targeting in DS given the broad effects they potentially have on a particular phenotype.

Next, we will discuss how DNA methylation could be involved in some important neurodevelopmental phenotypes in DS.

3.1. Epigenetic mechanisms underlying oxidative stress in DS

While excessive oxidative stress leading to mitochondrial dysfunction is a main feature of DS neurodevelopment, its effects on DNA methylation are not known. Currently no direct evidence demonstrates a role for oxidative stress in regulating DNA methylation changes in DS brain. However, DNA methylation studies from cancer seem to provide some clues. For instance, hydroxyl radicals generated from hydrogen peroxide can cause DNA damage including base modifications, deletions, and breakages, which could consequently interfere with normal function of DNMTs, leading to global hypomethylation in cancer cells [78]. 8-OHdG in CpG dinucleotides or the presence of O6-methylguanine could inhibit adjacent cytosine methylation [79-82] by inhibiting DNMTs or MBDs binding [83]. By extension, some of these same pathological mechanisms in cancer cells will likely be relevant in DS.

Methylation changes in the subset of DS genes involved in oxidative stress can contribute to similar phenotypes seen in DS development and disease. For instance, Dnmt1 conditional knockout in neural progenitor cells induced precocious astrogliogenesis through demethylation of *S100b, Gfap* and *Stat1* promoters and activation of the JAK-STAT pathway. Silencing of these genes occurs through Mecp2 mediated inactivation of chromatin remodeling [84], with demethylation resulting in an increase in S100B, GFAP and STAT1 expression. Enhanced expression of these genes further promotes oxidative stress, cell death and gliosis. HSA21 localized APP could also be regulated by promoter dependent DNA methylation. The methylation pattern in the APP promoter is different in different tissues and even in different brain areas [85]. Hypomethylation of APP is found in the cerebral cortex of aging people and AD patients [86, 87]; the methylation frequency of CpG sites on APP promoter in younger people (26%) is higher than that in older people (8%), suggesting an age related methylation difference [86]. Altered methylation patterns have also been implicated in deregulation of APP processing enzymes PS1 and BACE in AD [88]. Finally, APP can also regulate the expression of other genes such as *CTIF, NTX2* and *DDR2* through DNA methylation [89]. Overall, these studies suggest that DNMTs appear to play some role in regulation of neurogenesis and

http://dx.doi.org/10.5772/52807

neurodegeneration, and they do so by regulating several genes on HSA21 involved in oxidative stress. Moreover, HSA21 genes associated with oxidative stress can influence the methylation status of other genes.

3.2. Epigenetic mechanisms underlying neurogenesis in DS

DNA methylation regulates neurogenesis. Dnmts are broadly expressed in the brain and are dynamically regulated [90, 91]. For example, Dnmt1 is expressed in both dividing neuroprogenitors and postmitotic neurons [91, 92]. Dnmt3b is mainly expressed in neuroprogenitor cells during neurogenesis, whereas Dnmt3a is predominantly expressed in maturing brain (including neural precursors, neurons, astrocytes and oligodendrocytes). Dnmt3a expression peaks at three weeks after birth and then declines in adulthood [93, 94]. Dnmt3l directly regulates Dnmt3a and Dnmt3b but is weakly expressed in the brain and does not appear to disrupt normal cortical development. As for function, Hutnick et al used Emx1-cre to conditionally knockdown Dnmt1 exclusively in telencephalic precursors of mice, which induced hypomethylation in excitatory neurons and astrocytes of cortex and hippocampus. The methylation change increased neuronal apoptosis coupled with upregulation of apoptosis-related genes such as *Gadd45a*, *Casp4* and *Ngfr*. Loss of Dnmt1 also impaired neurogenesis, maturation, learning and memory and was associated with downregulation of layer specific gene such as *Lhx2*, neuronal channel genes such as *Kcnh5*, *Kcnj9* and *Scnn1a* [95]. Interestingly, Gadd45b could contribute to DNA demethylation of pro-neuronal genes such as *BDNF* and *FGF* [96]. Studies using postnatal neural stem cells (NSC) in Dnmt3a knockout mice suggest that Dnmt3a promotes non-promoter DNA methylation of neurogenesis genes such as *Dlx2*, *Gbx2* and *Sp8* by functionally antagonizing Polycomb repression, resulting in increased expression of these genes [77]. Finally, the expression pattern of Dnmt3b suggests that it may be important for the early phase of neurogenesis (Feng et al., 2005).

DNA methylation may directly effect neural progenitor development in DS. In normal development, Dnmt3l does not appear to have a significant phenotype in the developing mouse cerebral cortex, likely due to its relatively low expression levels in the brain [97, 98], (personal communications, Dr. Yi E. Sun, UCLA). DNMT3L, however, is located on chromosome 21 and its triplication results in aberrantly high levels of expression in DS neuroprogenitors (personal observations). Given that DNMT3L directly regulates both DNMT3A/B and both these proteins have been implicated in neural progenitor development, a pathological role for methylation genes such as DNMT3L in contributing to neurogenesis is likely.

3.3. Epigenetic mechanisms underlying synaptic formation, maturation and plasticity in DS

Several HSA21 genes can indirectly regulate epigenetic factors involved in synaptic function. For example, SWI/SNF (SWItch/Sucrose NonFermentable) is a nucleosome-remodeling complex that can destabilize histone-DNA interactions in an ATP-dependent manner. HSA21-localized *DYRK1A* binds the SWI/SNF complex and subsequently induces a coordinated deregulation of multiple genes that are responsible for dendritic growth [65]. Likewise, APP has been shown to alter CpG methylation in three target genes CTIF (CBP80/CBP20-dependent translation initiation factor), NXT2 (nuclear exporting factor 2), and hypermethylated DDR2

[89]. DDR2 is a tyrosine kinase that functions as a cell surface receptor for fibrillar collagen and regulates cell differentiation, remodeling of the extracellular matrix, cell migration, cell proliferation, and cell cycle progression. More evidences from DNA methylation changing synaptic function come from Dnmt transgenic mice. Dnmt1 and Dnmt3a knockout mice show reduced LTP, deficits in learning and memory and deregulated genes expression associated with synaptic plasticity [74]. Dnmt3a overexpression increases spine density in nucleus accumbens [75]. DNMT3B is the gene mutated in ICF syndrome. Its mutation in lymphoblastoid cell line from patients led to altered genes expression of several systems including regulators of neurogenesis and synaptic function, such as ROBO1, JPH4, FRY, MAP4K4, PCDHGC3, IGF1, SNCA, GABRA4 and BCHE [62]. Methyl-CpG binding protein 1 (MBD1), a member of the methylated DNA-binding protein family, whose mutation leads to reduced neurogenesis, decreased LTP and impaired spatial learning [99]. The involvement of Dnmts and Hdacs in synaptic function is further supported by pharmacological manipulations [100-102]. For instance, Dnmt inhibitors zebularine and 5-aza-2-deoxycytidine can alter DNA methylation at promoters for Reln and Bdnf, and block the induction of LTP in synapses of mouse hippocampus [103].

4. Global effects of DNA methylation in causing DS phenotypes

Several reports have shown global DNA methylation changes in DS [104, 105]. For example, individual proteins on HSA21 such as beta amyloid (the protein encoded by HSA21 localized APP) can induce global hypomethylation [106, 107]. Comparison of normal and DS methylation in DS leukocytes and T lymphocytes using microarray-based profiling (MSNP (single nucleotide polymorphism (SNP) chip-based method for profiling DNA methylation) identified a small subset of genes with altered methylation, specific to the DS cell population [104]. Among the genes identified, five candidates (*TMEM131, CD3Z, NOD2* and *NPDC1*) showed correlation with RNA expression, and the methylation changes could be recapitulated by exposing normal lymphocytes to the demethylation drug 5-aza-cytidine. These genes have known or predicted roles in lymphocyte development. In order to gain some insights into the DNA methylation deregulation in DS brain, we have performed some preliminary studies by comparing the methylation profiles of control (CON) and DS frontal cortex from 18 gestational weeks' fetal brain using Illumina 450 Infinium Beadchip assay. Approximately 4% of the CpG sites showed significant changes at the methylation level. When compared to CON baseline methylated and unmethylated states, more CON unmethylated CpG sites became methylated in DS than CON methylated states that became unmethylated. Moreover, there was overall greater global hyper versus hypomethylation in DS compared to CON across all chromosomes, except on HSA21. Chromosome 21 actually demonstrated a greater degree of hypo versus hypermethylation in DS (unpublished data). Hypomethylation generally results in increased gene transcription, whereas hypermethylation leads to the converse. Cross comparison of DNA methylation states with the differential mRNA expression genes from previous microarray studies, suggested epigenetic effects on several specific pathways (oxidative phosphorylation, insulin signaling and ubiquitination).

4.1. Oxidative phosphorylation

Oxidative phosphorylation involves cellular metabolism through oxidation to produce ATP. The broad methylation and gene expression changes in this pathway suggest its role as a primary consequence of DS genes' overdose effects. Plasma membrane NADPH oxidase is considered a major producer of ROS in neurons or astrocytes in brain and is activated by S100B through a RAGE-dependent pathway [108-111]. Over-expression of HSA21 genes such as *S100B* and *APP* likely promote this pathway and cause cell death in DS neurons [19]. Small amounts of superoxide anion and peroxide are also produced by the electron transport chain in mitochondria [112-114]. The global deregulation of enzymes in this mitochondrial pathway could thus disrupt the balance between oxidant generation and ATP production, result in enhanced ROS generation and lead to diminished ATP levels [115, 116]. Several DS genes have been implicated in this process. For instance, three HSA21 genes, *ATP5J*, *ATP5O* and *NDUFV3* are components of ATP synthase and NADH dehydrogenase, though their expression and regulation in DS brain are not known yet. In addition, other HSA21 genes may indirectly affect this pathway. Alternatively, HSA21 gene *S100B* may target mitochondrial proteins such as p53 and ATPase ATAD3A, thereby assisting the cytoplasmic processing of proteins for proper folding and subcellular localization [117-121]. Another HSA21 gene APP and its product beta amyloid can interact with import receptors to gain entry into mitochondrial compartment, where they accumulate and affect the normal function of this pathway [122, 123]. Finally, gene expression in mitochondrial oxidative phosphorylation may be modulated by DNA methylation. For instance, prenatal protein diet excess or restriction leads to hypomethylation of CpG sites in the cytochrome C *CYCS* gene promoter, including those representing putative transcription factor-binding sites. Elevation of this protein can alter electron transport chain function in mitochondria and initiate apoptosis [124]. Our preliminary studies suggest there is a broad change of DNA methylation and genes expression in this oxidative phosphorylation pathway. Given the importance of ATP/ROS metabolism in mitochondrial function, further studies will be needed to understand the epigenetic contribution to this pathway.

4.2. Insulin signaling

The insulin/insulin growth factor (IGF)-I pathway is a conserved pathway required for neurogenesis and neuroprotection. It acts through IR/IGF-IR, IRS, and RAS/MAPK or PI3K/AKT in regulating neurogenic cell fate [125]. Decreased levels of IGF-I have been found to associate with growth retardation in DS patients, which could be rescued by GH therapy [126, 127]. In addition, the insulin receptor knockout mouse suggests that neurons without insulin receptor exhibit significant reduction of Akt and Gsk3beta and increased tau hyperphosphorylation, characteristics of neurotoxicity in DS and AD [128]. Inhibition of the brain insulin signaling pathways have been report in AD brain, with decreased expression of IR, IRS1, IRS2, PI3K and AKT [129, 130]. This deficiency may, in part, involve DNA methylation changes, given reports of co-localization of Hdac2 with insulin signaling components (Ir, Irs) in postsynaptic glutamatergic neurons of the mouse hippocampus [131]. DNA methylation changes in human DS progenitors (personal observations Lu and Sheen) also suggest that the insulin-associated pathways may contribute to the DS endophenotype during development.

4.3. Ubiquitin proteolysis

The ubiquitin proteasome/lysome system (UPLS) is responsible for the removal of excessive proteins from multiple cellular compartments (especially mitochondria and synapses) in order to maintain normal cellular function [132, 133]. Progression in DS cognitive impairment is associated with accumulation of NF plaques and tangles, which have been shown to contain ubiquitin [134]. Dystrophic neurites in DS also contain ubiquitin and the UPLS-associated molecules PSMA5 and USP5 are upregulated in DS fetal brain [135]. Beta amyloid could regulate synaptic protein degradation and function through ubiquitin pathway [136, 137]. Moreover, several E3 ubiquitin ligases have been shown to promote APP degradation [138, 139]. Additionally, HSA21 located genes *AIRE* and *UBE2G2* are directly involved in the ubiquitin pathway and could contribute to the phenotype. Taken in this context, disruption of mitochondrial function (i.e. through S100B, APP, OLIG2 or disruption of the oxidative phosphorylation pathway) might consequently impair ubiquitin-dependent lysosomal and proteosomal clearance, because it is an ATP-dependent process. Finally, our preliminary studies suggest that DNA methylation may also directly impair ubiquitin function. Loss of ubiquitin function would have direct effects on synaptic function and structure (through beta amyloid or synaptic proteins) but would also possibly enhance oxidative stress and mitochondrial dysfunction. It is interesting to note that the high throughput DNA methylation screen in DS invoked changes in methylation involving three networks (oxidative phosphorylation, insulin signaling, and ubiquitin function), which are highly dependent on one another.

5. Possible functions of *DNMT3L* in DS

Given that DNMT3A and DNMT3B are involved in neurogenesis and synaptic plasticity, HSA21 localized *DNMT3L* regulates activities of *DNMT3A/3B*, suggesting that over-expression of this gene will have pathological implications in methylation patterns involved in neural development. Moreover, DNMT3L represses transcription by recruiting HDACs, which may also affect the neurodevelopment [140, 141]. *Dnmt3l* null mice do not demonstrate a neurological phenotype due to low levels of expression but rather exhibits defects in reproductive organs where it is highly expressed and leads to imprinting and differentiation defect in early stages of embryonic development [97, 98]. *DNMT3L (R271Q)* variant is associated with significant DNA hypomethylation at the subtelomeric region in healthy human, though it does not seem to cause any diseases [142]. On the other hand, over-expression of DNMT3L in Hela cells mimics the characteristics of iPS cells and carcinogenesis by upregulating SOX2, HOX genes and DNMTs including DNMT1 and DNMT3B expression, suggesting that DNMT3L over-expression may change the DNA methylation profile in later stages of embryo development through activating DNMT3A/DNMT3B when neurogenesis and synapse formation happen [143]. Interestingly, a recently developed DS model Dp(10)1Yey/+ mice harboring a duplication spanning the entire HSA21 syntenic region on mouse chromosome 10 (Mmu10), which contains Dnmt3l and S100b, did not show alterations in cognitive behaviors or hippocampal LTP [144]. However, other mouse transgenic studies with over-expression of select HSA21 genes (i.e. APP and S100b) have shown combinatorial effects in contributing to AD features in DS and neuronal survival [19, 145]. These observations would suggest combinatorial and interactive effects between these genes in contributing to the MR seen in DS. It remains to be seen whether DNMT3L effects on DNMT3A/B are responsible for the part of the preliminary methylation defects seen in the several pathways discussed above. It is also not known how the trisomy of HSA21 genes will effect methylation, but it is highly likely that DNMT3L alters at least a subset of genes. In this respect, it will be important to identify the causative methylation defects due to this single gene, as it will have implications for other DS phenotypes.

6. Possible targets for pharmaceutical interference

The epigenetic screens in DS predict involvement of several mutually interactive pathways in contributing to the neurological endophenotype in this disorder: oxidative phosphorylation, insulin signaling, and ubiquitination. Approaches for therapeutic intervention possibly involve either altering the methylation patterns or directly targeting specific pathways.

If global hypermethylation in DS neuroprogenitors is confirmed, then inhibition of DNMT or DNA deamination could be used to rescue or treat the pathological phenotypes. There are two clinical licensed DNMT inhibitors currently used in myelodysplastic syndrome, where they relieve the repression of tumor suppressor genes: 5-aza-cytidine (Vidaza®) and 5-aza-2'-deoxycytidine (Dacogen®) [59]. In addition, because of the occurrence of hypomethylation, especially on HSA21, it would be desirable to develop a more specific methylation inhibitor/activator or deamination activator/inhibitor in order to target specific promoters of genes in important pathways.

Dysfunction of the UPLS system causes protein accumulation or over-degradation in cellular organelles. Thus developing activator or inhibitor of proteasomes would have therapeutic meaning. Most currently available activators/inhibitors of the ubiquitin-proteasome pathway directly target the subunits of proteasome, the core of the proteolysis machinery, instead of targeting upstream ubiquitination and recognition of ubiquitinated protein substrates by more specific E3 ubiquitin ligases. Proteasome inhibitors such as Bortezomib, (Velcade®) are in clinical treatment for multiple myeloma [146, 147]. Proteasome activators including 11s activator, Blm10/PA200, and 19s activator are still under research.

Preservation of oxidative phosphorylation pathway and mitochondrial function can be achieved through a new investigational drug EPI-743, currently in phase 2B/3 pivotal clinical trials in Inherited Mitochondrial Respiratory Chain Disease [148]. EPI-743 is an orally absorbable small molecule that readily crosses into the central nervous system. It works by targeting an enzyme NADPH quinone oxidoreductase 1 (NQO1). Its mode of action is to synchronize energy generation in mitochondria with the need to counter cellular redox stress [149].

7. Conclusion

DS is a contiguous gene syndrome which gives rise to MR, dementia, and seizures. These clinical outcomes are mirrored by endophenotypes including increased oxidative stress, decreased neurogenesis and synaptic dysfunction. While these characteristics have largely been attributed to HSA21 gene dosage effects, recent progresses in epigenetic studies have raised the high likelihood that DNA methylation have significant effects on DS neurodevelopment. Methylome screening suggests disruption of pathways involving oxidative phosphorylation, ubiquitination and insulin signaling in DS. Candidate gene analyses suggest that DNMT3L is over-expressed in DS given its location on chromosome 21. Alternatively, other studies have implicated several HSA21 genes in altering methylation sites on genes involved in these same pathways. The pathways invoked through epigenetic regulation contribute directly to known pathological mechanisms identified on prior gene expression profiling such as oxidative stress, gliosis, and mitochondrial dysfunction. In this respect, the DS brain endophenotypes likely arise from the integration of various genetic and epigenetic factors on chromosome 21.

Acknowledgements

This work was supported by grants to V.L.S from NINDS 1R01NS063997 and NICHD 1R21HD054347.

Author details

Jie Lu and Volney Sheen*

*Address all correspondence to: vsheen@bidmc.harvard.edu

Department of Neurology, Beth Israel Deaconess Medical Center, Boston, MA, USA

References

[1] Capone G, Goyal P, Ares W, Lannigan E. Neurobehavioral disorders in children, adolescents, and young adults with Down syndrome. American journal of medical genetics Part C, Seminars in medical genetics. (Review). 2006 Aug 15;142C(3):158-72.

[2] Coe DA, Matson JL, Russell DW, Slifer KJ, Capone GT, Baglio C, et al. Behavior problems of children with Down syndrome and life events. J Autism Dev Disord. (Clinical Trial Controlled Clinical Trial). 1999 Apr;29(2):149-56.

[3] Gath A, Gumley D. Behaviour problems in retarded children with special reference to Down's syndrome. The British journal of psychiatry : the journal of mental science. 1986 Aug;149:156-61.

[4] Kent L, Evans J, Paul M, Sharp M. Comorbidity of autistic spectrum disorders in children with Down syndrome. Dev Med Child Neurol. (Case Reports). 1999 Mar;41(3): 153-8.

[5] Myers BA, Pueschel SM. Psychiatric disorders in persons with Down syndrome. J Nerv Ment Dis. 1991 Oct;179(10):609-13.

[6] Lott IT. Down's syndrome, aging, and Alzheimer's disease: a clinical review. Annals of the New York Academy of Sciences. (Research Support, U.S. Gov't, P.H.S. Review). 1982;396:15-27.

[7] Arya R, Kabra M, Gulati S. Epilepsy in children with Down syndrome. Epileptic Disord. 2011 Mar 11.

[8] Pueschel SM, Louis S, McKnight P. Seizure disorders in Down syndrome. Archives of neurology. 1991 Mar;48(3):318-20.

[9] Romano C, Tine A, Fazio G, Rizzo R, Colognola RM, Sorge G, et al. Seizures in patients with trisomy 21. American journal of medical genetics Supplement. 1990;7:298-300.

[10] Cortez MA, Shen L, Wu Y, Aleem IS, Trepanier CH, Sadeghnia HR, et al. Infantile spasms and Down syndrome: a new animal model. Pediatr Res. (Research Support, Non-U.S. Gov't). 2009 May;65(5):499-503.

[11] Coussons-Read ME, Crnic LS. Behavioral assessment of the Ts65Dn mouse, a model for Down syndrome: altered behavior in the elevated plus maze and open field. Behavior genetics. (Research Support, Non-U.S. Gov't Research Support, U.S. Gov't, P.H.S.). 1996 Jan;26(1):7-13.

[12] Hyde LA, Frisone DF, Crnic LS. Ts65Dn mice, a model for Down syndrome, have deficits in context discrimination learning suggesting impaired hippocampal function. Behav Brain Res. (Research Support, U.S. Gov't, P.H.S.). 2001 Jan 8;118(1):53-60.

[13] Reeves RH, Irving NG, Moran TH, Wohn A, Kitt C, Sisodia SS, et al. A mouse model for Down syndrome exhibits learning and behaviour deficits. Nature genetics. (Comparative Study Research Support, U.S. Gov't, P.H.S.). 1995 Oct;11(2):177-84.

[14] Westmark CJ, Westmark PR, Malter JS. Alzheimer's disease and Down syndrome rodent models exhibit audiogenic seizures. Journal of Alzheimer's disease : JAD. (Research Support, N.I.H., Extramural Research Support, Non-U.S. Gov't). 2010;20(4): 1009-13.

[15] Lu J, Sheen V. Combinatorial gene effects on the neural progenitor pool in Down syndrome. In: Dey S, editor. Down syndrome Book 1 Genetics and Etiology of Down Syndrome Rijeka, Croatia: InTech; 2011. p. 37-64.

[16] Vilardell M, Rasche A, Thormann A, Maschke-Dutz E, Perez-Jurado LA, Lehrach H, et al. Meta-analysis of heterogeneous Down Syndrome data reveals consistent genome-wide dosage effects related to neurological processes. BMC Genomics. (Meta-Analysis Research Support, Non-U.S. Gov't). 2011;12:229.

[17] Lott IT. Neurological phenotypes for Down syndrome across the life span. Prog Brain Res. (Research Support, N.I.H., Extramural). 2012;197:101-21.

[18] Esposito G, Imitola J, Lu J, De Filippis D, Scuderi C, Ganesh VS, et al. Genomic and functional profiling of human Down syndrome neural progenitors implicates S100B and aquaporin 4 in cell injury. Hum Mol Genet. 2008 Feb 1;17(3):440-57.

[19] Lu J, Esposito G, Scuderi C, Steardo L, Delli-Bovi LC, Hecht JL, et al. S100B and APP Promote a Gliocentric Shift and Impaired Neurogenesis in Down Syndrome Neural Progenitors. PLoS One. 2011;6(7):e22126.

[20] Sturgeon X, Le T, Ahmed MM, Gardiner KJ. Pathways to cognitive deficits in Down syndrome. Prog Brain Res. (Research Support, N.I.H., Extramural Research Support, Non-U.S. Gov't). 2012;197:73-100.

[21] Bambrick LL, Fiskum G. Mitochondrial dysfunction in mouse trisomy 16 brain. Brain research. (Research Support, U.S. Gov't, Non-P.H.S.). 2008 Jan 10;1188:9-16.

[22] Behar TN, Colton CA. Redox regulation of neuronal migration in a Down Syndrome model. Free Radic Biol Med. 2003 Sep 15;35(6):566-75.

[23] Brooksbank BW, Balazs R. Superoxide dismutase, glutathione peroxidase and lipoperoxidation in Down's syndrome fetal brain. Brain Res. 1984 Sep;318(1):37-44.

[24] Ishihara K, Amano K, Takaki E, Shimohata A, Sago H, Epstein CJ, et al. Enlarged brain ventricles and impaired neurogenesis in the Ts1Cje and Ts2Cje mouse models of Down syndrome. Cerebral cortex. (Research Support, Non-U.S. Gov't). 2010 May;20(5): 1131-43.

[25] Schmidt-Sidor B, Wisniewski KE, Shepard TH, Sersen EA. Brain growth in Down syndrome subjects 15 to 22 weeks of gestational age and birth to 60 months. Clin Neuropathol. 1990 Jul-Aug;9(4):181-90.

[26] Sweeney JE, Hohmann CF, Oster-Granite ML, Coyle JT. Neurogenesis of the basal forebrain in euploid and trisomy 16 mice: an animal model for developmental disorders in Down syndrome. Neuroscience. (Research Support, Non-U.S. Gov't Research Support, U.S. Gov't, P.H.S.). 1989;31(2):413-25.

[27] Wisniewski KE, Laure-Kamionowska M, Wisniewski HM. Evidence of arrest of neurogenesis and synaptogenesis in brains of patients with Down's syndrome. N Engl J Med. 1984 Nov 1;311(18):1187-8.

[28] Lu J, Lian G, Zhou H, Esposito G, Steardo L, Delli-Bovi LC, et al. OLIG2 over-expression impairs proliferation of human Down syndrome neural progenitors. Human molecular genetics. 2012 Mar 1.

[29] Joo Y, Ha S, Hong BH, Kim J, Chang KA, Liew H, et al. Amyloid precursor protein binding protein-1 modulates cell cycle progression in fetal neural stem cells. PLoS One. 2010;5(12):e14203.

[30] Scotto C, Delphin C, Deloulme JC, Baudier J. Concerted regulation of wild-type p53 nuclear accumulation and activation by S100B and calcium-dependent protein kinase C. Mol Cell Biol. 1999 Oct;19(10):7168-80.

[31] Park J, Oh Y, Yoo L, Jung MS, Song WJ, Lee SH, et al. Dyrk1A phosphorylates p53 and inhibits proliferation of embryonic neuronal cells. J Biol Chem. 2010 Oct 8;285(41): 31895-906.

[32] Bhattacharyya A, McMillan E, Chen SI, Wallace K, Svendsen CN. A critical period in cortical interneuron neurogenesis in down syndrome revealed by human neural progenitor cells. Dev Neurosci. 2009;31(6):497-510.

[33] Becker LE, Armstrong DL, Chan F. Dendritic atrophy in children with Down's syndrome. Annals of neurology. 1986 Oct;20(4):520-6.

[34] Marin-Padilla M. Pyramidal cell abnormalities in the motor cortex of a child with Down's syndrome. A Golgi study. The Journal of comparative neurology. (Research Support, U.S. Gov't, P.H.S.). 1976 May 1;167(1):63-81.

[35] Takashima S, Becker LE, Armstrong DL, Chan F. Abnormal neuronal development in the visual cortex of the human fetus and infant with down's syndrome. A quantitative and qualitative Golgi study. Brain research. (Research Support, Non-U.S. Gov't). 1981 Nov 23;225(1):1-21.

[36] Kleschevnikov AM, Belichenko PV, Salehi A, Wu C. Discoveries in Down syndrome: moving basic science to clinical care. Prog Brain Res. (Research Support, N.I.H., Extramural Research Support, Non-U.S. Gov't). 2012;197:199-221.

[37] Arai Y, Ijuin T, Takenawa T, Becker LE, Takashima S. Excessive expression of synaptojanin in brains with Down syndrome. Brain & development. (Research Support, Non-U.S. Gov't). 2002 Mar;24(2):67-72.

[38] Bahn S, Mimmack M, Ryan M, Caldwell MA, Jauniaux E, Starkey M, et al. Neuronal target genes of the neuron-restrictive silencer factor in neurospheres derived from fetuses with Down's syndrome: a gene expression study. Lancet. 2002 Jan 26;359(9303): 310-5.

[39] Cheon MS, Fountoulakis M, Dierssen M, Ferreres JC, Lubec G. Expression profiles of proteins in fetal brain with Down syndrome. Journal of neural transmission Supplementum. 2001(61):311-9.

[40] Downes EC, Robson J, Grailly E, Abdel-All Z, Xuereb J, Brayne C, et al. Loss of synaptophysin and synaptosomal-associated protein 25-kDa (SNAP-25) in elderly Down syndrome individuals. Neuropathol Appl Neurobiol. (Research Support, Non-U.S. Gov't). 2008 Feb;34(1):12-22.

[41] Weitzdoerfer R, Dierssen M, Fountoulakis M, Lubec G. Fetal life in Down syndrome starts with normal neuronal density but impaired dendritic spines and synaptosomal structure. J Neural Transm Suppl. 2001(61):59-70.

[42] Belichenko PV, Kleschevnikov AM, Masliah E, Wu C, Takimoto-Kimura R, Salehi A, et al. Excitatory-inhibitory relationship in the fascia dentata in the Ts65Dn mouse model of Down syndrome. The Journal of comparative neurology. (Research Support, N.I.H., Extramural Research Support, Non-U.S. Gov't). 2009 Feb 1;512(4):453-66.

[43] Belichenko PV, Kleschevnikov AM, Salehi A, Epstein CJ, Mobley WC. Synaptic and cognitive abnormalities in mouse models of Down syndrome: exploring genotype-phenotype relationships. The Journal of comparative neurology. (Research Support, N.I.H., Extramural Research Support, Non-U.S. Gov't). 2007 Oct 1;504(4):329-45.

[44] Belichenko PV, Masliah E, Kleschevnikov AM, Villar AJ, Epstein CJ, Salehi A, et al. Synaptic structural abnormalities in the Ts65Dn mouse model of Down Syndrome. J Comp Neurol. 2004 Dec 13;480(3):281-98.

[45] Benavides-Piccione R, Ballesteros-Yanez I, de Lagran MM, Elston G, Estivill X, Fillat C, et al. On dendrites in Down syndrome and DS murine models: a spiny way to learn. Prog Neurobiol. 2004 Oct;74(2):111-26.

[46] Di Filippo M, Picconi B, Tantucci M, Ghiglieri V, Bagetta V, Sgobio C, et al. Short-term and long-term plasticity at corticostriatal synapses: implications for learning and memory. Behav Brain Res. (Research Support, U.S. Gov't, Non-P.H.S. Review). 2009 Apr 12;199(1):108-18.

[47] Kurt MA, Davies DC, Kidd M, Dierssen M, Florez J. Synaptic deficit in the temporal cortex of partial trisomy 16 (Ts65Dn) mice. Brain Res. 2000 Mar 6;858(1):191-7.

[48] Levenga J, Willemsen R. Perturbation of dendritic protrusions in intellectual disability. Prog Brain Res. (Research Support, Non-U.S. Gov't). 2012;197:153-68.

[49] Perez-Cremades D, Hernandez S, Blasco-Ibanez JM, Crespo C, Nacher J, Varea E. Alteration of inhibitory circuits in the somatosensory cortex of Ts65Dn mice, a model for Down's syndrome. J Neural Transm. 2010 Apr;117(4):445-55.

[50] Pollonini G, Gao V, Rabe A, Palminiello S, Albertini G, Alberini CM. Abnormal expression of synaptic proteins and neurotrophin-3 in the Down syndrome mouse model Ts65Dn. Neuroscience. (Research Support, N.I.H., Extramural Research Support, Non-U.S. Gov't). 2008 Sep 22;156(1):99-106.

[51] Ahn KJ, Jeong HK, Choi HS, Ryoo SR, Kim YJ, Goo JS, et al. DYRK1A BAC transgenic mice show altered synaptic plasticity with learning and memory defects. Neurobiology of disease. (Research Support, Non-U.S. Gov't). 2006 Jun;22(3):463-72.

[52] Benavides-Piccione R, Dierssen M, Ballesteros-Yanez I, Martinez de Lagran M, Arbones ML, Fotaki V, et al. Alterations in the phenotype of neocortical pyramidal cells in the Dyrk1A+/- mouse. Neurobiology of disease. (Research Support, Non-U.S. Gov't). 2005 Oct;20(1):115-22.

[53] Kim Y, Park J, Song WJ, Chang S. Overexpression of Dyrk1A causes the defects in synaptic vesicle endocytosis. Neurosignals. (Research Support, Non-U.S. Gov't). 2010;18(3):164-72.

[54] Herault Y, Duchon A, Velot E, Marechal D, Brault V. The in vivo Down syndrome genomic library in mouse. Prog Brain Res. (Research Support, Non-U.S. Gov't). 2012;197:169-97.

[55] Bestor TH. The DNA methyltransferases of mammals. Human molecular genetics. (Research Support, Non-U.S. Gov't Research Support, U.S. Gov't, P.H.S. Review). 2000 Oct;9(16):2395-402.

[56] Jurkowska RZ, Rajavelu A, Anspach N, Urbanke C, Jankevicius G, Ragozin S, et al. Oligomerization and binding of the Dnmt3a DNA methyltransferase to parallel DNA molecules: heterochromatic localization and role of Dnmt3L. The Journal of biological chemistry. (Research Support, Non-U.S. Gov't). 2011 Jul 8;286(27):24200-7.

[57] Suetake I, Shinozaki F, Miyagawa J, Takeshima H, Tajima S. DNMT3L stimulates the DNA methylation activity of Dnmt3a and Dnmt3b through a direct interaction. J Biol Chem. 2004 Jun 25;279(26):27816-23.

[58] Hashimoto H, Vertino PM, Cheng X. Molecular coupling of DNA methylation and histone methylation. Epigenomics. (Research Support, N.I.H., Extramural Review). 2010 Oct;2(5):657-69.

[59] Carey N, Marques CJ, Reik W. DNA demethylases: a new epigenetic frontier in drug discovery. Drug Discov Today. (Review). 2011 Aug;16(15-16):683-90.

[60] Gopalakrishnan S, Van Emburgh BO, Robertson KD. DNA methylation in development and human disease. Mutat Res. (Research Support, N.I.H., Extramural Review). 2008 Dec 1;647(1-2):30-8.

[61] Sanchez-Mut JV, Huertas D, Esteller M. Aberrant epigenetic landscape in intellectual disability. Prog Brain Res. 2012;197:53-71.

[62] Jin B, Tao Q, Peng J, Soo HM, Wu W, Ying J, et al. DNA methyltransferase 3B (DNMT3B) mutations in ICF syndrome lead to altered epigenetic modifications and aberrant expression of genes regulating development, neurogenesis and immune function. Human molecular genetics. (Comparative Study Research Support, N.I.H., Extramural Research Support, Non-U.S. Gov't). 2008 Mar 1;17(5):690-709.

[63] Bakshi R, Hassan MQ, Pratap J, Lian JB, Montecino MA, van Wijnen AJ, et al. The human SWI/SNF complex associates with RUNX1 to control transcription of hematopoietic target genes. J Cell Physiol. (Research Support, N.I.H., Extramural). 2010 Nov; 225(2):569-76.

[64] Huang ZQ, Li J, Sachs LM, Cole PA, Wong J. A role for cofactor-cofactor and cofactor-histone interactions in targeting p300, SWI/SNF and Mediator for transcription. The EMBO journal. (Research Support, U.S. Gov't, Non-P.H.S. Research Support, U.S. Gov't, P.H.S.). 2003 May 1;22(9):2146-55.

[65] Lepagnol-Bestel AM, Zvara A, Maussion G, Quignon F, Ngimbous B, Ramoz N, et al. DYRK1A interacts with the REST/NRSF-SWI/SNF chromatin remodelling complex to deregulate gene clusters involved in the neuronal phenotypic traits of Down syndrome. Hum Mol Genet. 2009 Apr 15;18(8):1405-14.

[66] Reese BE, Bachman KE, Baylin SB, Rountree MR. The methyl-CpG binding protein MBD1 interacts with the p150 subunit of chromatin assembly factor 1. Molecular and cellular biology. (Research Support, U.S. Gov't, P.H.S.). 2003 May;23(9):3226-36.

[67] Ueda T, Postnikov YV, Bustin M. Distinct domains in high mobility group N variants modulate specific chromatin modifications. The Journal of biological chemistry. (Research Support, N.I.H., Intramural). 2006 Apr 14;281(15):10182-7.

[68] Keck-Wherley J, Grover D, Bhattacharyya S, Xu X, Holman D, Lombardini ED, et al. Abnormal microRNA expression in Ts65Dn hippocampus and whole blood: contributions to Down syndrome phenotypes. Developmental neuroscience. (Research Support, N.I.H., Extramural Research Support, Non-U.S. Gov't Research Support, U.S. Gov't, Non-P.H.S.). 2011;33(5):451-67.

[69] Kuhn DE, Nuovo GJ, Martin MM, Malana GE, Pleister AP, Jiang J, et al. Human chromosome 21-derived miRNAs are overexpressed in down syndrome brains and hearts. Biochemical and biophysical research communications. (Research Support, N.I.H., Extramural). 2008 Jun 6;370(3):473-7.

[70] Kuhn DE, Nuovo GJ, Terry AV, Jr., Martin MM, Malana GE, Sansom SE, et al. Chromosome 21-derived microRNAs provide an etiological basis for aberrant protein expression in human Down syndrome brains. The Journal of biological chemistry. (Research Support, N.I.H., Extramural Research Support, Non-U.S. Gov't). 2010 Jan 8;285(2):1529-43.

[71] Donkena KV, Young CY, Tindall DJ. Oxidative stress and DNA methylation in prostate cancer. Obstet Gynecol Int. 2010;2010:302051.

[72] Franco R, Schoneveld O, Georgakilas AG, Panayiotidis MI. Oxidative stress, DNA methylation and carcinogenesis. Cancer Lett. (Research Support, N.I.H., Intramural Research Support, Non-U.S. Gov't Review). 2008 Jul 18;266(1):6-11.

[73] Chedin F, Lieber MR, Hsieh CL. The DNA methyltransferase-like protein DNMT3L stimulates de novo methylation by Dnmt3a. Proceedings of the National Academy of Sciences of the United States of America. (Research Support, Non-U.S. Gov't Research Support, U.S. Gov't, P.H.S.). 2002 Dec 24;99(26):16916-21.

[74] Feng J, Zhou Y, Campbell SL, Le T, Li E, Sweatt JD, et al. Dnmt1 and Dnmt3a maintain DNA methylation and regulate synaptic function in adult forebrain neurons. Nature neuroscience. (Comparative Study Research Support, N.I.H., Extramural Research Support, Non-U.S. Gov't). 2010 Apr;13(4):423-30.

[75] LaPlant Q, Vialou V, Covington HE, 3rd, Dumitriu D, Feng J, Warren BL, et al. Dnmt3a regulates emotional behavior and spine plasticity in the nucleus accumbens. Nature neuroscience. (Research Support, N.I.H., Extramural). 2010 Sep;13(9):1137-43.

[76] Levenson JM, Roth TL, Lubin FD, Miller CA, Huang IC, Desai P, et al. Evidence that DNA (cytosine-5) methyltransferase regulates synaptic plasticity in the hippocampus. The Journal of biological chemistry. (In Vitro Research Support, N.I.H., Extramural). 2006 Jun 9;281(23):15763-73.

[77] Wu H, Coskun V, Tao J, Xie W, Ge W, Yoshikawa K, et al. Dnmt3a-dependent non-promoter DNA methylation facilitates transcription of neurogenic genes. Science. (Research Support, N.I.H., Extramural Research Support, Non-U.S. Gov't). 2010 Jul 23;329(5990):444-8.

[78] Wachsman JT. DNA methylation and the association between genetic and epigenetic changes: relation to carcinogenesis. Mutat Res. (Review). 1997 Apr 14;375(1):1-8.

[79] Hepburn PA, Margison GP, Tisdale MJ. Enzymatic methylation of cytosine in DNA is prevented by adjacent O6-methylguanine residues. The Journal of biological chemistry. (Research Support, Non-U.S. Gov't). 1991 May 5;266(13):7985-7.

[80] Tan NW, Li BF. Interaction of oligonucleotides containing 6-O-methylguanine with human DNA (cytosine-5-)-methyltransferase (published erratumm appears in Biochemistry 1992 Aug 4;31(30):7008). Biochemistry. (Research Support, Non-U.S. Gov't). 1990 Oct 2;29(39):9234-40.

[81] Turk PW, Laayoun A, Smith SS, Weitzman SA. DNA adduct 8-hydroxyl-2'-deoxyguanosine (8-hydroxyguanine) affects function of human DNA methyltransferase. Carcinogenesis. (Comparative Study Research Support, Non-U.S. Gov't Research Support, U.S. Gov't, P.H.S.). 1995 May;16(5):1253-5.

[82] Weitzman SA, Turk PW, Milkowski DH, Kozlowski K. Free radical adducts induce alterations in DNA cytosine methylation. Proceedings of the National Academy of Sciences of the United States of America. (Research Support, U.S. Gov't, P.H.S.). 1994 Feb 15;91(4):1261-4.

[83] Valinluck V, Tsai HH, Rogstad DK, Burdzy A, Bird A, Sowers LC. Oxidative damage to methyl-CpG sequences inhibits the binding of the methyl-CpG binding domain (MBD) of methyl-CpG binding protein 2 (MeCP2). Nucleic acids research. (Research Support, Non-U.S. Gov't Research Support, U.S. Gov't, P.H.S.). 2004;32(14):4100-8.

[84] Fan G, Martinowich K, Chin MH, He F, Fouse SD, Hutnick L, et al. DNA methylation controls the timing of astrogliogenesis through regulation of JAK-STAT signaling. Development. 2005 Aug;132(15):3345-56.

[85] Rogaev EI, Lukiw WJ, Lavrushina O, Rogaeva EA, St George-Hyslop PH. The upstream promoter of the beta-amyloid precursor protein gene (APP) shows differential patterns of methylation in human brain. Genomics. (Comparative Study Research Support, Non-U.S. Gov't). 1994 Jul 15;22(2):340-7.

[86] Tohgi H, Utsugisawa K, Nagane Y, Yoshimura M, Genda Y, Ukitsu M. Reduction with age in methylcytosine in the promoter region -224 approximately -101 of the amyloid precursor protein gene in autopsy human cortex. Brain Res Mol Brain Res. (Research Support, Non-U.S. Gov't). 1999 Jul 5;70(2):288-92.

[87] West RL, Lee JM, Maroun LE. Hypomethylation of the amyloid precursor protein gene in the brain of an Alzheimer's disease patient. J Mol Neurosci. (Comparative Study Research Support, Non-U.S. Gov't Research Support, U.S. Gov't, P.H.S.). 1995;6(2): 141-6.

[88] Fuso A, Seminara L, Cavallaro RA, D'Anselmi F, Scarpa S. S-adenosylmethionine/homocysteine cycle alterations modify DNA methylation status with consequent deregulation of PS1 and BACE and beta-amyloid production. Molecular and cellular neurosciences. (Research Support, Non-U.S. Gov't). 2005 Jan;28(1):195-204.

[89] Sung HY, Choi EN, Ahn Jo S, Oh S, Ahn JH. Amyloid protein-mediated differential DNA methylation status regulates gene expression in Alzheimer's disease model cell line. Biochemical and biophysical research communications. (Research Support, Non-U.S. Gov't). 2011 Nov 4;414(4):700-5.

[90] Feng J, Fouse S, Fan G. Epigenetic regulation of neural gene expression and neuronal function. Pediatr Res. (Research Support, N.I.H., Extramural Review). 2007 May;61(5 Pt 2):58R-63R.

[91] Goto K, Numata M, Komura JI, Ono T, Bestor TH, Kondo H. Expression of DNA methyltransferase gene in mature and immature neurons as well as proliferating cells in mice. Differentiation. (Research Support, Non-U.S. Gov't). 1994 Apr;56(1-2):39-44.

[92] Brooks PJ, Marietta C, Goldman D. DNA mismatch repair and DNA methylation in adult brain neurons. The Journal of neuroscience : the official journal of the Society for Neuroscience. 1996 Feb 1;16(3):939-45.

[93] Feng J, Chang H, Li E, Fan G. Dynamic expression of de novo DNA methyltransferases Dnmt3a and Dnmt3b in the central nervous system. Journal of neuroscience research. (Comparative Study Research Support, N.I.H., Extramural Research Support, U.S. Gov't, P.H.S.). 2005 Mar 15;79(6):734-46.

[94] Watanabe D, Uchiyama K, Hanaoka K. Transition of mouse de novo methyltransferases expression from Dnmt3b to Dnmt3a during neural progenitor cell development. Neuroscience. (Comparative Study In Vitro Research Support, Non-U.S. Gov't). 2006 Oct 27;142(3):727-37.

[95] Hutnick LK, Golshani P, Namihira M, Xue Z, Matynia A, Yang XW, et al. DNA hypomethylation restricted to the murine forebrain induces cortical degeneration and impairs postnatal neuronal maturation. Hum Mol Genet. 2009 Aug 1;18(15):2875-88.

[96] Ma DK, Jang MH, Guo JU, Kitabatake Y, Chang ML, Pow-Anpongkul N, et al. Neuronal activity-induced Gadd45b promotes epigenetic DNA demethylation and adult

neurogenesis. Science. (Research Support, N.I.H., Extramural Research Support, Non-U.S. Gov't). 2009 Feb 20;323(5917):1074-7.

[97] Arima T, Hata K, Tanaka S, Kusumi M, Li E, Kato K, et al. Loss of the maternal imprint in Dnmt3Lmat-/- mice leads to a differentiation defect in the extraembryonic tissue. Developmental biology. (Research Support, Non-U.S. Gov't). 2006 Sep 15;297(2):361-73.

[98] Bourc'his D, Xu GL, Lin CS, Bollman B, Bestor TH. Dnmt3L and the establishment of maternal genomic imprints. Science. (Research Support, Non-U.S. Gov't Research Support, U.S. Gov't, P.H.S.). 2001 Dec 21;294(5551):2536-9.

[99] Zhao X, Ueba T, Christie BR, Barkho B, McConnell MJ, Nakashima K, et al. Mice lacking methyl-CpG binding protein 1 have deficits in adult neurogenesis and hippocampal function. Proceedings of the National Academy of Sciences of the United States of America. (Research Support, Non-U.S. Gov't Research Support, U.S. Gov't, P.H.S.). 2003 May 27;100(11):6777-82.

[100] Lubin FD, Roth TL, Sweatt JD. Epigenetic regulation of BDNF gene transcription in the consolidation of fear memory. The Journal of neuroscience : the official journal of the Society for Neuroscience. (Comparative Study Research Support, N.I.H., Extramural Research Support, Non-U.S. Gov't). 2008 Oct 15;28(42):10576-86.

[101] Miller CA, Campbell SL, Sweatt JD. DNA methylation and histone acetylation work in concert to regulate memory formation and synaptic plasticity. Neurobiol Learn Mem. (Research Support, N.I.H., Extramural Research Support, Non-U.S. Gov't). 2008 May; 89(4):599-603.

[102] Miller CA, Sweatt JD. Covalent modification of DNA regulates memory formation. Neuron. (Research Support, N.I.H., Extramural Research Support, Non-U.S. Gov't). 2007 Mar 15;53(6):857-69.

[103] Levenson JM, Qiu S, Weeber EJ. The role of reelin in adult synaptic function and the genetic and epigenetic regulation of the reelin gene. Biochimica et biophysica acta. (Review). 2008 Aug;1779(8):422-31.

[104] Kerkel K, Schupf N, Hatta K, Pang D, Salas M, Kratz A, et al. Altered DNA methylation in leukocytes with trisomy 21. PLoS Genet. (Research Support, N.I.H., Extramural). 2010 Nov;6(11):e1001212.

[105] Loudin MG, Wang J, Leung HC, Gurusiddappa S, Meyer J, Condos G, et al. Genomic profiling in Down syndrome acute lymphoblastic leukemia identifies histone gene deletions associated with altered methylation profiles. Leukemia. (Research Support, N.I.H., Extramural Research Support, Non-U.S. Gov't Validation Studies). 2011 Oct; 25(10):1555-63.

[106] Chen KL, Wang SS, Yang YY, Yuan RY, Chen RM, Hu CJ. The epigenetic effects of amyloid-beta(1-40) on global DNA and neprilysin genes in murine cerebral endothelial cells. Biochemical and biophysical research communications. 2009 Jan 2;378(1):57-61.

[107] Mastroeni D, Grover A, Delvaux E, Whiteside C, Coleman PD, Rogers J. Epigenetic changes in Alzheimer's disease: decrements in DNA methylation. Neurobiology of aging. (Randomized Controlled Trial Research Support, N.I.H., Extramural Research Support, Non-U.S. Gov't). 2010 Dec;31(12):2025-37.

[108] Anantharam V, Kaul S, Song C, Kanthasamy A, Kanthasamy AG. Pharmacological inhibition of neuronal NADPH oxidase protects against 1-methyl-4-phenylpyridinium (MPP+)-induced oxidative stress and apoptosis in mesencephalic dopaminergic neuronal cells. Neurotoxicology. (Research Support, N.I.H., Extramural). 2007 Sep; 28(5):988-97.

[109] Donato R, Sorci G, Riuzzi F, Arcuri C, Bianchi R, Brozzi F, et al. S100B's double life: intracellular regulator and extracellular signal. Biochimica et biophysica acta. (Research Support, Non-U.S. Gov't Review). 2009 Jun;1793(6):1008-22.

[110] Glass MJ, Huang J, Oselkin M, Tarsitano MJ, Wang G, Iadecola C, et al. Subcellular localization of nicotinamide adenine dinucleotide phosphate oxidase subunits in neurons and astroglia of the rat medial nucleus tractus solitarius: relationship with tyrosine hydroxylase immunoreactive neurons. Neuroscience. (Comparative Study Research Support, N.I.H., Extramural). 2006 Dec 1;143(2):547-64.

[111] Serrano F, Kolluri NS, Wientjes FB, Card JP, Klann E. NADPH oxidase immunoreactivity in the mouse brain. Brain research. (Research Support, U.S. Gov't, P.H.S.). 2003 Oct 24;988(1-2):193-8.

[112] Finkel T, Holbrook NJ. Oxidants, oxidative stress and the biology of ageing. Nature. (Review). 2000 Nov 9;408(6809):239-47.

[113] Raha S, McEachern GE, Myint AT, Robinson BH. Superoxides from mitochondrial complex III: the role of manganese superoxide dismutase. Free Radic Biol Med. (Research Support, Non-U.S. Gov't). 2000 Jul 15;29(2):170-80.

[114] Raha S, Robinson BH. Mitochondria, oxygen free radicals, disease and ageing. Trends Biochem Sci. (Research Support, Non-U.S. Gov't Review). 2000 Oct;25(10):502-8.

[115] Echtay KS, Roussel D, St-Pierre J, Jekabsons MB, Cadenas S, Stuart JA, et al. Superoxide activates mitochondrial uncoupling proteins. Nature. 2002 Jan 3;415(6867):96-9.

[116] Kadenbach B, Ramzan R, Vogt S. Degenerative diseases, oxidative stress and cytochrome c oxidase function. Trends in molecular medicine. (Research Support, Non-U.S. Gov't). 2009 Apr;15(4):139-47.

[117] Donato R. Intracellular and extracellular roles of S100 proteins. Microsc Res Tech. 2003 Apr 15;60(6):540-51.

[118] Gilquin B, Cannon BR, Hubstenberger A, Moulouel B, Falk E, Merle N, et al. The calcium-dependent interaction between S100B and the mitochondrial AAA ATPase ATAD3A and the role of this complex in the cytoplasmic processing of ATAD3A. Mol Cell Biol. 2010 Jun;30(11):2724-36.

[119] Leclerc E, Sturchler E, Vetter SW. The S100B/RAGE Axis in Alzheimer's Disease. Cardiovasc Psychiatry Neurol. 2010;2010:539581.

[120] Lin J, Blake M, Tang C, Zimmer D, Rustandi RR, Weber DJ, et al. Inhibition of p53 transcriptional activity by the S100B calcium-binding protein. J Biol Chem. 2001 Sep 14;276(37):35037-41.

[121] Mihara M, Erster S, Zaika A, Petrenko O, Chittenden T, Pancoska P, et al. p53 has a direct apoptogenic role at the mitochondria. Mol Cell. 2003 Mar;11(3):577-90.

[122] Devi L, Anandatheerthavarada HK. Mitochondrial trafficking of APP and alpha synuclein: Relevance to mitochondrial dysfunction in Alzheimer's and Parkinson's diseases. Biochim Biophys Acta. 2010 Jan;1802(1):11-9.

[123] Manczak M, Anekonda TS, Henson E, Park BS, Quinn J, Reddy PH. Mitochondria are a direct site of A beta accumulation in Alzheimer's disease neurons: implications for free radical generation and oxidative damage in disease progression. Hum Mol Genet. 2006 May 1;15(9):1437-49.

[124] Altmann S, Murani E, Schwerin M, Metges CC, Wimmers K, Ponsuksili S. Somatic cytochrome c (CYCS) gene expression and promoter-specific DNA methylation in a porcine model of prenatal exposure to maternal dietary protein excess and restriction. Br J Nutr. (Comparative Study Research Support, Non-U.S. Gov't). 2012 Mar;107(6): 791-9.

[125] Bateman JM, McNeill H. Insulin/IGF signalling in neurogenesis. Cell Mol Life Sci. (Review). 2006 Aug;63(15):1701-5.

[126] Anneren G, Tuvemo T, Carlsson-Skwirut C, Lonnerholm T, Bang P, Sara VR, et al. Growth hormone treatment in young children with Down's syndrome: effects on growth and psychomotor development. Arch Dis Child. (Clinical Trial Controlled Clinical Trial Research Support, Non-U.S. Gov't). 1999 Apr;80(4):334-8.

[127] Barreca A, Rasore Quartino A, Acutis MS, Ponzani P, Damonte G, Miani E, et al. Assessment of growth hormone insulin like growth factor-I axis in Down's syndrome. J Endocrinol Invest. (Clinical Trial Controlled Clinical Trial Research Support, Non-U.S. Gov't). 1994 Jun;17(6):431-6.

[128] Schubert M, Gautam D, Surjo D, Ueki K, Baudler S, Schubert D, et al. Role for neuronal insulin resistance in neurodegenerative diseases. Proceedings of the National Academy of Sciences of the United States of America. (Research Support, Non-U.S. Gov't Research Support, U.S. Gov't, P.H.S.). 2004 Mar 2;101(9):3100-5.

[129] Liu Y, Liu F, Grundke-Iqbal I, Iqbal K, Gong CX. Deficient brain insulin signalling pathway in Alzheimer's disease and diabetes. J Pathol. (Research Support, N.I.H., Extramural Research Support, Non-U.S. Gov't). 2011 Sep;225(1):54-62.

[130] Rivera EJ, Goldin A, Fulmer N, Tavares R, Wands JR, de la Monte SM. Insulin and insulin-like growth factor expression and function deteriorate with progression of

Alzheimer's disease: link to brain reductions in acetylcholine. Journal of Alzheimer's disease : JAD. (Research Support, N.I.H., Extramural). 2005 Dec;8(3):247-68.

[131] Yao ZG, Liu Y, Zhang L, Huang L, Ma CM, Xu YF, et al. Co-location of HDAC2 and Insulin Signaling Components in the Adult Mouse Hippocampus. Cell Mol Neurobiol. 2012 Jun 26.

[132] Livnat-Levanon N, Glickman MH. Ubiquitin-proteasome system and mitochondria - reciprocity. Biochimica et biophysica acta. (Research Support, Non-U.S. Gov't Review). 2011 Feb;1809(2):80-7.

[133] Mabb AM, Ehlers MD. Ubiquitination in postsynaptic function and plasticity. Annu Rev Cell Dev Biol. (Research Support, N.I.H., Extramural Research Support, Non-U.S. Gov't Review). 2010 Nov 10;26:179-210.

[134] Mattiace LA, Kress Y, Davies P, Ksiezak-Reding H, Yen SH, Dickson DW. Ubiquitin-immunoreactive dystrophic neurites in Down's syndrome brains. Journal of neuropathology and experimental neurology. (Research Support, U.S. Gov't, P.H.S.). 1991 Sep; 50(5):547-59.

[135] Engidawork E, Juranville JF, Fountoulakis M, Dierssen M, Lubec G. Selective upregulation of the ubiquitin-proteasome proteolytic pathway proteins, proteasome zeta chain and isopeptidase T in fetal Down syndrome. Journal of neural transmission Supplementum. (Research Support, Non-U.S. Gov't). 2001(61):117-30.

[136] Roselli F, Livrea P, Almeida OF. CDK5 is essential for soluble amyloid beta-induced degradation of GKAP and remodeling of the synaptic actin cytoskeleton. PloS one. (Research Support, Non-U.S. Gov't). 2011;6(7):e23097.

[137] Roselli F, Tirard M, Lu J, Hutzler P, Lamberti P, Livrea P, et al. Soluble beta-amyloid1-40 induces NMDA-dependent degradation of postsynaptic density-95 at glutamatergic synapses. The Journal of neuroscience : the official journal of the Society for Neuroscience. (Research Support, N.I.H., Extramural Research Support, Non-U.S. Gov't). 2005 Nov 30;25(48):11061-70.

[138] Kaneko M, Saito R, Okuma Y, Nomura Y. Possible involvement of ubiquitin ligase HRD1 insolubilization in amyloid beta generation. Biol Pharm Bull. (Research Support, Non-U.S. Gov't). 2012;35(2):269-72.

[139] Watanabe T, Hikichi Y, Willuweit A, Shintani Y, Horiguchi T. FBL2 Regulates Amyloid Precursor Protein (APP) Metabolism by Promoting Ubiquitination-Dependent APP Degradation and Inhibition of APP Endocytosis. The Journal of neuroscience : the official journal of the Society for Neuroscience. 2012 Mar 7;32(10):3352-65.

[140] Aapola U, Liiv I, Peterson P. Imprinting regulator DNMT3L is a transcriptional repressor associated with histone deacetylase activity. Nucleic Acids Res. 2002 Aug 15;30(16):3602-8.

[141] Deplus R, Brenner C, Burgers WA, Putmans P, Kouzarides T, de Launoit Y, et al. Dnmt3L is a transcriptional repressor that recruits histone deacetylase. Nucleic Acids Res. 2002 Sep 1;30(17):3831-8.

[142] El-Maarri O, Kareta MS, Mikeska T, Becker T, Diaz-Lacava A, Junen J, et al. A systematic search for DNA methyltransferase polymorphisms reveals a rare DNMT3L variant associated with subtelomeric hypomethylation. Human molecular genetics. (Research Support, Non-U.S. Gov't). 2009 May 15;18(10):1755-68.

[143] Gokul G, Ramakrishna G, Khosla S. Reprogramming of HeLa cells upon DNMT3L overexpression mimics carcinogenesis. Epigenetics. (Research Support, Non-U.S. Gov't). 2009 Jul 1;4(5):322-9.

[144] Yu T, Liu C, Belichenko P, Clapcote SJ, Li S, Pao A, et al. Effects of individual segmental trisomies of human chromosome 21 syntenic regions on hippocampal long-term potentiation and cognitive behaviors in mice. Brain research. (In Vitro Research Support, N.I.H., Extramural Research Support, Non-U.S. Gov't). 2010 Dec 17;1366:162-71.

[145] Mori T, Koyama N, Arendash GW, Horikoshi-Sakuraba Y, Tan J, Town T. Overexpression of human S100B exacerbates cerebral amyloidosis and gliosis in the Tg2576 mouse model of Alzheimer's disease. Glia. 2010 Feb;58(3):300-14.

[146] Huang L, Chen CH. Proteasome regulators: activators and inhibitors. Curr Med Chem. (Research Support, N.I.H., Extramural Review). 2009;16(8):931-9.

[147] Stadtmueller BM, Hill CP. Proteasome activators. Molecular cell. (Research Support, N.I.H., Extramural Review). 2011 Jan 7;41(1):8-19.

[148] Enns GM, Kinsman SL, Perlman SL, Spicer KM, Abdenur JE, Cohen BH, et al. Initial experience in the treatment of inherited mitochondrial disease with EPI-743. Mol Genet Metab. (Clinical Trial Research Support, N.I.H., Extramural Research Support, Non-U.S. Gov't). 2012 Jan;105(1):91-102.

[149] Shrader WD, Amagata A, Barnes A, Enns GM, Hinman A, Jankowski O, et al. alpha-Tocotrienol quinone modulates oxidative stress response and the biochemistry of aging. Bioorg Med Chem Lett. 2011 Jun 15;21(12):3693-8.